THE INTERNATIONAL CAMPAIGN AGAINST LEPROSY

JO ROBERTSON

The International Campaign Against Leprosy

1948–2005

HURST & COMPANY, LONDON

First published in the United Kingdom in 2021 by
C. Hurst & Co. (Publishers) Ltd.,
New Wing, Somerset House, Strand, London, WC2R 1LA

Copyright © Jo Robertson, 2021

Printed in Great Britain by Bell and Bain Ltd, Glasgow

Distributed in the United States, Canada and Latin America
by Oxford University Press, 198 Madison Avenue, New York,
NY 10016, United States of America.

A Cataloguing-in-Publication data record for this book is
available from the British Library.

ISBN: 9781787385498

www.hurstpublishers.com

CONTENTS

CONTENTS

DEDICATION

To all the people silenced by leprosy, all the people named and
unnamed who have worked tirelessly against the disease,
and finally to those who continue to call attention to
the human rights of people who still suffer
from the disease.

ACKNOWLEDGEMENTS

This long journey has had two distinct stages. The first was when I worked on the International Leprosy Association's Global Project on the History of Leprosy, based at what was then the Wellcome Unit for the History of Medicine at Oxford. The second was when I was researching and writing this book, at the Institut d'Histoire de la Médecine et de la Santé, Centre Médicale Universitaire (CMU) at the University of Geneva.

I could not have done either without the funding provided by both the Nippon Foundation and the Sasakawa Health Foundation. Originally provided by the Nippon Foundation through WHO, the International Leprosy Association, and the University of Oxford, this funding enabled me to seek out records created in the work done against leprosy under the auspices of the International Leprosy Association's Global Project on the History of Leprosy. Funding from the Nippon Foundation subsequently enabled me to carry out the research at WHO.

I am grateful for this unique opportunity that took me to so many far-flung places: old leprosy asylums, sanatoria, and colonies all over the world, where pockets of people bearing the physical damage caused by the disease were still living. Most of all, the funding gave me tremendous autonomy, for never at any stage was I put under any pressure about what to write or even when to deliver. Many thanks to the Nippon Foundation and to the Sasakawa Health Foundation for their graciousness over all of those years. In the midst of all of that, I owe a debt of gratitude to Mr Yohei Sasakawa, who told me about his vision for the human rights of people affected by leprosy, and Mrs Kay Yamaguchi, who provided enthusiastic support and expertise.

This journey has taken such a long time that some of those who began with me are no longer here. It is with the greatest sadness that I remember Dr Yo Yuasa, Emeritus Professor Baron Michel Lechat, Dr Colin McDougall, and Professor Kenzo Kiikuni, all uniquely dedicated to the pursuit and elimination of leprosy. We spent so much time together in various parts of the world, and I miss them every day. To Dr S. K. Nordeen, who I also miss so much, thank you for the benefit of your generous, finely honed intelligence, drive, passion, and integrity. I'll always remember when we went to Haldia, to the Indian Leprologists Conference, driving through the night in a car full of distinguished Indian leprosy medical men. You'll have to forgive me for falling short of your and Dr Yuasa's vision.

I will always be grateful to all of those who so willingly taught me about leprosy. My first encounter with leprosy outside Australia was in India, in 2001, at the Adams Wylie hospital in Bombay. The old bungalow had been built in 1902, when plague had flared up in the city. There I met Dr Hari Bulchand, who was working for Bombay Leprosy Project (BLP) under the authority of Dr R. Ganapati, Dr C. R. Revankar, and Mr Pai. BLP had taken over the Adams Wylie Hospital in 1979 to look after people with leprosy in need of hospital care. He told me about the current treatment and introduced me to some of the patients, and then took it upon himself to take me on a three-day tour of Bombay, undeterred by increasingly bemused phone calls from BLP. Thank you, thank you for the adventure, Dr Hari.

On that same trip, I met the only other woman in the world, it seemed at the time to both of us, who was studying something about the history of leprosy (although we did wonder what university Dr Jane Buckingham was based at – this was before her book – did Canterbury mean the UK, or perhaps it was NZ?). Shubhada S. Pandya had already had one perfectly valid career. She had been a neurophysiologist, but she was also the trusted historian of leprosy in India. Everyone I met in Bombay told me, "Oh, history of leprosy, have you met Shubha Pandya?" It turned out that we were destined to fly to Wardha, in central India, to visit Gandhi's ashram in Sevagram, to go to Orissa with Mr Jayadev Sahu, to go to the old Leprosy Mission asylums from Purulia, down the Coromandel Coast to Salur, Vadthorasalur, and then again north to Faizabad. Thank you to Jayadev Sahu who accompanied us around the old leprosy places of Orissa. And to Chandi Prasad Nanda for all of his assistance in Orissa.

Thank you too to the Leprosy Mission India and to all of the superintendents throughout India who welcomed me as a guest. Thank you to Joyce Missing and June Nash at the Leprosy Mission International, in Brentford, London, with the most wonderful repository that spans the years of their organisation. My delighted thanks too to the Raoul Follereau Foundation (*La Fondation Raoul Follereau*) for welcoming me to their office in Paris, to M. Récipon (who is sadly no longer with us), and to Brigitte de Bellefon for all of her assistance. I also had the pleasure of being let loose in the Damien Foundation archives in Brussels and the ILEP archives, which were at that time in London. Thank you to everyone for this privilege and freedom.

ACKNOWLEDGEMENTS

One of the outstanding and most instructive experiences in this journey took place when, at the invitation of Dr Artur Cunanan, I went with Nao Hoshino to Culion, in the Palawan group of islands in the Philippines, where Dr Windsor Wade had conducted his research and where generations of leprosy-affected people had been isolated. The museum on Culion, part of the heritage of the nation, now speaks of those people. I had the privilege of being there when leprosy-affected people turned it into a living exhibition by telling their stories beside the artefacts that bore testimony to their experiences.

My odyssey is bookended by two of the brightest, most supportive, and most intellectually engaged people anyone could ever have the good fortune to meet. My doctoral supervisor, Professor Helen Tiffin, was there for me in the beginning and never failed to reassure me when I doubted the value of what I was doing. At the other end of the journey, Dr Chris Tiffin stepped up with his fine eye for editing and added a degree of finesse beyond my capabilities, when it seemed that this book would never get published. My debt of gratitude to both is immense.

I am grateful to my family for getting on with their lives while I was absent, my benignly indifferent children – Dominic, Anna, Brian, and David – who were thankfully grown up enough to do without me. I am proud of how they have forged themselves into functioning adults in the world, with, of course, the support of my husband, James.

Finally, to Bill Malo, June Bertelsen, Hilarion Guia, and the many people whose names have been eroded by history, your sacrifice has been immense and nothing can ever compensate you.

LIST OF ABBREVIATIONS

ALM	American Leprosy Missions
APD	Les Amis du Père Damien
BCG	Bacillus Calmette-Guérin
BELRA	British Empire Leprosy Relief Association
BI	Bacterial Index
BMJ	*British Medical Journal*
Bulletin WHO	Bulletin of the World Health Organization
Chronicle	Chronicle of the World Health Organization
DAHW	Deutsche Aussätzigen Hilfwerk
ELEP	European Federation of Anti-Leprosy Organizations
GA	General Assembly
GAEL	Global Alliance for the Elimination of Leprosy
GPZL	Global Partnership for Zero Leprosy
GRECALTES	Greater Calcutta Leprosy Treatment and Health Education Scheme
IJL	*International Journal of Leprosy and Other Mycobacterial Diseases*
ILA	International Leprosy Association
ILEP	International Federation of Anti-Leprosy Associations
IMMLEP	Research on the Immunology of Leprosy
IMR	Institute for Medical Research
JSIF	Japan Shipbuilding Industry Foundation
LEC	Leprosy Elimination Campaign
LEP	Leprosy Unit of WHO
LEPRA	British Leprosy Relief Association
LR	*Leprosy Review*

LIST OF ABBREVIATIONS

LWM	Leonard Wood Memorial for the Eradication of Leprosy
MDT	Multidrug Therapy
MI	Microbial Index
MLEC	Modified Leprosy Elimination Campaign
PLM	Philippine Leprosy Mission
SEARO	South East Asian Region
SMHF	Sasakawa Memorial Health Foundation
THELEP	Scientific Working Group on Chemotherapy of Leprosy
TNF	Nippon Foundation
TUB	Tuberculosis Unit
UNDP	United Nations Development Program
UNICEF	United Nations International Children's Emergency Fund
USPHS	US Public Health Service
WPRO	Western Pacific Region
WHA	World Health Assembly
WHO	World Health Organization

LIST OF TABLES

PROLOGUE

ORDINARY PEOPLE

When I started my research, I was shocked to discover how those with leprosy had been treated. In colonial Queensland, for example, several Chinese people had been exiled to a remote island in the Torres Strait. They were put ashore with materials to build shelters little more substantial than grass huts. A steamer was supposed to visit regularly with food, but its schedule was interrupted by bad weather. They quickly fell into a weakened and debilitated condition and within a matter of months died, almost certainly from starvation and exposure.[1]

If you were diagnosed with leprosy anytime from the nineteenth century onwards, the law demanded that you be detained and isolated for the rest of your life, for there was no hope of a cure. Your fate would be plain to see on the faces and the bodies of those who had been isolated like you. No exception was made if you were a child. Admittedly, there were differences in the policies and procedures and in the degrees of isolation and segregation depending upon the country in which you lived. Not everyone was isolated from society. In India, for example, people would wait outside an asylum in the hope of being admitted. Not everyone was segregated. In Hawaii, men, women, and children all dwelt together. In Australia, not only were people isolated, they were segregated by ethnicity. In Brazil and Colombia, people were isolated in places laid out like small townships, but not segregated. If you lived in a colony without segregation, you may have had children. Your children may have in turn become infected with leprosy, or they may have been taken away from you before they became infected. In the Philippines and in Malaysia, many children were removed from their parents as early as possible to avoid infection. If you were in Japan and you chose a partner in the sanatorium, you could marry on condition that you were sterilised. Even today, you may still be yearning to find those lost children or the children you never had.

Then, when doctors discovered they could use the sulphones against leprosy, the asylums were emptied out, as indeed Foucault writes. Only, they weren't. There was nowhere to go, for if you were disabled and unable to support yourself, you would be an unwelcome burden for your family.[2] If you were in Japan, you would not be released until after 1996.

From the 1950s and up until the 1980s, the walls of the asylum did slowly melt away, and you could be treated in your home or as an outpatient. But, as quickly became evident, the medication was only bacteriostatic, so you needed to continue with it for your whole life, only to face the fact that you had become resistant to it and your symptoms had not subsided.

But things changed for the better after 1981, when an effective chemotherapy became available. Disability was no longer inevitable, provided you were diagnosed in time and the loss of sensitivity associated with the disease had not led you to damage your hands and feet. You did not necessarily have to be physically marked by leprosy, if you did not experience any reaction to the medication. It seemed that leprosy had been defanged, provided you could be treated in time.

June Bertelesen was the first person who had suffered from leprosy that I ever met. On diagnosis as a young married woman, she was immediately removed to Peel Island, a small island in Moreton Bay off the coast of Brisbane, in Queensland, Australia. She barely had time to bid farewell to her children or her husband. Needless to say, when she was finally released from isolation, those family bonds were forever disrupted. Her marriage was over. She was estranged from her children. People found her bitter and full of complaints, but there was no remedy for the violence done to her in the name of public health.

The next place I met people affected by the disease was in Bombay at the Adams Wylie Hospital, a beautiful, old colonial bungalow built for plague victims in the early 1900s, probably now demolished. There in the large, dark, open room, Dr Hari Bulchard introduced me to several men, all lying in hospital beds, one with a face so infiltrated with the bacillus that it was crumpled and resembling a lion's: leonine facies, a description introduced by the Greeks to describe one of the effects of the disease. The doctor remarked wryly that WHO said this sort of infection no longer occurred. The men were all clearly curious about my presence, but they also seemed subdued and sad.

I met another man in the south of India several years later who told me that he was a Bengali, a teacher with a university degree, who on diagnosis had packed up his life and left everything out of shame and consideration for his family. He severed all ties and never looked back, making a new life for himself by joining a leprosy organisation in the south. To be diagnosed with leprosy was to lose status and caste.

I have since met people with leprosy all over the world – some of whose names I know, some whose names I never discovered. These were people in many countries: from the UK to the United States, Hawaii, China, India, Nepal, Japan, Brazil, the Philippines, South Africa, Nigeria, and Ghana. There is nothing special about them. They are just like you and me.

The woman I met in England agreed to meet me on condition that I did not talk about the disease. She wanted to put it behind her. She wanted to meet me on equal terms – not as an object of curiosity defined by leprosy. The man I know from the United States is full of purpose. He gives public addresses, edits a famous newsletter, has published a book. His life has been defined by leprosy, but in a way that he controls. His profession is to be an advocate for others. The people that I met in China lived in a remote leprosy village in Anhui, one of the poorest provinces in China. My visit was hosted by the mayor of the province, and we were heralded with firecrackers as we entered the village. The people were lined up along the front entrance, many on their crutches, many profoundly marked by the disease. I went to each and greeted them by shaking their mutilated hands – I did not speak Chinese, so this was my only means of communicating. As I walked into the courtyard, I could see in the shadows at the far end, the torso of a man propped up in an open doorway. He didn't have a hand for me to shake.

In my travels, I met Bill Malo from Hawaii. He told me that when he was a child, his mother had hidden him to avoid his being sent away to the leprosy settlement on Molokai. In spite of her attempts to protect him, he was finally discovered and sent off. He told me he blames himself for his brother's subsequent infection. If he had left home earlier, his brother may have been spared. In spite of his regrets, Bill had a hearty appreciation of life that triumphed over any setbacks. He had married several times in his life. He had no fear of the reaction of people to his disabled hands. He told me how he would go to the shops prepared for the first shocked response from the person who was serving him. This, in his view, was perfectly natural. He would make a joke of it, and the next time he went they would not be so shocked. Before long, their attention would be on him and his ebullient personality, not on his hands. Bill belongs to an advocacy organization, IDEA, the International Association for Integration, Dignity and Economic Advancement. Before he passed away, he would tell people about his experiences with leprosy, reassuring them that it didn't make a difference to who he was.

I also met Hilarion Guia on Culion in the Philippines, and he told me how he too had been diagnosed as a child and sent to the faraway island in the Palawan group for the rest of his life. He spoke of the sadness of his condition, but he concluded that it was the best thing that could have happened. To start with, instead of being hidden away, he had other children to play with openly, just like him. Then he received a Jesuit education, went on to be a teacher, and took up a position in the municipal council. If he had stayed in his village, none of this would have been available to him.

These are people just like you and me, different only in their cultures. True, they have suffered in ways that most of us can barely imagine, even though we all have our unique burdens. But in a time of widespread narcissism, when physical appearance has increasingly come to define who we are, these people have been forced to produce themselves and their identities in more complex ways. They have been forced to be explicit about their identities, to proclaim that they were more than their bodies. I will never forget the Christian minister on Robben Island who was adamant that he was more than his physical body and the social worker from Brazil who refused to be defined by her illness, by having to constantly "recount her story".

A moment of triumph sticks in my mind when in 2006, as a conclusion to the centennial celebrations on the island of Culion, the former leprosy colony, beautiful young women – Culion-born descendants of the people who had been isolated there – took part in a beauty contest. The final question to decide the winner was "what do you say to people when they ask you where you come from?" The winner was the one who could say without shame that they had been born on the island that had been known as "the isle of the living dead".

So much has been written about people with leprosy that is highly emotive and sensational. I refuse to write about these people in this way. They are the same as you and me, only they have been infected by a mycobacterium that has affected their body and may have changed their physical appearance, although that is not a given with the current medication. Physicians who have worked in this field have long been at pains to bill leprosy as a disease like any other. Who has been called by the name of their illness? If I am afflicted with cancer, do I become a "cancerite"? Why, if I am infected with *M. Leprae*, should I be called a leper?

INTRODUCTION

There is hardly anything on earth, or between it and heaven, which has not been regarded as the cause of Leprosy; and this is but natural, since the less one knows, the more actively does his imagination work. And since all that was known of Leprosy was that it was a loathsome disease, search was made everywhere for a cause.[1]

— Gerhard Henrik Armauer Hansen and Carl Looft

Mycobacterium leprae was identified by G. H. Armauer Hansen in 1873 to be the bacillus consistently present in the nodes of leprosy patients.[2] But this was far from the last word on the disease, for this entity still continues to puzzle histologists, pathologists, geneticists, and clinicians. This powerful and elusive bacterium that stalked through mediaeval Europe, inexplicably disappearing in the West and reappearing at the end of the nineteenth century in the colonies, still defies researchers. Medically, it is the aristocrat of diseases — the oldest, and the most aloof. Its ancient genome is described as degenerate since it has discarded many of its pathways and pared itself down to only what it needs to survive. Its effects depend more upon the reaction of the host than upon the action of the invader.[3] Its stages and categories have always been subject to confusion and debate. How it enters the body and is transmitted to others are still unknown. Its history is also shrouded in an uncertainty that is heightened by the confusion and debate surrounding its naming. Its progress within the body is still only partly understood. It has managed to maintain its huge reputation despite an economy of effort: by multiplying slowly, infecting only a few.

Persistent efforts have been made to understand, treat, and even eliminate this disease. This book charts those efforts from a number of different perspectives: the experiences of the patients, the evolution in understanding of what the disease was and how it might be contained, the ingenious science deployed to advance knowledge of the bacterium, the sources of funding of the fight against the disease, and the complex politics underlying

1

international attempts to systemise the attempt to control and even eliminate the disease. First, though, I discuss the cultural freight of leprosy, a disease recorded in classical and biblical times, which over the centuries accreted a symbolic potency that continued to be felt in some measure even to the present. The focus of the book is on the development of treatment regimens from approximately 1948 to 2005, the period when scientific discoveries, international post-war politics, and changes in sources of funding all contributed to a reassessment of what a "cure" of leprosy meant, and how and where patients should be treated. I introduce the story by describing the partial understanding of the disease and its appropriate treatment in the first half of the twentieth century. No effective cure was known, and some of the attempted treatments such as ingestion of chaulmoogra oil created nothing but enormous distress for the patient.

The true complexification of the history, however, occurs as the aspirations, treatment practices, scientific collaboration, and funding become international, with the consequent confusions and tensions that the conjunction of many powerful voices introduced. Chapter 1 explores a clear turning point in the transition to the international phase of leprosy research and treatment. In 1949, a delegation of medical and political figures from the newly independent republic of India petitioned the World Health Organization (WHO) to include leprosy in its programme. The chapter shows how treating leprosy had already figured in Mahatma Gandhi's national development programme, and analyses some of the political and financial constraints that the Indian initiative had to overcome. It also shows how the International Leprosy Association came into relationship with WHO in the interest of forming a determined strategy to ensure that leprosy be included in the programme of works in order to ensure the public health of those exposed to the disease.

Chapter 2 discusses one of the most important developments in the way the treatment of leprosy was conceived and implemented. For early-twentieth-century missionary workers, leprosy treatment had consisted of isolating and nursing the leprosy sufferer. As effective drug treatments started to be discovered and national and international bodies took over the leadership in treatment regimens, large-scale anti-leprosy campaigns became the norm, and leprosy was seen as a disease that could be treated under the rubric of public health. The decolonisation of much of the African and Asian world in this period inflects the story significantly.

Chapter 3 describes the unique culture of the long-standing, benevolent anti-leprosy organisations that federated in order to coordinate fundraising and assistance to workers and affected people and their ongoing relationship with WHO, brokered by the federation's Medical Commission.

Chapter 4 gives a short account of the reasons why laboratory scientists found it so difficult to discover the processes of leprosy infection, and documents their extraordinary inventiveness in trying to propagate leprosy bacilli in the laboratory to enable more vigorous research. It also examines the extent of international cooperation between scientists and the newly available air transport systems for the circulation of infected leprotic material for research. The resulting breakthroughs confirmed the fears of emerging drug resistance, both secondary and primary, and the phenomenon of bacterial "persisters". As the mass campaigns against leprosy lost steam, and faced with the threat of drug resistance, the Leprosy Unit at WHO arrived at a crisis point.

Chapter 5 describes the arrival of the Japanese delegation from the Sasakawa Memorial Health Foundation to WHO to offer substantial and much-needed funding support to the work against leprosy, and the ways in which this galvanised anti-leprosy work and research.

Chapter 6 describes how drug resistance provoked recourse to a standardised multidrug therapy that was adopted with a sense of urgency before trials were completed.

Chapter 7 marks the WHO's turn to primary healthcare at the precise moment that multidrug therapy was to be implemented. It argues that the Leprosy Unit's response to primary healthcare was pragmatic, especially in the face of the stigma associated with the disease amongst general medical professionals. It traces varying approaches to the implementation of multidrug therapy through primary healthcare in the Philippines, China, India, and Brazil.

Chapter 8 tells of the World Health resolution on the elimination of leprosy, noting that the difficulties with the resolution were apparent from the beginning in the debates before the executive board and the assembly.

Chapter 9 describes the reality of the work towards the elimination of leprosy as the failure to reach the target became apparent.

Chapter 10 recounts the formation and fracturing of the Global Alliance for the Elimination of Leprosy.

Chapter 11 describes the evaluation of the Global Alliance for the Elimination of Leprosy and the end of the elimination campaign that succeeded in resituating the Leprosy Unit in Delhi, much to the satisfaction of the benevolent anti-leprosy organisations.

Chapter 12 brings the narrative to a conclusion by arguing that the persistent and emerging voices of leprosy-affected people today, against all odds, have begun to be heard. They are taking on the power to represent themselves and reclaim their human rights, and in so doing reconcile that bifurcation between the two approaches to a cure: the public health approaches to the disease and the rehabilitation of the whole person. It argues that this reconciliation is accomplished in the politicised, proactive bodies of the people affected by the disease. The history concludes by offering three possible and possibly overlapping interpretations of the events that it has recounted. Each interpretation invokes a specific perspective and perhaps a corresponding label: bureaucratic, triumphalist, elitist. None of the versions exists independently of the other. None of the versions is without credit and none is to the complete credit of all involved. Anne-Emanuelle Birn argues the significance of the role of the historian of medicine:

> If policymakers tailor historical arguments to suit particular agendas (an obvious sign of political engagement) it strikes me that the historian's role is two-fold: first, to provide evaluation of the events or policies in question based on analysis of historical sources; and second, to demonstrate the selectivity and subjectivity of "historical" references and to show how this selectivity is related to particular goals and ideologies. Through this effort, the historian may offer an illuminating, if at times troubling, perspective on contemporary debates about the shaping of international/global health paradigms, priorities and programs. Policymakers in turn, may need to interact further with historians and examine the history of the field comprehensively if they wish to extract real "lessons" from the past in defining what could and should constitute success in this field.[4]

The story of anti-leprosy work as part of the international health initiatives that took place from 1948 onwards has been driven by competing agendas to the extent that events as they occurred can be explained in ways that are difficult to reconcile. Birn's description of the task that awaits me could not be more apposite. This history seeks to evaluate the events or policies around anti-leprosy work over eight decades, based on extensive analysis of historical sources. This history of the international politics of leprosy resonates with other historical analyses of international health initiatives. Accounts of anti-disease efforts in the post-World War II era emphasise over-investment in technologies such as DDT or antibiotics, to the neglect of the social and economic circumstances of people living in developing countries.[5] Except for smallpox, investment in a magic bullet approach to international health has not ended well. Transmission has not been interrupted, and resistant strains of disease have proliferated.

Superficially, international anti-leprosy work seems to fit into the same pattern as efforts against malaria and tuberculosis, but anti-leprosy efforts also demonstrate some differences. It is far too simplistic to argue that, as with malaria, hubris and overreach characterised those efforts. To start with, up until the availability of the sulphones, in spite of the efforts of a few, the field of anti-leprosy work was barely secularised, let alone professionalised. Workers were as marginalised by the general medical profession as those who suffered from the disease. Unlike malaria and tuberculosis, there was no widespread international enthusiasm for anti-leprosy work. Consequently, those who worked in leprosy saw the inclusion of anti-leprosy work into the international health agenda as an advance in its recognition and status.

Neither were there any assumptions around the absolute efficacy of the treatment. For while the sulphones finally offered the prospect of a treatment for leprosy, the medical experts remained cautious, constantly acknowledging the need for further research. In fact, in the hope that they could diminish transmission, medical administrators calculated the public health benefits of mass treatment against the uncertain prospects of a complete cure for the individual when they distributed the medication in mass campaigns. There was no hubris, only determination to get leprosy on the same agenda as other diseases and to deliver people from a lifetime of isolation in leprosy asylums.

Medical historians record WHO's declining influence in the 1970s and 1980s so that voluntary donations became increasingly important and influential in determining its programme. The story of leprosy's donors partially shows the same trajectory with differences in timing and ideology. International anti-leprosy work was initially conducted in collaboration with the International Federation of Leprosy Associations (ILEP). Some of these anti-leprosy organisations in the Federation dated from the late nineteenth century, when few wanted to have anything to do with people affected by the disease. Historically, these organisations were financed by tiny public donations that added up to a substantial resource for anti-leprosy work that WHO hoped to channel towards what the organisation saw as priorities.

Then two newcomers, the Nippon Foundation (TNF) and the Sasakawa Memorial Health Foundation (SMHF), both founded by the controversial Ryoichi Sasakawa – through making substantial and sustained donations and through the hands-on influence of the medical director of the Sasakawa Memorial Health Foundation, Dr Yo Yuasa – came to drive the WHO leprosy programme. This coincided with the appearance of dapsone resistance and was counterpointed by new knowledge about *M. leprae*. The significant funds provided to the programme by TNF, SMHF, and the ILEP organisations made research and extensive anti-leprosy work possible, but at the cost of an arm's-length approach and at variance to the WHO policy for voluntary donations.

In this era, without question, work done against leprosy was designed to bring credit to the international reputation of Japan, and personal credit to Ryoichi Sasakawa. Those committed to anti-leprosy work knew this, but, like all of those who had gone before them, did not resile from the opportunity presented by the funding. The substantial funds provided to the programme and the newly standardised multidrug therapy provided the rationale for a World Health resolution on the elimination of leprosy by the year 2000. Under pressure of the elimination deadline, and at a time when the aspirations of primary healthcare changed ideas about the delivery of healthcare, work against leprosy was redefined in operational ways that were controversial to those who feared that the elimination of the disease was being confected statistically (by both WHO and TNF) for the sake of declaring success.

Superficial comparisons in the later decades could also obscure important differences between anti-leprosy work and work against diseases such as malaria and tuberculosis. In the 1990s, with Gro Harlem Brundtland's reinvention of the WHO, public–private partnerships with wealthy donors such as the World Bank increasingly dictated public health policy founded on a neoliberal economic model of cost-effectiveness that calculated what work against which diseases would reward investment. At this time, WHO attempted to break the influence of the donors with drug donations from Novartis, and the Global Alliance for the Elimination of Leprosy (GAEL) partnership was launched under the umbrella of public–private partnerships. But the differences between ideologies in the ILEP approach to the disease and the WHO approach shattered the alliance and delivered a mortal blow to the final stages of the elimination campaign. Yet when we review and compare the history of anti-leprosy work to anti-malaria and anti-tuberculosis efforts, the contested ownership of work against leprosy did not halt the work of people on the ground who orchestrated large, community-led leprosy elimination campaigns as big as the state of Tamil Nadu, in India.

The standard historical narrative of international health also tells of a descent into cost-efficient disease-control efforts, and this might appear to be the case if only a jaundiced view is taken of the WHO advocacy of multidrug therapy in the elimination campaign. Yet in spite of the fears of a confected disappearance of the disease, in spite of premature and misleading public relations announcements from WHO, in spite of suspicions about the agenda of the donors, in spite of the contested politics around fieldwork procedures and indicators of success, those who had both funded the work and also worked against the disease always continued their efforts against leprosy. Collaborations between WHO, TNF, SMHF, and ILEP organisations at the country level and World Bank-funded campaigns that were community driven succeeded in robbing leprosy of its stigma and prompting people to present themselves for early treatment. The drugs themselves had a role to play in the effectiveness of this. Yet, like malaria and tuberculosis, transmission of *M. leprae* has not been interrupted, and the bacillus is managing to hang on. While fewer people than ever are being infected, all eyes are turned to new research that promises to reveal more about the mysteries of transmission.

The symbolic power of leprosy

Leprosy has been recognised in many different cultures. It has long generated a symbolic freight that obscures and dominates the facts of its pathology, even to generating its own myths of origin. For example, a legend from the Tang Dynasty (618–906 CE) invokes the power of leprosy as a social signifier:

> According to this folk story, during the middle of the Tang Dynasty the reigning emperor was engaged in a war with a powerful war-lord named An Lui-Shan who laid siege to the capital and forced the emperor to flee in the company of his favorite courtesan, Yang Kwei Fei. She was a lady of legendary beauty and was responsible for the emperor's misfortune, having caused him to neglect affairs of state to the extent that discontent was rife among his people and his lords. While the emperor and his retinue, accompanied by the remnants of his army, were in flight, his immediate guards suddenly refused to proceed farther unless he first permitted the execution of Yang Kwei Fei. To save his own life, the emperor issued the order and her body was left lying by the roadside as a witness to the accompanying army that she had finally been deposed. As the convoy passed, some soldiers, charmed by the beauty of the body, had improper relations with it. The legend states that all the soldiers who committed this misdemeanor subsequently developed leprosy as a punishment from Heaven and that thus the disease originated.[6]

Although the final sentence locates the cause of leprosy as divine punishment for necrophilia, the situation in which this act takes place is elaborately detailed. The legend tells of a kingdom in internal disarray and threatened from without. The emperor has neglected his responsibilities as a ruler, seduced by his favouritism and private desire for his courtesan. Ironically, the attempt to rectify this state of affairs further compounds the decay of the kingdom. Yang Kwei Fei, the woman who is the seeming cause of the disruptions, is executed. The rule of order and chain of authority are disrupted to such an extent that her execution takes place in response to the demands and threats issued on the king's life by his own guards, whose role it is to defend him. The king's moral fibre and integrity are so weakened that he cannot even be loyal to her, and he has her executed in order to preserve his own life. Even in death, her body is a source of danger. Her betrayal by the man who loved her so much that he was prepared to neglect his kingly responsibilities for her, and her violation by the passing soldiers, encapsulates the calamity and disorder that has led to this point. The corruption of the king and orderly rule together with the unnatural sexual acts of the soldiers underlie the appearance of leprosy. Leprosy is not conceived of as an "innocent" disease to be accepted fatalistically. It is presented as a retributive result of sexual and political indulgence.

This legend is related by Olaf Skinsnes in a comparison of early responses to leprosy in Chinese, Japanese, Indian, and pre-Christian Mediterranean and Middle Eastern writings.[7] These comparative studies clearly indicate that in countries not influenced by the Judeo-Christian tradition there is "some unique intrinsicality relating to leprosy that makes it subject to society's opprobrium".[8] Significantly, the myths and commonplaces attached to leprosy convey a sense of it as a catastrophe, as something that could have occurred only as the result of some serious infringement of the moral order. They also convey a sense of the disease as something that is transmitted at a level of intimacy that is forbidden.

These negative overshadowings of the disease continue to the present day. Just as leprosy still manages to infect over 200,000 new cases in the world every year, its traces persist in our lexicon and in our cultural heritage, easily summoning up the past and amplifying its burden of signification. I wish to explore some of the reasons for the obdurate and unyielding imaginings attached to the disease, bearing in mind that these have very real consequences for people with leprosy.

A long and hard battle has been fought against the stigma attached to leprosy. A significant milestone was reached when the word "leper" was written out of medical and organisational usage and "Hansen's disease" became the standard medical nomenclature.[9] Nonetheless, leprosy's negative representational history continues. The idea of the disease triggers a whole range of extremely complex associations. Not only is leprosy abhorred, it is also sentimentalised, exoticised, romanticised, and orientalised. In addition, leprosy is appropriated to different discourses, often for political purposes, so that the representational force of leprosy shifts, merges with other diseases and discourses, may seem to vanish, but inevitably re-emerges reinforced with revivified symbolic resonance.

To an extent, the appropriation of the language of disease is not exclusive to leprosy, but I argue that this representational circularity finds itself intensified with leprosy. In *Illness as Metaphor* and *AIDS and Its Metaphors*, Susan Sontag struggles to uproot the metaphoric function of the language of disease and illness because it is so permeated with blame. She writes:

> My subject is not physical illness itself but the uses of illness as a figure or metaphor. My point is that illness is not a metaphor, and that the most truthful way of regarding illness – and the healthiest way of being ill – is one most purified of, most resistant to, metaphoric thinking. Yet it is hardly possible to take up one's residence in the kingdom of the ill unprejudiced by the lurid metaphors with which it has been landscaped. It is toward an elucidation of those metaphors, and a liberation from them, that I dedicate this inquiry.[10]

This metaphoric function of disease is Janus-faced. Metaphors of disease are used to represent experience. At the same time, specific illnesses become enshrouded with a metaphoric potency, and what they are taken to represent is often in excess of their materiality. Metaphors of disease thus assume an autonomy from the specific illness and bring themselves to focus on diverse phenomena, but return to their specific illnesses replete with associations. These metaphors mediate the reality of the illness and in turn, in combination with everything that they take from and bring to the illness, mediate completely unrelated events. Sontag traces this Janus-faced metaphoric power:

> Any important disease whose causality is murky, and for which treatment is ineffectual, tends to be awash in significance. First, the subjects of deepest dread (corruption, decay, pollution, anomie, weakness) are identified with the disease. The disease itself becomes a metaphor. Then, in the name of the disease (that is, using it as a metaphor), that horror is imposed on other things. The disease becomes adjectival. Something is said to be disease-like, meaning that it is disgusting or ugly.[11]

But in writing that "the disease becomes a metaphor", she fails to realise the power of this metaphoric function; she fails to notice how separate the metaphor actually is from the material illness. The metaphor takes on a separate life and gathers to itself its own associations – it departs from the illness and returns to it with new connotations. It *is* already liberated from the illness in a way that Sontag does not acknowledge. The metaphoric function of disease forms its own autonomous discourse.[12] Scheper-Hughes and Lock, medical anthropologists, write:

> Sickness is not just … an unfortunate brush with nature. It is a form of communication – the language of the organs – through which nature, society, and culture speak simultaneously. The individual body should be seen as the most immediate, the proximate terrain where social truths and social contradictions are played out, as well as a locus of personal and social resistance, creativity, and struggle.[13]

Sontag's thesis has been critiqued as being unrealistic and overemphasising the responses of cancer sufferers to their illness. I think she is right in so far as the meanings associated with a disease profoundly and insidiously affect the responses of many (not all) to their illness: for example, to be diagnosed with cancer is to "change" how one views oneself. Everything that has circulated culturally and socially about cancer converges on one's own body. This is even more the case with leprosy, as millennia of sufferers have experienced. To be told that one had leprosy was to become "a leper", as the accounts in Betty Martin's and June Berthelsen's writings indicate.[14] And this is still the case to differing degrees in many cultures.

While the redesignation of leprosy as Hansen's disease has made leprosy almost invisible in the Western world, I argue that the associations attached to leprosy refuse to be repressed or purged. History demonstrates that no matter how hard one attempts to control the accumulated meanings of leprosy, the more resistant these meanings become. They circulate endlessly. They may seem to disappear, but they reappear in different clothing with their old familiar aspect. I am thinking of an example in Australia when failed army recruits were referred to as lepers, and one who suffered a physical disability took his own life. The way leprosy is represented, and the way leprosy is used to represent things unrelated to leprosy, has a powerful autonomy that has no respect for the lived experience of illness.

I want to explore some of these associations and point to a possible reason for their persistence. To return to my opening myth of origin which connected leprosy with personal and political disorder, I set against it another account of the origin of leprosy. It is claimed that Alexander the Great's soldiers on their victorious return from India in 327–6 BCE brought leprosy to the eastern Mediterranean.[15] The troops returned with Asian women whom they publicly married. Shortly after this, the earliest descriptions of leprosy appear in Alexandria.

This is another story of leprosy coming to the kingdom as a result of the actions of a king. And although Alexander seems to be the very opposite of the irresponsible emperor in the first story, it is another story of the boundaries of the body politic being permeated. The incursion into India "crosses" the boundary between the West and the Orient. The story also conceals a reversal of the natural order of authority. Although the union with the women takes place by his authority, Alexander's incursions into India came to a halt because his soldiers refused to go any further. The publicly orchestrated mass marriage of his soldiers with the women from the East becomes an icon of intermingling of East and West, the product of which is physical contamination and a legacy of leprosy, a disease that is an attack on identity and the defining boundaries of the body. In this narrative of origin, recounted by Mark, leprosy demonstrates the consequences of "going beyond" the known world and intermingling with exotic women. Leprosy thus becomes an index of orientalism and a cautionary tale against miscegenation.

Whether these narratives of the origin of leprosy have any truth is immaterial; the fact that they are repeated contributes to the historical representation of leprosy. This representational history encapsulates connections between the political and the personal. Violations in one sphere have consequences in the other, and leprosy is used to express both the connections between the spheres and the magnitude of the consequences. The effectiveness of these stories relies on leprosy having a certain identity involving its effect on the body. In her study of witchcraft and leprosy, Mary Douglas suggests that the freight of associations and the recurring stigma attached to leprosy were employed as fundamental "controlling" mechanisms in society.[16]

In times of social disruption, the assigning of leprosy to a particular group enabled society to cast that group off and realign itself. So, in the Chinese legend, what is really important is that whoever was "accused" of leprosy was linked to a corrupt regime, hence their exclusion from the newly organised society. In the times of Alexander the Great, whoever was accused of leprosy was connected to a campaign that introduced the corrupting influences of the East to the West. They had been irreparably orientalised, and to exclude them was to exclude something that was suspect and potentially corrupt. Douglas uses this argument to suggest that the assigning of leprosy in the Middle Ages had more to do with those who were disenfranchised by social change than those who actually had the disease.

Douglas takes this one step further when she suggests that "the idea of contagious leprosy was used to solve social dilemmas by shifting legitimacy into a new pattern".[17] While leprosy expressed the violation of boundaries, it was also used to reconfigure them. She suggests that leprosy may be used as a mode of social control in three different ways. In the first case "the arrow points up, against the office holders attempting to abuse their privileges" (for example, the Chinese king, in the first legend). In the second case, "it points down, against the disfranchised majority" (for example, the poor, who were the victims of social dislocation in the Middle Ages in Europe). In the last case, it points outwards, "against the outsiders who threaten the tight beleaguered community" (in the case of the Asian women who were married to Alexander the Great's soldiers).[18] If it is an accurate analysis, it suggests that the stigma associated with leprosy is most apparent in times of economic and social stress, or whenever a society is undergoing upheaval.

The scholarly historical research that has been conducted on leprosy, I believe, adds dimensions to my argument. In the case of Megan Vaughan's research, we see how the missionary work done on leprosy in Africa is simultaneously directed at the reconstruction of African communities, African society, and African identity. This work took place within the context of a widespread perception of disintegration and a "breakdown of tribal authority". Vaughan highlights this when she writes that in Africa "Theories of leprosy causation also came to reflect not only Christian concerns but wider colonial concerns over social change and social order."[19] The energy expended on leprosy epitomised the reconstruction of the body politic. She writes that leprosy settlements including mission-run ones reflected the larger colonial society and systems of control, and stood as microcosms of the British colony.

This work becomes focused on individual African identities. Vaughan describes the recreation of village communities for people with leprosy as "a place where a new identity and a new community could be forged".[20] A British Empire Leprosy Relief Association (BELRA) report of the time describes leprosy as erasing identity: "Men, women and children became molded into that ghastly form, in which personality, sex, and age are blotted out, and the victim becomes a mere caricature of humanity."[21] In the place of this loss of identity, "an alternative identity as a 'leper' was what some missionaries appeared to be advocating in their settlements". This replacement of identity was the precursor to a larger project: "Leprosy offered to the missionaries the possibilities of engineering new African communities, isolated from, and expunged of, all those features of African society which they saw as impeding the development of Christianity."[22]

There seems to be no end to the use of leprosy to make connections between the body and the body politic. Rita Smith Kipp's study of missionary leprosy work in colonial Sumatra, then a part of the Dutch East Indies, supports this history of representation. Her exploration of the evangelistic opportunity afforded by leprosy in an era of segregation touches on the symbolic purposes to which leprosy is put. She writes that "In many of the tropical colonies, the ancient scourge became a symbol of backwardness, inferiority, and filth of those requiring control." In the leprosarium of Lau si Momo, an artificial village was created which offered "an enclosed and relatively insular new world".[23]

> Lau si Momo stood out as a successful oasis in a mission field that struggled for half a century in a desert of failure, presenting European donors and the colonial government with an irresistible before-and-after vision – the most wretched of outcasts transformed into church-going, soccer-playing natives who lived in a village that was the "model" of Dutch hygiene and order. Laui si Momo was the colonial dream come true in microcosm. The efficacy of Western medicine was vindicated here, but quite beyond that, within the confines of this one village, space, time, and the social world had been moulded successfully according to a "rational" design.[24]

Warwick Anderson's "Leprosy and Citizenship" makes connections between the American colonial project and the Culion leprosarium. He writes, "To understand the American colonial project it is necessary to study Culion, for the leper colony had become an allegory of the prospects of the macrocolony ..."[25] Diana Obregón's work examines the connections between the representation of Colombia as a modernising nation and the energy devoted to leprosy. She describes the historical irony of a country that made much of its leprosy in order to demonstrate its attention to the modernising project, but then found itself in the paradoxical situation of having to revise its reputation as a nation afflicted by leprosy, in order to continue to represent itself as a modern nation.[26]

My own earlier research focuses upon concerns about the spread of leprosy in colonial Queensland in the 1890s. In political cartoons, the colony of Queensland is represented as a woman with leprosy. Around her the premier of the colony and his imported indentured, leprosy-infected "scab" labourers dance in a parody of the children's nursery rhyme that recalls the signs of the plague. They are dancing to her tune, and they are dancing off to the lazarette. The body politic is threatened because those responsible for its government are looking after their own interests, rather than those of the people. The ruling elite continue to employ cheap labour, rather than employ workers according to union conditions; consequently, they are importing disease into the colony. The body politic is threatened literally with disease from imported labour, but it is also figuratively corrupt and diseased. And that trope of corruption associated with Queensland's politics persists even today.

Leprosy is used to contain and express social disruption and reorganisation. So the representation of leprosy and the use of leprosy for representation indicate leprosy's connection to fundamental social processes. Trying to contain the representation of leprosy, that is, trying to control the way it is used, is a never-ending and ultimately futile task. In a historical sense, work done on the body of the person with leprosy is never done naively. It always takes place in the context of the body politic. So in this narrative, the work being done on leprosy-affected bodies served differing agendas for different political purposes, some of which would inevitably come into conflict.

Early scientific approaches to leprosy

In their struggle to understand, contain, and control the disease, the physicians of the late nineteenth century mapped the occurrence of the disease in a variety of ways in order to investigate the enabling conditions for transmission. They drew up family trees to investigate transmission by inheritance. They recorded case studies to investigate transmission by contagion, inoculation, and vaccination. They searched for commonalities in disease patterns across race, gender, class, region, topography, diet, religious and denominational grouping, standards of personal hygiene, and morality. They mapped these commonalities country by country and colony by colony, looking for a pattern to prove their particular hypotheses.

Formal medical knowledge at the time was filtered through a Greek, Roman, and Arabian inheritance. In 1846, Francis Adams produced *The Seven Books of Paulus Ægineta*, which included a commentary on all medical and surgical knowledge and descriptions and remedies from the Romans, Greeks, and Arabs.[27] His contribution to the multitude of meanings clustered around the disease was to secure more tightly the completely erroneous and confusing connection between the disease and syphilis.

In 1875, Ferdinand Hebra and Moriz Kaposi's *On the Diseases of the Skin Including the Exanthemata* began a discussion of leprosy with a litany of the names identifying the disease in various countries throughout the world.[28] They also noted the variety of names used to describe symptoms of the disease, the confusion encountered in Adams (described above), as well as the confusion between the Hebrew *zaraath* and its misleading translation as lepra.[29] They then set about distinguishing between "Lepra Arabum-Elephantiasis Graecorum", "Elephantiasis Arabum", and "Lepra Graecorum", words which, they noted, had been used indiscriminately to denote different diseases occurring in the same region or in the same individual, or used in place of some other skin afflictions, including syphilis. Finally, they described how almost any "rare, disfiguring, incurable, or exotic diseases" had been diagnosed as leprosy, contributing to the confusion over what precisely the disease was. They concluded that this persisting terminological and diagnostic confusion made regional comparisons and thus clear identification even more difficult: "Owing to the conflicting views, everyone was quite at a loss to determine whether, and in what manner, certain diseases, supposed to be endemic, such as the Radesyge of Norway, the Morbus Dithmarscicus, the Sibbens of Scotland, the Falcadina of Istria, were connected with lepra."[30]

In their view, the Norwegians Daniel Cornelius Danielssen (1815–94), from St Jørgen's Hospital in Bergen, and Carl Wilhelm Boëck (1808–75), professor of the Faculty of Medicine in Oslo, supplied the first clear description of its pathology.[31] Danielssen and Boëck's account was based on extensive and systematic analysis of leprosy's effects on the body through autopsies and comparisons with the disease in southern parts of Europe.[32] They believed that leprosy was an inheritable dyscrasia of the blood that was capable of latency and would emerge in unfavourable living conditions. Based on their observations of clusters of families, they concluded that leprosy was a constitutional condition that would develop in those with a hereditary disposition.[33]

Hebra and Kaposi therefore felt empowered to pronounce that this much was known: "that wherever lepra exists, at the present time, it always presents the same characters, and that the lepra of all countries is identical". In addition, differences in symptoms in various localities are not significant and did not represent different varieties of the disease. Therefore,

> in consequence of this discovery, all the names hitherto applied to the disease which are derived from its geographical position … must be given up, and one designation, founded on the history of the disease, and which may be understood by the physicians of all countries, must be substituted for them, once for all.[34]

The elusive disease was named and attached to a set of symptoms. But this was only the beginning of controversy. Danielssen's son-in-law, Gerhard Henrik Armauer Hansen (1841–1912), held a different view of the disease. He is credited with discovering, in 1873, that leprosy was a distinct nosological entity and that *Mycobacterium lepra* (*M. leprae*) was the specific cause of the disease.[35]

As processes of naming and describing had produced difficulty and confusion, so the effects of the disease observed on the body were protean.

The body's response to *M. leprae* results in a variety of symptoms that seem to vary depending on ethnicity and location. Over the next 100 years, clinicians and researchers exhaustively debated these differences in an attempt to arrive at a universal nomenclature that would be useful both in the field and in the laboratory. Table 1 below maps some of those changing categorisations from the publications of Danielssen, Boëck, and Hansen, through to those created by the various meetings on classification at International Leprosy Congresses in Berlin (1897), Bergen (1909), Cairo (1938), Havana (1948), and so on …

Table 1: Changing Categorisations of the Symptoms of Leprosy

1848	Danielssen and Boëck	Nodular and Anaesthetic
1895	Hansen and Looft	Tuberosa (nodular) and Maculoanaesthetic
1903	Neisser	Lepra tuberosa Lepra cutane Lepra nervorum
1905 1923 1934	Jadassohn Darier Wade	Tuberculoid
1931	Manila classification (Leonard Wood Memorial Conference)	Cutaneous, Neural, and Mixed
1939	Cairo classification (International Leprosy Conference)	Lepromatous Neural (neuromacular simple, neuromacular tuberculoid, neuro-anaesthetic)
1946	Pan-American Classification (Second Pan-American Leprosy Conference, Rio de Janeiro)	Lepromatous Tuberculoid Uncharacteristic
1948	Havana Classification (International Leprosy Congress, Havana)	Indeterminate instead of Uncharacteristic
1952	World Health Organization Expert Committee	Lepromatous Tuberculoid Borderline Indeterminate

1955	Indian Association of Leprologists (All India Leprosy Workers Conference)	Lepromatous Tuberculoid Maculoanaesthetic Borderline Polyneuritic Indeterminate

1953	Madrid Classification (International Leprosy Congress, Madrid)	Lepromatous Type (L)
		  Macular
		  Diffuse
		  Infiltrated
		  Nodular
		  Neuritic, pure
		Tuberculoid Type (T)
		  Macular (Tm)
		  Minor tuberculoid (Tt)
		  Major tuberculoid (TT)
		  Neuritic, pure (Tn)
		Indeterminate Group (I)
		  Macular (Im)
		  Neuritic, pure (In)
		Borderline (Dimorphous)
		Group (B)
		  Infiltrated
		  (Others?)

These changing systems of categorisation resulted from fierce debates that consumed the energy and intellectual oxygen at international gatherings well into the twentieth century. The typological wrangling was less a testament to the contentiousness of the participants than to the elusiveness of *M. leprae* and the way it reveals itself clinically through the response of the host's immune system – something that was not discovered until the 1960s. For leprosy persisted in presenting a diverse spectrum of symptoms in individuals and in specific cohorts of the population from different parts of the world, complexifying attempts to understand the essential characteristics and pathology of the disease.[36]

Treatment

At the end of the nineteenth century, physicians were so impressed at the large quantities of bacilli shed from the skin and in the nasal mucous membranes of those infected with *M. leprae* that they declared leprosy sufferers to be a danger to their neighbours. And although they conceded that leprosy did occur amongst those "in the higher social circles", they perceived the real danger to be amongst the lower classes, who when infected were especially dangerous to their family and fellow workers.[37] When leprosy declined in Norway towards the end of the nineteenth century, the Norwegian isolation measures appeared to have been vindicated.

From the 1890s, and hastened by the first Leprosy Conference in Berlin in 1897, legislation was introduced in many countries to segregate leprosy sufferers.[38] After every new international congress – in Bergen in 1909, Strasbourg in 1923, and Cairo in 1938 – successive bursts of legislation to confine sufferers and to construct leprosy asylums, colonies, or sanatoria precipitated modernising approaches to the disease in different countries throughout the world.

Institutions for isolation and segregation varied widely in character and in the degree of compulsion exerted on those who were detained.[39] Once leprosaria were established, they brought their own unique set of complex and ultimately irresolvable problems. People did not die from leprosy, and many lived out their entire lifetimes in a leprosy institution. Once people with the disease were confined, segregation of the sexes, control of sexual activity, and sometimes forced sterilisation and abortion militated against the birth of children. However, in spite of all precautions and policing, children were born within these institutions, and this problem was addressed by removing babies from their mothers, establishing orphanages, organising adoptions, and training children to work in leprosy asylums as nursing attendants and paramedical workers. As well as the practical problem of what to do with children born to the leprosy-affected, there was a growing concern that leprosy was communicated in childhood; therefore, children born to those with the disease and in primary contact with carriers of *M. leprae*, were not only considered particularly susceptible but also important subjects for scientific observation.[40]

Sir Leonard Rogers and Ernest Muir demonstrated some of the persisting and tenacious uncertainties around leprosy in the first half of the twentieth century in their manual on leprosy, which was in its third edition in 1946. They picked through leprosy's tangled history and geographical mapping, through the as yet uncertain field of epidemiology, in which the conditions influencing the prevalence of leprosy could only be hypothesised, and through various theories of causation and communicability, to arrive at a passionate argument against absolute segregation in favour of early detection and outpatient treatment. The writers concluded that leprosy was "a communicable disease" whose dissemination was favoured by insanitary conditions, especially in a hot, humid climate. Infection from the disease was aided by insanitary contact: defective and overcrowded houses, sexual promiscuity, and social customs connected with communal sleeping, eating, and smoking. It flourished where there was an absence of fear of the disease.

Environmental explanations for the spread of the disease were also racialised. The authors explained that the tropical countries where the disease was most prevalent were "mainly inhabited by coloured races in a low stage of civilization, living in primitive, small, generally one-roomed, overcrowded houses".[41] Additionally, the spread of leprosy was associated with miscegenation: "The great majority of cases of cohabiting occurred in tropical countries, where men have frequently been attacked with leprosy during or within the common incubation period of the disease after living with leprous native women."[42]

In summary then, if a culture did not share any natural caution against leprosy, close contact with infective persons guaranteed its propagation, and little effort would be made to prevent the disease. Additionally, people who suffered from poor nutrition were particularly vulnerable. Most susceptible to infection, however, were children and young adults up to twenty years of age, so detecting and treating these early cases before they progressed beyond hope of successful treatment and before other people were infected was of paramount importance.[43]

Early treatment for leprosy was based on chaulmoogra or hydnocarpus oil, which had traditionally been recognised as a cure for leprosy in India, Burma, and China.[44] The oil had been introduced into Western medicine, when it was "discovered" by Frederic John Mouat in 1854, when he was Professor at the Bengal Medical College.[45] Originally, chaulmoogra oil had been given orally, but it was extremely nauseating, and people were reluctant to take it and unable to tolerate it. Physicians then injected it, but it was absorbed slowly. Subsequently, attempts were made to produce mixtures that would reduce the irritation caused by the painful injections and also assist its rapid absorption.[46] These could be given intramuscularly, subcutaneously, intradermally, or intravenously, and physicians were advised to begin with small doses and increase them gradually, for a patient's tolerance varied with their physical condition, weight, and age. In addition, immediately after treatment, they could experience a "negative phase" which was, once again, dependent upon their condition.[47]

A Public Health Service Report from 1930 reveals details of sixty-five patients who had received chaulmoogra treatment at the Carville

Leprosarium in the United States over a ten-year period.[48] These were people who had been released from the hospital because the progress of the disease had been judged to be arrested, bacilli had disappeared, and most of their symptoms had subsided.[49] In spite of the sparse details provided in each of these case studies, it is possible to read between the lines and gain a sense of the outlook for people at this time, and also perhaps gain some insight into the hopes, uncertainties, and frustrations clustered around the treatment and the possibility of a cure.

A glance at individual cases leaves the lasting and shocking impression that the disease ate up the subjects' lives.[50] One 30-year-old man had suffered from leprosy for fifteen years, and although he had spent only nine months in hospital, during which time he had consumed 144 cubic centimetres of the ethyl esters of chaulmoogra oil, he had returned after three years with symptoms of active leprosy.[51] After ten years suffering from leprosy, a 32-year-old woman spent eleven years in hospital while experiencing the loss of her hair on her eyebrows and forearms, experiencing the contraction of her toes on her left foot, and consuming more than five litres of chaulmoogra oil.[52] Another, a man of forty-three years, after ten years of symptoms spent fifteen years in hospital, "improving slowly", while consuming four litres of chaulmoogra oil, taking strychnine sulphate for two years, receiving 167 cubic centimeters of intravenous mercurochrome, and undergoing the amputation of his right foot.[53] A 32-year-old man, who had spent twenty years in hospital, was blind, and his hands, feet, and face suffered from mutilations. His total anaesthesia and blindness locked him into complete sensory exclusion; nonetheless, the report optimistically records that after only palliative treatment his symptoms had not yet reappeared, six months later.[54] A woman, who was nineteen on admission, was hospitalised for twenty-four years.[55] A young girl, who was thirteen on admission, was subsequently hospitalised for 33 years.[56] A 16-year-old male was hospitalised for sixteen years.[57]

Treatment of leprosy oscillated erratically between what had seemed for so long an inviolable truth and what now seemed like a possible albeit elusive goal: the divinely ordained incurability of the disease on the one hand and a possible scientific discovery of a cure on the other. The concept of "cure" always had to be qualified, however; patients were only ever "paroled", not pardoned, with all of the psychologically negative connotations of infringement left intact. The disease was "active" or "quiescent", but the prospect of "relapse" was constantly present, always overshadowing the possibility of "cure". The status of the disease in the individual was subject to bacteriological examination, the results of which could either be negative or positive; but a negative result would have to be repeated consistently over a set period before the patient could be considered eligible for parole.

In 1930, the investigations of the Secretary for the Leprosy Commission of the League of Nations, Etienne Burnet, provided an interesting insight into the instability of knowledge around treatment and cure.[58] He reported that there were the "keenest discussions" about the efficacy of the then current treatment. People's views were polarised: some stated openly that it was "mere humbug"; others declared that to be "lukewarm" about it was "as great a crime as to refuse quinine to a malaria patient". There were also those who believed that "you can't cure, you can only bleach, and not for long", but others who argued that "If by bleaching the danger of infection disappears for a period of months or years, this represents a medical improvement from the leper's standpoint and an immense progress in the matter of prophylaxis."[59]

There was also a great deal of blame attached to failures: advocates of the various forms of treatment responded to detractors by saying that "if it fails to produce the best results, this is because the treatment has been too slight, too short and irregular, and has been administered without conviction".[60] All agreed, however, on the need for the earliest possible treatment, support for which was drawn from observing early and successful treatment of children.[61] But even when people were treated and apparently "cured", doctors were reluctant to discharge the patient, explaining that it was necessary to maintain sanitary supervision for an indefinite period.

This instability around the notion of cure impacted on the idea of the "leprosarium" so that the ideal institution was constantly being reinvented. If leprosy was indeed curable, then segregation measures could be gradually reduced until the leprosarium would be simply a home for "advanced cases, aged invalids and incurables". Treatment could be given via dispensaries and to people in their homes. Alternatively, if the disease could not be successfully treated, then "isolation and measures of constraint" would continue to be "imperative".[62]

In the 1930s, there was an attempt to move away from the older notions of segregation to a preferable idea of "isolation" under "sanatorium" conditions, like the tuberculosis sanatorium, founded on hygienic living, early treatment, good food, rest, temporary isolation, and "common-sense" approaches to building physical health.[63] It became a mantra that compulsory confinement of people in leprosaria led only to concealment, which meant that infectious cases went undetected and continued to spread the disease. Segregation measures and "older therapeutic measures" were opposed to "modern hygienic measures" and "advanced therapeutic measures". In the overheated debates, segregationists were opposed to anti-segregationists; "constraint" was opposed to "liberty"; and "regulationists" were opposed to "abolitionists". Outpatient dispensaries were developed as an alternative to leprosaria, especially by those who espoused the value of early treatment using hydnocarpus injections.[64]

This change impacted catastrophically upon the person with the disease. There seemed to be hope, but it all depended upon one's ability to tolerate litres and litres of a nauseating treatment or, even worse, to subject oneself to extremely painful intramuscular injections or the countless pinpricks of intradermal injections. Then there were the unfortunate ones who were subjected to Sir Leonard Rogers's intravenous injections and who could count themselves lucky if they were not killed by a fatty embolism.[65] As is often the case where there are so many uncertainties, responsibility was placed upon the patient who had to shoulder not only the burden of the disease but also some of the blame if they were not cured. Their mental condition was commonly acknowledged as having a part to play in their cure: "Patients must be encouraged to exert their will power in the direction of getting better. If any improvement is to be effected, the co-operation of the patient is most important."[66] Patients were to be warned that the treatment would be protracted and "that the chance of final recovery must depend to a large extent on the energy and persistence with which they carry out their part".[67] Many people who wrote of their experience tell of the heartbreak of waiting for the pathology results that would take them one step further towards discharge, only to fall short of the required number of negative results when they seemed so near to health and freedom.

Stanley Stein, one of the more articulate and proactive leprosy-affected inmates of Carville in the United States, graphically describes his experience with chaulmoogra injections. His oft-quoted words are that

> Whether I was to take the oil externally, internally or – as someone once said – eternally was up to me. The oral doses were nauseously given out in the cafeteria at mealtime. The injections were administered in what was to me a distressingly public manner … The spectacle of several dozen patients with trousers at half-mast, standing in line to bare their rumps to the doctor, had startled me.[68]

By his account, at Carville patients could choose between hydnocarpus ethyl esters or chaulmoogra oil with olive oil and benzocaine. He describes the administration:

The technique for both was more or less the same – a sharp jab into the gluteal muscles, regardless of the farmer's daughters stories which some of the doctors told in an effort to ease the impact of the needle. However, the after effects were sometimes frightful – painful, suppurating abscesses which the chaulmoogra oil would generate in the patient's backside. The sight of a man with a pillow under his arm, on his way to sit down somewhere, was quite common. In my own case, I was hospitalized several times with chaulmoogra-induced, rear-end ulceration.[69]

The responses of people to treatment were varied. Stein tells of a man who seemed to consume an extraordinary quantity of chaulmoogra oil, but who confessed that he was using it to lubricate a machine. Then there were the many others who were consuming suspiciously large quantities and were in fact sending part of their allocation home to a member of the family who was in hiding with the disease.[70] Nonetheless, people were not passive recipients of treatment. They were well informed, and they wanted to be treated. Burnet commented that they "simply ask that the treatment shall not be too painful; they read the papers, never miss any item dealing with leprosy and are on the look-out for the newest remedies."

Remarkably, a chief cause of objection was insufficiently energetic treatment.[71] Stein also tells that the newspaper which he published at Carville, *The Star*, would report on any experimental therapy being conducted in other parts of the world "in the hope that our own medical staff would be encouraged to look beyond the chaulmoogra rut".[72] He also describes how patients would seek out their own cures and administer them surreptitiously.[73] People were desperate for a "cure", and they were prepared to tolerate extreme measures, nauseating treatments, and painful procedures in the hope of a reprieve from leprosy.

Hope

The powerful antibacterial compound, sulphanilamide, had been synthesised by Paul Gelmo in Vienna in 1908, but it was not until 1932 that a derivative, Prontosil, was discovered to be effective against streptococcal infection in mice in the laboratory of Gerhard Domagk.[74] This discovery represented an extraordinary moment in medical science, if only for the impact that it had on the lives of women who would otherwise have died of puerperal fever, a fatal infection that developed after childbirth.[75] French researchers at the Pasteur Institute in Paris – Jacques and Therese Tréfouël, Daniel Bovet, and Federico Nitti – discovered in 1935 that sulphanilamide was the active molecular component in the diazo compound Prontosil. This discovery succeeded in avoiding the patent that had been put on Prontosil, which would otherwise have limited the availability of the drug and also the subsequent research that was to prove to be so important.[76]

In the same year that Gelmo described sulphanilamide, Emil Fromm, who was the professor of chemistry in the medical faculty of the University of Freiburg im Breisgau in Germany, described another compound related to the sulphonamides: this was diaminodiphenylsulphone or dapsone (DDS). No one recognised the potential of this compound until 1937, when Gladwin A. H. Buttle and his colleagues at the Wellcome Laboratories and Ernest Fourneau and the researchers at the Institut Pasteur simultaneously found that dapsone was ten times as potent against streptococcal infection in mice and about a hundred times as toxic as sulphanilamide.[77] As Greenwood states, "Like sulphanilamide, dapsone's antibacterial potential had lurked unsuspected in the chemical literature."[78] But there was a catch, for while DDS was much more effective than sulphanilamide in pneumococcal infections, it was highly toxic.[79] George Brownlee, who was then at Wellcome Laboratories, would later explain the problem of the toxicity of DDS, as it was perceived at the time:

> As soon as the efficiency of DDS against pneumococci in animals was discovered in these laboratories here [Wellcome Laboratories] that substance was pressed into service in man. The blood level which was necessary to eliminate the pneumococcus in animals, i.e., somewhere about 5 to 7.5 microgrammes per cent is indeed toxic in man – terribly toxic. Doses of 1 to 3 gm daily produced an acute haemolytic crisis on the third day, followed later by signs of central (cerebral) irritation.[80]

So, as James Doull states so succinctly, "DDS was introduced – and abandoned – as a chemotherapeutic agent in human infections without having been tried in either tuberculosis or leprosy."[81] Chemists then searched for a related compound that would be less toxic, and hence Promin, 4,4'-diaminodiphenyl-sulfone-N, N' di-(dextrose sodium sulfonate), was synthesised by substituting the two amino groups in dapsone with complex, but symmetrical, chemical groupings. Tillitson synthesised Promin at the laboratories of Parke-Davis in the United States on 6 August 1937.

In the same year, Dr Guy Faget, who had studied tuberculosis, decided to use sulphanilamide at the National Leprosarium in Carville to treat secondary infections in leprosy and also to see if the drug had any effect on the disease itself. He knew of sulphanilamide's bacteriostatic effect against tuberculosis in guinea pigs, and he also knew that its toxic effects produced a diverse array of responses such as headaches, dizziness, nausea, vomiting, cyanosis, drug fever, and drug rashes. Most seriously, he knew that it could produce hepatitis because of its toxic effect upon the liver.[82] The challenge was to administer the drug in sufficient quantities to maintain effective concentration in the blood but not produce toxic effects in the recipients.

The drug was administered in two trials. The first was for nine patients, only two of whom completed it without toxic effects. The second trial was with twenty patients, including six from the first group two months later, with a reduced dosage. Only six patients completed the entire course, and twelve had to be hospitalised for toxic reactions. Faget observed that the toxic complications were more frequent and more severe than had been reported. They also produced lepra reactions.[83] At the same time, six out of the twenty patients did show some improvement of their leprous lesions. He concluded that sulphanilamide therapy was effective in treating secondary infections and in healing secondarily infected leprous ulcerations, but it could not be regarded as a curative agent for leprous lesions.[84]

Betty Martin, who was at Carville at the time, tells how her husband Harry was one of Guy Faget's first nine patients. She describes the desperation of the Carville residents who were eager to try anything if it made a difference. At the same time, she had been reading everything she could about the sulphone drugs and had decided that they were "too toxic and too dangerous". Harry, on the other hand, was willing to take the risk. She describes what happened:

> Harry became nervous, tense, and extremely sensitive to noise. Still, his mouth condition and nasal passages improved. After a few more weeks he had to be hospitalized for "red eye". By this time six others of the nine were in the hospital with high fevers and other complications; one had developed jaundice, and his body was so clammy and cold many of us were certain he could not pull through, but after several injections of glucose and saline he recovered. Several of the other patients showed temporary improvement, but the drug was too toxic to continue for any length of time. Only two of the nine patients were able to complete the course without toxic manifestations. In Harry's case the drug was discontinued … the improvement in his mouth and nasal passages was lost. Gradually his condition reverted to its former stage.[85]

Once again, it seemed that a vestige of hope for that elusive "cure" had been snatched away.

Then in the same year, as a result of a random series of encounters and communications, Faget also started a trial of Promin. In a chance meeting on a train on 29 December 1939, Walter M. Simpson, who belonged to the Kettering Institute in Dayton, Ohio, suggested to E. V. Cowdry from Washington University, St Louis, that he try Promin in rats infected with rat leprosy. Rat leprosy had developed from transmission of mycobacterium by inoculation from rat to rat, but the bacillus has become specialised in the rat in the same way that bovine tuberculosis has become specialised in cows.

Meanwhile, two other researchers at the Mayo Foundation, Hindshaw and Feldman, had received a supply of Promin from E. A. Sharpe at Parke-Davis to use in a trial against postoperative infections and for studies in experimental tuberculosis. Their published results prompted Faget to write to Sharpe enquiring about this and any other related experiments in acid-fast diseases. He also asked for information about the toxicity of Promin. Sharpe told Faget about Cowdry's work on murine leprosy, offering to supply ampoules if Faget were interested, and he recommended that Promin not be given orally, but intravenously. He supplied Faget with 150 ampoules of 2g and 5g of Promin, and in the meantime Faget learnt from Cowdry that although he had not achieved spectacular results using Promin in the rats, their nodules seemed to be slightly reduced and they did not experience adverse reactions.[86]

Faget delayed the trial with Promin until March 1941 because of an outbreak of influenza amongst the patients. Within a month, he needed more Promin. He did not publish his results until 1943, although in the May 1942 issue of *Public Health Reports* he wrote about several new experiments with various sulphonamide drugs with encouraging results, especially for secondary infection, but added cautiously, "Whether some of the newer sulphonamide derivatives have therapeutic action in leprosy remains to be proved."[87] By 1943, there is a detectable note of delight in his paper: "in our experience promin is the best of the sulphonamide derivatives, including sulphanilamide, sulfathiazole, sulfapyridine, and sulfadiazine, which have been used in the treatment of leprosy at the National Leprosarium." These were, in his view, "the most encouraging experimental treatment ever undertaken" and "an advance in the right direction".[88]

Today, the results of this trial provide a striking contrast to the results with chaulmoogra ten years earlier. It is impossible not to be profoundly moved by the changed prospects for those who had been prepared to try anything. On 10 March 1941, the volunteers received their injections.[89] One 59-year-old man had extensive chronic ulceration of his extremities and was confined in the infirmary because his nasal obstruction was gradually suffocating him. He was a short step away from a tracheotomy. After treatment, he could get up and move around, and his ulcers had all healed except for two small ones on his leg.[90] A 28-year-old man, who had had leprosy since he was eighteen, was losing his sight and had to be led into a room for his injections. After treatment, he was reading normally.[91] A 28-year-old man with lepromatous leprosy, who had suffered from the disease for twelve years and been hospitalised for nine, appeared to be "entirely free of leprous lesions" and after two years of treatment his skin smears were bacteriologically negative.[92] For another young man, his facial nodules had become smaller and less prominent, and a nasal obstruction that had hindered his breathing had cleared up. He was thirty-six. He had suffered from "far-advanced" lepromatous leprosy for twelve years, and his general health had improved so much that he was able to play baseball.[93] A 34-year-old man with lepromatous leprosy since he was seventeen found that the ulcers on his lips, mouth, nose, and legs had all healed. Those on his legs had been four centimetres in diameter and two millimetres in depth. The infiltration of bacteria on his face, which would have distorted his facial features, had subsided, and despite some temporary complications in his white blood cell count that could be treated with injections of liver extract, he had objectively and definitely improved.

Fifteen improved, six were stationary (using the most uncompromising criteria), and one was worse. Five had become bacteriologically negative. Although Faget was at pains to point out that spontaneous remission could occur in leprosy, and this made it difficult to determine the success of the trial, the numbers showing improvement enabled him nonetheless to claim that "it is evident that Promin produced improvement in the majority of treated patients" and that the improvement increased in proportion to the duration of treatment. He had already begun to treat forty-six additional patients.[94] He would not claim that Promin was a specific for leprosy, but he believed that it was an advance in the right direction. He urgently recommended further trials before more definite conclusions could be made, but as far as he was concerned, "Promin can be considered to have opened a new avenue in the chemotherapy of mycobacterial diseases." He concluded his paper with the hope that "further synthesis of sulfa compounds may produce a substance which will succeed in saving countless lives in this still dark field of medicine".[95]

Once again Stanley Stein described the experience of this ground-breaking trial from an insider's point of view. Before starting, Faget had consulted his staff, and there was some trepidation amongst the doctors. Dr Johansen, the clinical chief, was sensitive to the use of patients "as guinea pigs" and to the many false hopes that they had experienced; nonetheless, he conceded that if the treatment did prove to be better than anything else "it would be a crime not to use it". According to Stein, Faget began tentatively, "He was exploring a new world and the pitfalls were many. How was the new drug to be administered? In what dosage?" Once again, he had to find the balance between the concentration of the drug in the blood that would be sufficient for it to have an effect on the bacillus and the dosage that an individual could tolerate. At first, he tried it orally in spite of Sharpe's recommendations, perhaps because intramuscular injections had been so painful for the patients. In the end, he administered it intravenously. Effects were not seen immediately, and Stein recounts that "the original volunteers grew discouraged until Dr Raymond C. Pogge arrived at Carville". He was very popular with the patients because of his freshness and youthfulness. He invented what they call the "Pogge Cure-all Cocktail" which contained Promin with glucose, calcium, Vitamin B and penicillin. Stein says that the patients "flocked to try it. His confident optimism and enthusiasm was contagious and the experimental sulfone program gained momentum."[96]

The lives of the patients were turned around. Stein describes their gradual but dramatic awakening to the power of the treatment:

> Results were slow but dramatic. Early cases cleared up remarkably in six months; nodules and blemishes disappeared, even when bacteriological tests still registered positive. Older cases showed marked improvement in two or three years. The effect on the patients' morale was even more striking. Chaulmoogra oil had been nothing like this.[97]

Betty Martin tells how after two months her husband Harry pulled back from the brink: "This was our miracle." After that, "every injection of promin added to Harry's energy and strength".[98] Betty Martin started on the treatment herself, and despite complications she also experienced its benefits: "we began to take a new lease on life. We no longer made ourselves do things, we felt like doing them, and we put wholehearted efforts into doing them."[99] Sadly, Faget did not live to enjoy the acclaim that was his due. He died on 17 July 1947, in tragic and puzzling circumstances. His health had been failing, and his body was discovered beneath the open window of his office.[100]

There were two more key events that would enhance the potential for a practical and inexpensive treatment against leprosy, hence driving the need for further research. The first was Robert Cochrane's successful use of DDS, the active component of the sulphone drug Promin that had been so effectively trialled at Carville. The second event was the successful administration of DDS orally, in spite of all the indications that the drug was highly toxic. This was carried out by John Lowe at Uzuakoli in Nigeria.[101]

Both steps would make it possible to produce a treatment that was cheap, effective, and deployable on a mass scale.

The sulphone derivatives like Promin were too expensive for Robert Cochrane to use at the Lady Willingdon Leprosy Settlement in Chingleput, outside of Madras. He needed to find a cheaper form of the drug if he was going to administer on a large scale. On a visit to the United Kingdom, in early 1946, he learned that DDS or dapsone was being used by Dr John Francis at Imperial Chemical Industries at Wilmslow, Cheshire, to treat mastitis in cows. Returning to India, he tried administering a 25% suspension of DDS in arachis (peanut) oil, using a needle inserted into the subcutaneous tissue. After preliminary trails, he set up an experimental treatment group early in 1947, although he remained cautious of the toxic effects of the drug.[102] John Francis also left some DDS with the British Empire Leprosy Relief Association (BELRA) in London, and when Dr John Lowe, who had worked as a medical missionary at Dichpali in Hyderabad and also in Calcutta, joined BELRA at the end of 1947, Ernest Muir suggested that he try it at the leprosy colony Uzuakoli in Nigeria. Against all advice, Lowe says, he decided that logic, to say nothing of local conditions, indicated that the trials should be administered orally.[103]

Lowe's decision to use DDS in this way was carefully reasoned. To begin with, he noted Buttle's experience with doses of 1–2g a day, which they found alarmingly toxic.[104] Lowe realised that he needed to determine "the therapeutic blood-level needed in man or the dosage necessary to produce that level".[105] He wondered "whether the more complex sulphones exert their antibacterial action in the form in which they are given or only when they are broken down to DDS in the body?" If they had to be broken down to the active form of the compound, where did this occur, in the gut before the drug was absorbed or in the body fluids or cells after it had been absorbed by the gut? Or was it broken down in the tissues? When Promin was injected, nearly all of it was able to be recovered in the urine, which meant that very little had been either broken down or absorbed. By contrast, when the drug was given orally, only 30% of it could be recovered from the urine and some of that had been broken down into DDS. This led Lowe to conclude that Promin had been changed into DDS in the gut either before or while it was being absorbed. Hence, it must be much more effective when administered orally than by injection.

At the same time, he also concluded that much of the Promin given by mouth was not absorbed at all, and, even more importantly, when it was injected it hardly broke down at all. While up to 15g of Promin could be injected, only 1–3g could be tolerated by mouth, so that, although intravenous injections were not as toxic, they had a greatly reduced therapeutic activity. Lowe and Smith compared the administration of, and absorption of, Promin and other derivatives of DDS: diasone and sulphetrone. They concluded that "complex sulphones possibly or probably act by being hydrolysed to DDS, though with some of the complex sulphones, the amount of this hydrolysis is very small".[106] On the basis of previous research, he estimated that the "minimum therapeutic blood-level of DDS itself in leprosy was perhaps one mg per one hundred ml, or even less". The next step was to determine what concentration of DDS he could produce in the blood without causing toxic effects.

Between October and December 1948, Lowe started nine patients on 100mg a day of DDS for two weeks. He then increased this to 200mg a day for two more weeks and so on, every two weeks. At doses of 400mg daily, by seven and eight weeks, he started to get some signs of toxic reactions in the blood (haemolysis, or the destruction of red blood cells, which produces haemolytic anaemia). When the patients were receiving 300mg of DDS a day, their blood showed the requisite concentration of 1mg per 100mL, and they showed no ill effects. The results of the trial showed that "with 300 mg of DDS a day the blood level was comparable to that attained with doses of diasone or sulphetrone five to ten times greater". They found that DDS or dapsone was almost completely absorbed by the gut and slowly eliminated from the kidneys. This also explained why the earlier and much higher doses of DDS had been so alarmingly toxic when administered.

Lowe then selected fifty and eventually ninety people with very severe lepromatous leprosy and put them on the same regimen. After nearly a year, they were all in good general condition and none had suffered any toxic effects. He stated: "The experiment has thus amply proved the safety of oral administration of DDS by the method here outlined." He stressed the importance of slowly increasing the dosage until it reached 400–500 mg a day where it could be maintained without toxic effects.[107] He found that the basic compound was as effective and perhaps acted more rapidly in lepromatous cases than the complex proprietary sulphones. Additionally, this form of the sulphone was also rapid and effective in tuberculoid forms of leprosy. He concluded that

> The change in outlook produced by sulphone treatment is one of the most striking achievements of modern medicine. The full action of sulphone treatment in severe cases is very slow but amazingly certain. The physician can now feel absolute confidence that an active case of leprosy, no matter

how severe, will respond to sulphone treatment; that the disease will cease to progress from the time when the treatment is begun and that the lesions already present will slowly subside and the infection gradually die out.

This made it possible to treat "vast numbers of patients in tropical countries".[108]

Joseph Chukwu recounts the patient's side of the story of this first chemotherapeutic breakthrough. Apparently, before Lowe administered dapsone orally, he also tried it by the conventional methods with catastrophic results:

> Some ninety patients volunteered and he started trials. He also used rabbits, goats, cattle. Chemotherapy research is painstaking, rigorous risky business. During those days it was common to see patients (the volunteers) about the hospital, carrying bottles. Every drop of their urine had to be collected and examined. So was the urine of the animals. He tried this compound, side by side with RO4, Etisul and so on. Traditionally, a sulphonamide regimen is usually started with a high dose, which is gradually tapered off. Lowe naturally worked with the scientific assumptions. Tragedy. The patients began to die in their numbers. Ten to twenty patients died every day. When they took the high dose of dapsone, the next day, they developed skin eruption (ex-foliative dermatitis). Their skin peeled off. Then they caught infections and died of septicaemia. Other patients became psychotic.
>
> ... Lowe was now left to his own devices. He resorted to the unconventional. And it worked! He administered in reverse order the same sulphone compounds to another set of patients. They presented none of the violent reactions described earlier. Instead their conditions began to show marked improvement.[109]

Lowe's *Lancet* publication on the administration of DDS by mouth did not appear until January 1950, but the results were known before then. The editor of the *International Journal of Leprosy* (*IJL*) stated, before the *Lancet* publication, that this was the beginning of "an experience which, by all accounts, holds promise of being an important new advance in leprosy therapy". Most importantly, the cost of DDS per patient, per year, was about 14s, against £10–15 for the derivative.[110] For the editor of the *IJL*, this was momentous: for "where only limited numbers of patients now receive the benefit of treatment with the proprietary derivatives perhaps twenty times as many can be treated with DDS under the same budget".[111] Suddenly there was hope for people. They had an affordable treatment at little cost.

By the end of the 1940s, then, the landscape of leprosy treatment had changed dramatically. Significant issues such as the infectiousness of different forms of leprosy were being conceptualised and explored. The transition from palliative care leprosarium to research centre had commenced. Researchers in different parts of the world were collaborating. Something like a scientific method was the rule rather than the exception in trials that were being conducted in the scattered research outposts. Drugs that seemed to offer genuine remission from the disease were becoming available, although, as we shall see in subsequent chapters, not all the early promise was realised. One element of the full story was still missing, however: the international coordination of the campaign against leprosy. The next chapter discusses the first steps towards that.

1

WINNING PRIORITY FOR LEPROSY
AT THE WORLD HEALTH ORGANIZATION

It had taken the trauma of war to demonstrate that disadvantage and deprivation in one state could ultimately destabilise all states. The United Nations (UN) and the World Health Organization (WHO) were international bodies designed in 1945 to heal the unimaginable horrors of two World Wars by addressing themselves, symbolically at least, to "disease that knew no frontiers". The beginnings of the WHO were marked by a call for a "new spirit" that would be fundamentally different from anything that had gone before. Instead of the preoccupation with the protection of nation–states that characterised the war years, the new perspective would sweep across national borders, and at the same time focus upon the peoples within those national boundaries. This marked a renewed sense of connectedness between nation–states in which "world action" would ensure that all nations would benefit equally and no nation would be deprived.[1]

Equally, this broad and sweeping perspective was accompanied by a more focused perception. Health was no longer "merely the absence of disease or infirmity", it was defined in positive terms as "a state of complete physical, mental and social well-being".[2] The energy that had been unable to halt the war was now redirected to attaining a utopia of complete physical, mental, and social well-being. Albert Camus produced an allegory of war using the language of disease in his novel *The Plague*; these new organisations reversed this allegory by making disease their battleground and imagining their narratives in metaphors of warfare.

In the opening address to the first World Health Assembly (WHA), the Director of the UN European Office spoke of the trauma out of which these new institutions emerged: "War devastated not only towns, factories, villages, homes and so on, but also the health of millions of people; and – I should like to emphasise – not only the health of the body but also that of the soul."[3] The aspirations of the UN and the WHO were captured in the address by the Head of the Department of the Interior of the Swiss Federation when he told the attendees at the first WHA that they were "assuming the magnificent task of weaving closer relations between mankind and between the different nations, in the service of peace, and for the welfare of all".[4] The idealism and the high-flung rhetoric betray an unexamined paternalism and a new-found faith in Western medicine that would undergo many readjustments in the decades to come. However, the aspirations expressed were in deadly earnest because their activities were conducted in the shadow of the very real prospects of biological warfare, nuclear holocaust, and the annihilation of humanity.[5]

In setting out the programme for the WHO and delineating the fields "in which international action may be expected to yield the best results", the Interim Commission, influenced by the experience of the League of Nations' Health Organization, decided that diseases such as cancer and leprosy did not "lend themselves easily to international action".[6] The Commission argued that "Nothing really useful can be done to fight these diseases at the present stage of medical knowledge, nor even to promote scientific research, which costs so much that the Organization's entire budget would be merely a drop in the ocean."[7] In view of the massive task ahead and the tight budgetary constraints, malaria, tuberculosis, and venereal disease were much more realistic targets because the new insecticides and the newly discovered sulphonamides and penicillin enabled mass diagnosis and treatment, while leprosy would require a huge effort beyond the limits of the budget and the available technologies.

The delegation from India

Not content with this determination, on 1 June 1949 a delegation from the government of India approached the Second World Health Assembly (WHA) in Rome with a memorandum on leprosy. They hoped to persuade the World Health Organization (WHO) to make leprosy one of its priorities. The delegation was led by Rajkumari Amrit Kaur, as both Minister for Health in the new Indian Cabinet and former Vice President of the First World Health Assembly.[8] But behind Amrit Kaur and authorising her representation to the World Health Assembly were a cast of luminaries beginning with the inspiring "Bapu" – Mahatma Gandhi.

Gandhi's awareness of leprosy went back to his time in South Africa. He mentions in his book *Experiments With Truth* that a leprosy-affected immigrant labourer had sought shelter in his home in Durban and, although the man stayed for a time, Gandhi found that he "lacked the will to keep him".[9] Later,

Gandhi met Parchure Shastri, a Sanskrit scholar with leprosy, when they were in Yeravada Jail. In response to Shastri's request to live out the rest of his life in the ashram at Sevagram, Gandhi willingly assented and personally nursed him there on a daily basis.[10] Gandhi was also deeply impressed by Manohar Diwan's Dattapur leprosy colony, which he praised in the Constructive Program for the new nation.[11] Amrit Kaur emphasised Gandhi's wishes and interest in leprosy work in a letter written five months after the delegation to the WHA. She confessed a sense of "special responsibility towards the cause of leprosy not only because I knew Bapu's mind about it and would like to do something tangible for it, but also because I have brought it before WHO and my proposal received a most favorable reception in Rome last June".[12]

While Gandhi provided moral and financial support for anti-leprosy activities, in his philosophy, leprosy – like salt and *kadhi* – assumed political, as well as symbolic, significance in India's struggle for independence.[13] People with the disease were situated symbolically in an overarching national strategy which contrasted physical leprosy to "moral leprosy". Care for and acceptance of people with leprosy were to be an index for the health of the Indian body politic. When Gandhi revised his Constructive Program, he drew attention to the odium in which leprosy was held in India, and the "studied neglect" of those with the disease:

> Leper is a word of bad odour. India is perhaps a home of lepers next only to Central Africa. Yet they are as much a part of society as the tallest among us. But the tall absorb our attention though they are least in need of it. The lot of the lepers who are much in need of attention is studied neglect. I am tempted to call it heartless, which it certainly is, in terms of non-violence.[14]

In his view, working against leprosy provided an inspirational pathway to building the nation and gaining independence:

> If India was pulsating with new life, if we were all in earnest about winning independence in the quickest manner possible by truthful and non-violent means, there would not be a leper or beggar in India uncared for and unaccounted for. In this revised edition I am deliberately introducing the leper as a link in the chain of constructive effort. For, what the leper is in India, that we are, if we will, but look about us, for the modern civilized world. Examine the condition of our brethren across the ocean and the truth of my remark will be borne home to us.[15]

The social neglect and marginalisation of leprosy-affected people revealed the urgent need for social responsibility. Simultaneously, the place of India in the "modern" world was expressed through an analogy with leprosy, something that was later extended by Amrit Kaur in correspondence when she discussed the delegation, saying: "Now if India does not redouble its efforts, it will be in the nature of a stigma on us."[16]

Leprosy workers were quick to capitalise on this moment.[17] *Leprosy in India*, which was edited by the Indian Council for the British Empire Leprosy Relief Association, hailed Gandhi's introduction of leprosy into the programme for the nation, saying that it was heartening to see that "national leaders are also becoming alive to this very important matter" and forecasting that it would stimulate public opinion.[18]

Two other strong personalities who played a role in drawing attention to the need for anti-leprosy work in India and who both directly contributed to placing it upon the international stage had also previously made themselves known to Gandhi. Just over four years before, in February 1945, a bright, erudite Tamil Brahmin, T. N. Jagadisan, who had suffered from leprosy from childhood and actively sought out ways of bringing social justice for leprosy-affected people, and the already-mentioned Robert Cochrane, a British medical missionary whose anti-leprosy work will be central to this narrative, visited the Sevagram ashram in the hope of an interview.[19] They wanted Gandhi's support for a new leprosy centre in South Arcot for affected women and children. Although Gandhi was observing a day of silence, he wrote, "You have preached to the converted. My interest in the leper problem is as old as my residence in South Africa ... I would like you to send a detailed plan with expenditure to the Board."[20]

It is impossible to know Cochrane's precise motive in accompanying Jagadisan, but it is tempting to imagine that he feared that, with India's approaching independence and the end of British influence in India, the work against leprosy might suffer. He certainly expressed anxiety about the direction in which medical work would go in India after independence when he was in London in 1947. He told *Lancet* readers of his fear of a loss of "scientific standards" as a consequence of "the backward pull of Eastern medicine", and a weakening of "professional integrity" accompanying "any weakening of the Christian ethic".[21] His 1945 visit to Gandhi, then, may have been a precautionary attempt to ensure ongoing efforts against the disease after independence.

In this novel milieu of the burgeoning nation's attention to leprosy, the initiative to take a delegation to the World Health Assembly came from two All-India Workers Conferences. The first, convened by the Maharogi Seva Mandal, was held at Wardha in the Central Provinces, 30 October to

1 November 1947. Photographs of the attendees show Gandhians standing with leprosy workers, some Indian, some Western (including missionaries).[22] The eighty delegates included medical men and women engaged in leprosy work, social workers connected with leprosy and other activities in Gandhi's Constructive Program, and some "veteran leaders and associates of Gandhiji" like Thakkar Bapa, Shri Jajuji, and Shri Kaka Kalelkar.[23]

The conference called for a "popular movement" against the disease. Symbolism, nationalism, populism, political activism, and medical activity converged. The same energies and ideals that had fuelled a popular movement against the British were being harnessed against leprosy.[24] This was evident in Shrikrishnadas Jaju's welcome address which emphasised what was to be a common theme for the conference: the need for a popular organisation with a focus on the village, for "Leprosy seems to be a rural disease. Its eradication is necessary for the uplift of the villager."[25] Thakkar Bapa also placed responsibility for future efforts at the feet of the people, by calling for a movement within which experts, laymen, doctors and social workers could work together, animated by a "missionary spirit" directed at a "village disease".[26]

The successful gathering and its international ambitions were reported in a newspaper in Madras. The author noted that it was fitting that so soon after the "birth of our freedom", and in the midst of the "terrible upheavals in the country following the partition of India", the first All-India Leprosy Workers Conference should have met. The conference had led to "a new movement in the country for the relief and control of leprosy", and now "the question of anti-leprosy work figured prominently on India's Health Program." After the second conference held in Calcutta, the participants "looked beyond cure to the departure from Bombay to the World Health Conference at Rome", for "India was greatly concerned about the prevention of leprosy in the country and would like to urge the World Health Organization to give its major attention to combat this disease."[27]

That the delegation would bring leprosy to the attention of the World Health Assembly illustrates the culmination of one of the more outstanding periods in which adventitious uses have been made of leprosy, when those who have worked in the field have entered into an alliance of interests for the long-term aim of attracting support to overcome the disease.

The International Leprosy Association

While the Indian delegation would make a direct approach to the World Health Assembly, the International Leprosy Association (ILA) played a crucial and complementary role in getting leprosy into the WHO programme. The ILA had been formed at a conference held by the Leonard Wood Memorial for the Eradication of Leprosy (LWM) and the League of Nations in Manila in January 1931, with Victor Heiser as the first president and Robert Cochrane as the secretary.[28] When the League of Nations instituted its inquiry into leprosy, Dr Herbert Windsor Wade was the chair for the LWM conference. Wade was the pathologist and acting chief physician at the large leprosy settlement on Culion Island in the Philippines. He was quick to see the opportunities for research that the colony presented, and it is quite astonishing that Wade's study of the disease, in one of the most remote places in the world and in pursuit of a field in which few people had any interest, would be influential at the very centre of international organisations such as the League of Nations and the WHO.[29] Initially, he formed the Culion Medical Society in 1924 to draw on, share, and disseminate reports on the many clinical opportunities presented by the island colony. From this the International Leprosy Association developed.

As a professional organisation, the International Leprosy Association functioned in the name of a cohort of workers with both professional and vocational commitments to leprosy work in diverse and usually extremely marginal parts of the world. Their main outlet for communication was the *International Journal of Leprosy (IJL)*, which Wade edited from Culion for thirty years.[30] He also served as President of the International Leprosy Association until 1963. By sheer dint of his personality and dedication to leprosy-related research, and with the support of the Leonard Wood Memorial, he shifted the focus of leprosy investigation and policy from protecting Europe against leprosy-bearing immigration to research based in tropical medicine, especially in the Pacific.[31] When Wade was at Culion, the colony was reputed to be a model for leprosy colonies, and people interested in leprosy came from all over the world to see it. When Wade relinquished the post of chief physician, he returned to his primary interest of pathology and spent the rest of his life on Culion, pursuing research in his laboratory until he died there in 1968.

The other key figures in the ILA who secured the acceptance of leprosy by the WHO programme were James Doull, Ernest Muir, and Roland Chaussinand. James Angus Doull was probably the most influential of all, as a prominent epidemiologist and editor. Doull had begun an intensive epidemiological study in 1933 centred on Cordova on Mactan Island in the Philippines, work that produced major findings about the contagiousness of lepromatous leprosy. Doull also developed the first scientific method for determining the effectiveness of chemotherapy through double-blind trial. Additionally, during the five years of World War II when Wade was unable to continue editing the *IJL* because the country was under Japanese occupation, Doull kept the journal going as acting editor.

Doull's influence in the international sphere began from 1930, when as Professor of Hygiene and Public Health at Western Reserve University in Cleveland he conducted surveys on public health in various parts of the world for the Surgeon General of the United States Public Health Service, Dr Thomas Parran. He subsequently involved himself in what might be termed medical diplomacy, serving with the US delegation to the United Nations Conference on International Organizations in San Francisco in 1945, out of which was created the United Nations. As Chief of the Office of International Health Relations of the USPHS and participant in the Advisory Health Group, Doull belonged to the taskforce that mapped out the plans in 1946 at the International Health Conference for the new organisation that would become the WHO.[32]

Ernest Muir was also influential as someone whose expertise bridged the missionary activity of the nineteenth century and the "scientific approach" of the twentieth century. He was a founding member of the ILA from 1931, secretary–treasurer and secretary–general of the International Leprosy Congresses in Cairo (1938) and Havana (1948), and an honorary vice president of the ILA. He was also vice president of the Leprosy Mission between 1949 and 1951. Like Cochrane and Lowe, he was simultaneously missionary and physician, as well as an expert on leprosy in the anglophone world.[33] As Jagadisan characteristically put it, "He had the unique privilege of working in the dark night of leprosy for the coming of the dawn, and also to work in the bright days of better drugs, better knowledge and improved outlook."[34]

Roland Chaussinand, a French doctor and medical researcher, was one of the key figures at the International Leprosy Conference at Strasbourg in 1923, and from 1931 to 1946 he worked for the Pasteur Institute in Saigon as director of the Leprosy Service. Then, in 1946, he became the director of the Leprosy Service at the Pasteur Institute in Paris.[35] A member of the Consultative Commission to the Overseas French Ministry, a member of the Permanent Commission on Hygiene (Leprosy Section) in the Ministry of Public Health and Population, the Secretary and Treasurer of the Western Section of the International Leprosy Association, and the associate editor of the *International Journal of Leprosy*, he liaised between the ILA and WHO. He became a consultant at WHO headquarters, and his efforts ensured that the crucial First Expert Committee on Leprosy became a reality.

Medical people who worked in leprosy did not enjoy much institutional status and often felt as marginalised as those with the disease. Many came from missionary backgrounds and had worked in the field when there was little hope of a cure. British doctors Ernest Muir, Robert Cochrane, and John Lowe had begun work in India with the Mission to Lepers. As work in leprosy became secularised and professionalised, these doctors made the transition to become medical researchers, inhabiting several fields simultaneously. They maintained their connections with the Mission to Lepers (later the Leprosy Mission) and were driving forces in the British Empire Leprosy Relief Association (BELRA), which established itself as a secular, philanthropic organisation with the journal *Leprosy Review* as its voice. Many of the small missionary leprosaria enjoyed the support of both the Mission to Lepers and BELRA, their religious affiliation not debarring them from receiving small sums from both organisations to advance their medical work and their research.

Americans like Herbert Windsor Wade and James Doull came from a more secular background as clinicians and medical researchers, bringing their own level of "new world" professionalism. All of these then came together under the auspices of the International Leprosy Association.[36] These were men with a shared passion for work against leprosy. This is not to say that they were not ambitious, both personally and on behalf of their specialisation, but although they received a great deal of acknowledgement in their own area, in the eyes of the larger medical and scientific community, they would have gained little status from lifetimes dedicated to their work. In this sense, they were truly missionary.

At the same time, working in the field of leprosy yielded a type of reward less tangible and more ambiguous than institutional status. Paradoxically, the stigma associated with leprosy enhanced the reputation of anyone who dedicated their life to this sort of work. Since the time of Father Damien, tropes of martyrdom and sainthood lay just below the surface of accounts of the endeavours of leprosy workers in the missionary tradition. The ILA was deeply suspicious of this sort of framing and sought to demystify the disease and purge its theological connotations. All their energies were directed to medicalising leprosy.

Importantly, although the ILA was an association, it had no physical headquarters. Rather, it occupied an imaginary space through its voice, the *IJL*, and through its congresses, which took place once every five years and were held in different geographical sites, increasingly in places where intensified national attention to leprosy was required. Both of these sites, the journal and the international congress, authorised medical and scientific utterances and provided an arena within which debates were conducted.

Equally, the WHO was both an empowering and a constraining site from which individuals could speak only as representatives of member states or as representatives of affiliated NGOs within specific limits. Although the World Health Assembly and the Executive Board meetings were fora at which resolutions could be passed to influence the activities of the same member states, these would occur only on the basis of consensus, and the organisation itself could act only upon the wishes of its member states. The ILA had to find how to act within these limits. Even if the influence that was available to it seemed considerable, it had to learn how to speak within this new organisation in an appropriate bureaucratic discourse so that it would be persuasive. It had to learn what was possible and what was outside the remit of the WHO. It had to learn how to work through national entities, and, judging by what was expressed in the *IJL*, it found this process of negotiation extremely frustrating, although ultimately productive. The ILA was eager to explore an alliance with the WHO so as to gain a level of influence for leprosy work equivalent to the one it had achieved with the League of Nations.[37] It expected to share in that official information on leprosy that the Organization would collect for the benefit of the "especially interested element of the medical profession".[38] It was also quite open about its wanting to be the WHO's official consulting body on leprosy problems.

When the members of the ILA met at the International Leprosy Congress in Havana in 1948, they wanted to know what needed to happen for them to come under the aegis of the WHO.[39] They were advised to secure an invitation to send a representative to the first Assembly and to ensure, unobtrusively but effectively, that the delegates of the various governments to WHO were familiar with the ILA and its stated aims.[40] The organisation had to be concerned with matters that "fell within the competence of WHO" and conform to the "spirit, purposes and principles of the Constitution of the WHO". At the same time, it had to have "recognized standing" and be sufficiently representative of people who participated in the same field so that it was authorised to speak on their behalf, internationally. Wade told the members that to attain this status, the ILA had to show that it represented the organisations involved in anti-leprosy work.

The war years had been difficult for the International Leprosy Association; its financial support base had been weakened, despite the Leonard Wood Memorial meeting all the publication expenses of the journal.[41] In order to seek more representative status, it had to develop alliances. It had no constituent branches, but it could affiliate with organisations in different countries that had worked against leprosy for many years, such as the Mission to Lepers which had both British and American branches, BELRA, and the Leonard Wood Memorial (LWM).[42] There were also professional and social relief organisations in South America, particularly Brazil and Argentina, that could be considered potential allies. Groundwork for establishing the affiliation between WHO and the ILA had already been prepared by Roland Chaussinand. Earlier in the year (on 12 April 1948), he had met with representatives of nine medical organisations in Paris to formulate plans for coordinating medical congresses under joint WHO–UNESCO auspices, and had made contacts that would be useful.

Getting leprosy onto the WHO programme

The "News and Notes" section of the *IJL* kept members in touch with the strategy for affiliation. James Doull was present at the Assembly as an alternate delegate of the United States, and "presumably as a result of his interest" a section on leprosy had been proposed for the programme. It stated that the "WHO should consider continuing the international work on leprosy, including investigations on epidemiology, treatment and prophylaxis in co-operation with the ILA and other organizations". Doull had made sure at the Committee on Program for the first WHA, in July 1948, that the provisional agenda contained leprosy in the category of "Special Endemic Diseases", which entrusted leprosy to the Epidemiological Division.[43] If he had not been able to achieve this, further efforts would have been pointless. In response to a request from Dr Bonne, who was to be the Chief of the Division of Epidemiological Studies, Chaussinand and Muir prepared two reports on leprosy to provide both Anglo-Saxon and French points of view.[44] Chaussinand estimated that there were probably at least 5 million people in the world with the disease.[45]

In November of the same year, the ILA learnt that it had been formally affiliated with WHO.[46] Brock Chisholm, the Director–General of WHO, wrote to the ILA with the good news.[47] But while leprosy had been included in the programme, it did not have a budget; worse, it suddenly seemed that the work of the ILA would be used as a reason not to dedicate further resources to leprosy-focused activities. The *IJL* commented acerbically: "Regarding leprosy, we are informed, the only action taken up was to assign to the secretariat (Epidemiological Section) the task of collecting, compiling and distributing statistics."[48]

The ILA was not content to leave matters at that, and a letter of inquiry elicited an expression of regret "that, owing to budget insufficiencies, the work on leprosy envisaged by the First World Health Assembly could not be carried out so far in 1949". In fact, most of the intended programme had to be deferred, and was to be presented again at the Second World Health Assembly. This problem was not unique to leprosy; it was also budgetary, for the first three Assemblies ran into problems reconciling the cost of the recommended programmes and the actual contributions available from the member states. Their next recourse was to make representation through the member nations. International Leprosy Association members learnt that "several delegations would press actively for development of the work in leprosy, which might mean requesting special specific information from governments and leprosy experts" at the Second WHA. So it was that the Indian delegation brought leprosy to the attention of the World Assembly.[49]

The arguments of the Indian delegation

The delegation argued that leprosy was a public health problem and an international health problem affecting some of the poorest people in the world in places that were least equipped to deal with any disease, let alone leprosy. Five million people suffered from leprosy in both tropical and subtropical regions, and the prevalence of the disease was so high in certain countries in Asia and Africa that it should receive the "highest priority" in the "national health program" of those countries.[50] Rajkumari Amrit Kaur told the assembly that this ancient disease from which millions suffered ostracised not only the individual but the family as well. Leprosy deserved the same level of attention as malaria and tuberculosis, for "intensive and coordinated research, which will lead to its cure, control and ultimate elimination".[51]

Leprosy was not like cholera, smallpox, or plague, for it was transmitted only after sustained close contact over a long period. As a result, children in close contact with family members were more susceptible to infection than adults. There was a great need for more knowledge about the aetiology and pathology of the disease.[52] Additionally, the administrative and social problems were immense. For isolation measures to be effective, the most infectious people would require segregation in institutions or special leprosy colonies over lengthy periods of time: an undertaking that caused severe social disruption to people from their families and their communities. Countries where leprosy was an important public health problem did not have the resources or the health services to take such measures.

The delegation urged haste: "WHO should begin to concentrate attention on this disease as early as possible and to promote international studies on a large scale." An Expert Committee could guide and coordinate leprosy work and investigate problems about therapy, epidemiology, pathology, surgery, social assistance, rehabilitation, occupational therapy, and social welfare. Experts could provide technical advice to countries. Fellowships would ensure trained "personnel". A World Center for Research was needed. Finally, the high cost of sulphones or any other forms of treatment had to be reduced, "in the interests of leprosy patients all over the world."[53] Delegates from the UK, Australia, Belgium, South Africa, and Brazil all supported the proposal which was adopted with amendments. The first Expert Committee would be organised in the following year, and international exchanges of workers in 1950. Countries could request the advice of consultants.[54] In confirmation, the WHO publication *The Chronicle* stated that "cogent arguments" had been made by the delegation for an international campaign to combat the disease.[55]

But while the Indian delegation had won a significant alteration to the agenda of the WHO, something that it would hold the Assembly and the Organization to, it would quickly become apparent that even if the WHO expressed the will to carry out work against leprosy, there was no way for this to happen immediately.[56] Several equally debilitating diseases were competing for scarce financial support, and the discrepancy between what the WHO resolved to do and what it had the means to achieve dawned slowly upon all interested parties, prompting a great deal of frustrated disillusionment.[57] After the Second World Health Assembly, the ILA members were told that "never before has there been assembled such a detailed review of the world's most urgent health problems, yet in spite of this, leprosy had not been mentioned even though the August–September issue of the *Chronicle* indicated that it was in the program".[58] Leprosy was only one of thirty diseases considered worthy of study and for which a campaign might be conducted. Worse still, the programmes in the group of diseases that included leprosy were in the supplemental budget so that it was even possible that some would "remain in abeyance".[59]

The *IJL* cloaked its disappointment in sarcasm, pointing out that "those responsible for the actual work of WHO" expressed a "courteous desire that the work advocated by those concerned with the leprosy problem might be undertaken" but regretted that "funds for it are lacking". There was "no reason" to believe that "leprosy has a high priority", the editor continued, for it was placed "between the diphtheria-and-whooping cough item and the brucellosis item".[60] Although the Communicable Diseases Division did intend to correspond with a select panel of experts on leprosy, the international coordination on the scale envisaged by the ILA was really only a remote possibility to be pursued when, and if, an opportunity arose.[61] If the urgently needed research was to find a place in the international programme, further pressure was clearly necessary at the next World Health Assembly.

At the following year's WHA, it seemed at first that nothing was going to change. The programme committee discussed communicable diseases, and the Director for the Division of Epidemiology, Dr Biruad, emphasised the "sad truth" that although the Second Assembly had recommended a dozen expert committees, most had to be put on the supplemental budget and only one of those had been convened in 1950.[62] For 1951, the budget could only stretch to two more expert committees: insecticides and yellow fever. But another delegation, this time from the Philippines, made a further energetic request for work on leprosy. Dr Rodriguez, the representative, like Cochrane and Chaussinand could speak with the authority of a national and international expert and with the conviction and confidence that only work in the field could bring. He also spoke as a representative of the Philippine Ministry of Health, for the government dedicated a large proportion of its health budget to leprosy control, a heavy burden which prevented initiatives on other equally pressing health issues. He pleaded for urgent advice about the new treatment for leprosy, emphasising the importance of including an Expert Committee on Leprosy in the budget for 1951.[63] After lengthy discussion, a resolution was passed to secure funding for the promised expert committee from the regular budget.[64]

In order to ensure that the expert committee met sooner, rather than later, the Philippines delegation also asked at the Executive Board meeting for support for a worldwide symposium on the disease.[65] The strategy was to maintain a tenacious and increasingly specific request for an international gathering of experts to produce technical consensus on treatment and leprosy control.[66] Rodriguez outlined the medical and technical issues that urgently needed to be clarified, and the meeting was informed there was no money for a symposium, unless the Executive Board made a special recommendation for a supplementary appropriation for that purpose.[67] The Board was asked to choose between tropical ulcer and leprosy, because the budget would not allow for both. They voted for leprosy, and a resolution was presented on 29 January 1951, with an agenda for a forthcoming Expert Committee on leprosy.[68]

Progress had indeed been achieved because the WHO budget for 1952 for leprosy also included funds for consultants from the technical assistance budget (TAED) for leprosy surveys in Burma (now Myanmar), Ceylon (now Sri Lanka), Thailand, and Indonesia.[69] The technical assistance funds were special supplemental programme funding from the United Nations and part of the general programme of technical assistance for economic development in underdeveloped countries.[70] Dharmendra, a well-known leprologist in India who had been present at that inaugural All-India Workers Conference at Wardha in 1949, was commissioned as a short-term consultant to Burma, and Robert Cochrane went as a consultant to Ceylon.[71]

Ethiopia was the first country to request assistance with leprosy control; Afghanistan asked for a consultant to conduct a leprosy survey; and Iraq requested the services of a leprosy expert. In the Americas, Dr Lauro de Souza Lima – an authoritative leprologist from Brazil – was commissioned to conduct surveys in Paraguay, Bolivia, Peru, and Ecuador. The names of the members selected to be on the WHO panel of experts were also published.[72] All were key figures who had been instrumental in the recent work against leprosy; most had had some role in promoting that work internationally; and all were members of the ILA. The *IJL* told members that Dr W. M. Bonne, the Chief of the Coordination of Research Section in the Division of Epidemiological Services, had maintained close contact with representatives of the ILA throughout the whole process.[73]

The ILA seemed mollified that matters were finally proceeding satisfactorily. The affiliation between the ILA and WHO was beginning to be productive, and Chaussinand explained to members that the ILA was one of the few NGOs recognised by the WHO. He also gave a glimpse of the intense lobbying that had taken place: "In this capacity our Association has stressed during recent WHAs the urgent need for WHO to take action against leprosy." As a result, he had been appointed as a WHO consultant and as the secretary of the Expert Committee on Leprosy.[74]

In a constrained economic climate for international health, the International Leprosy Association had managed to make a place for leprosy. It looked forward to an Expert Committee which drew heavily from its own membership, and it had managed the appointment of one of its most proactive and diplomatically skilled members as a WHO consultant and advisory secretary to the Expert Committee-to-be. This appointment was well received because members had confidence in Dr Chaussinand's "experience in leprosy work and his well-balanced critical spirit".[75] In April 1952, the relationship between the WHO and the ILA was reviewed and universally acknowledged to be successful.[76] Wade wrote to the Assistant Director–General, Dr P. Dorolle, emphasising the value of the cooperation between the two bodies. He cited the consultancy services and the panel of leprosy experts, both drawn from the ILA membership and benefiting from its body of expertise, as examples of outstanding services that demonstrated the result of WHO and ILA's cooperation. He also directly credited the ILA, "together with efforts of official delegates of the Assemblies who are also members of the Association", for pushing for anti-leprosy work to be included in the World Health Organization programme.[77] There was no question, he concluded, that the recognition of the ILA by the WHO had been of "real and mutual benefit".

The ILA had representatives attend nearly all the subsequent WHAs and Executive Board meetings, or it organised the attendance of national delegates who were ILA members over the next ten years. Cochrane was at the Third Assembly in 1950, Dr Wilson Rae was designated to represent the ILA at the Fourth Assembly in 1951, and Dr Ernest Muir was present at the Fifth Assembly in 1952.[78] There was no representation at the Sixth Assembly in 1953.[79] In that period, the delegates from India (returning in the context of their initial intervention) and also delegates from the Philippines (led by José Rodriguez, Wade's and Doull's research colleague and fellow ILA member) would be decisive in securing material and technical support to conduct large-scale work or mass campaigns in various countries, drawing upon ILA expertise.

An overview of the history of WHO shows that efforts to control leprosy were influenced by the overall trajectory of the organisation just as much as any other disease control effort, something not always appreciated by those immersed in anti-leprosy work. Yet while this trajectory determined what happened to international work against leprosy, the uniqueness of the history of leprosy calls for a degree of nuance to some of the usual debating points in the critical literature.

Much of the critical literature to do with the history of international health measures since World War II is, not without reason, underpinned by a critique of international paternalism and the narrow technological view of medicine.[80] These scholarly works see the biomedical (magic bullet) models of disease control of the 1950s and 1960s being supported at the expense of a more holistic approach to international health that would take into account the social, cultural, economic, and political conditions in which people live.[81] Packard argues that "International Health interventions during most of the twentieth century have focused on preventing the transmission of infectious agents and on treating those who are infected with specific curative agents."[82] He emphasises the focus of tropical medicine on the health of populations in underdeveloped but richly resourced colonised nations, citing the efforts of the Rockefeller Foundation in the 1920s and 1930s against yellow fever and malaria in Latin America, and demonstrates how these connections became even more pronounced after World War II.[83]

The case of leprosy is a little different. While arguments for international leprosy initiatives that were initially made to the World Health Assembly did indeed rely on the logic of cost to nations and societies of having permanently disabled people, leprosy also presents another perspective on third-world poverty. To be afflicted with leprosy could cause disability and make it difficult for people to earn a living, but the stigma associated with the disease inevitably brought about a loss of both social and economic status. So addressing the early onset of the disease with medication (the magic bullet of DDS) could prevent people from slipping out of their place in society. If all went well, they could even continue to make a contribution to their and their family's livelihoods. Equally, the biomedical model or magic bullet of medication made a difference to stigma. When people were confident that there were medications to deal with the disease, the disease was demystified. Improving a leprosy-affected person's social and economic conditions robbed the disease of its communal imaginary power.

2

THE MOBILE LEPROSY CAMPAIGN
FROM A LIFETIME IN A LEPROSARIUM TO A
LIFETIME OF TREATMENT

"Cars, bicycles, horses, camels and canoes were used for transport, and when none of these could be used, journeys were made on foot"[1]

In the next two decades, a whole new approach to leprosy was developed under the rubric of "leprosy control", and although there was some continuity with what had gone before, this approach, based on the therapeutic efficacy of DDS, was profoundly innovative in several ways.[2] These changes were apparent in terms of the spaces covered, the numbers treated, and the period of time thought necessary for treatment. They had a profound impact on people with leprosy who, until that time, could look forward only to a lifetime within a leprosarium. With the new treatment, a person suffering from leprosy came to be understood increasingly in medical terms as a "case" rather than as a "leper", a term increasingly proscribed as derogatory, marginalising, and dehumanising.[3]

Equally, the person working in leprosy was happily faced with new ways of imagining leprosy work in multiple dimensions: spatial, numerical, and temporal. At the same time, a new goal of "social rehabilitation" became accepted. The promise of treating people, surgically redressing the deforming effects of the disease, and then reinserting the patients into social relations and economic productivity emerged as the desirable and attainable outcome of leprosy work. Eventually and, perhaps, inevitably, leprosy control – which aimed at introducing and establishing a new public health face of the disease – and rehabilitation – which aimed at reversing the physical, social, and psychological effects of the disease on individual lives – would increasingly and inexplicitly come to compete with each other for scarce financial resources.

This chapter focuses on the changing meanings of a "cure" as work against leprosy began to be placed within the domain of public health, and ideas about and practices of leprosy control underwent a dramatic change when the site of leprosy work, the leprosaria, gradually faded into the multiple sites of the leprosy campaign. This change took place within the context of new initiatives in international health that found it necessary to prioritise diseases and juggle budgets in order to meet the requests of member nations. The landscape of Cold War politics and the shift from colonial regimes to newly independent African nations also played into the choice of which disease campaigns to support in which country. In this economic and political context, leprosy control through mass campaigns became strategically viable. As these changes took place, the prospect of a "cure" for leprosy served as a public health strategy to entice individual cases to present themselves for treatment to reduce the burden of infection in the populace, although even in the early 1950s those responsible for the policies openly admitted that treatment of the individual could take a whole lifetime. By 1973, at the 100-year anniversary of the discovery of the bacillus, as the reality of a "cure" for leprosy became increasingly problematic, mass campaigns modified their ambitions by prioritising who should be treated. And as the science of epidemiology evolved, the work against leprosy lost ground.

UNICEF and mass leprosy campaigns

The WHO turned to the United Nations International Children's Emergency Fund (UNICEF) for financial support against leprosy, but while the WHO–UNICEF joint committee was slow to be convinced that anti-leprosy efforts would be rewarded, international politics came into play. Between 1950 and 1953, the future of UNICEF was particularly uncertain. The United States wanted to wind up the organisation, reasoning that it had served its purpose by caring for refugee children in the aftermath of the war. Those involved in running UNICEF were only too aware of the acute need for their work to continue, so the strategy pursued by those who saw a continuing role for UNICEF involved meshing it more securely with the operations of WHO, particularly by focusing on needs in developing countries and on work against communicable disease. This strategy was designed to fend off criticism that UNICEF was developing into a rival of the other international organisations. By supplying urgently needed materials to developing countries, especially and increasingly to the newly independent African nations, UNICEF could fill a gap for which WHO, as an advisory organisation, did not have the resources, or for that matter a mandate to intervene.[4] Countries affected by diseases such as tuberculosis, syphilis, yaws, and leprosy presented as appropriate recipients of UNICEF support, although initially leprosy was not included.

The arguments to secure support for leprosy presented to the joint UNICEF–WHO committee once again made much of the long-term economic costs of leprosy to the health budgets of nations in contrast to the short-terms costs of dealing with it immediately. The first attempt to secure support was for drug production in member countries, and out of this initial attempt the idea of the full-blown mass leprosy campaign emerged. WHO envisaged geographically limited campaigns that could serve as a model for subsequent extended campaigns on a national and then international scale. Logistically, this was expected to be quite complicated, although treatment itself was astonishingly cheap. It cost less than US$3 to treat a patient for a year with DDS. Depending on what was suitable for a particular country, there would have to be a network of dispensaries to which people could come for diagnosis, treatment, and follow-up. Mobile dispensaries would seek out people and treat them in their local area, in their villages, and even in their homes. Specially trained auxiliary personnel would diagnose and treat those identified. Intensive health education for infected people, "contacts", and the general public would break down the prejudice that prevented people from seeking diagnosis and treatment.

When the first approach for support was made, the joint committee was sceptical of the value of a campaign against leprosy because it was unsure of the value of the new treatment.[5] The next year, with the report of the First Expert Committee on Leprosy in hand, WHO once again asked for assistance.[6] This time it conceded that treatment took time before clinical results could be achieved, and even longer before "bacteriological clearance" could be hoped for. In fact, the medication "may have to be administered during many years", and perhaps indefinitely, for a case to be no longer dangerous as a source of infection. Offsetting this obvious disadvantage, treatment was "cheap", and because it could be administered easily patients could be treated in their own homes by auxiliary staff. People would therefore be more willing to seek out treatment because they did not run the risk of being isolated in an institution: "Securing the willingness of patients to report for treatment would probably compensate for the slowness of bacteriological clearance following sulphone therapy."[7]

WHO argued that a chain reaction would occur as more and more patients asked for treatment earlier and earlier, and "the sources of infection in the community would be progressively reduced in number and the period of their infectiousness reduced in duration".[8] It asked UNICEF to supply drugs; equip dispensaries to diagnose and treat people; improve the conditions of leprosaria; supply transport for paramedical workers who would treat people; provide training facilities and fellowships for doctors and auxiliary personnel; and send consultants, when requested, to carry out surveys and to advise governments.[9]

Still reluctant about funding mass campaigns, the Committee requested copies of the newly released Report of the First Expert Committee on Leprosy, which cautiously outlined the significance of mass campaigns in a limited area and also the vulnerability of infants and children to infection.[10] This latter observation may have been influential. In the debate that followed, the committee decided to limit its support so that it was in concert with that given to other mass campaigns. UNICEF would provide drugs, equipment for dispensaries, improvements to health education, and training for health professionals, as in the tuberculosis and yaws campaigns. It stopped short at leprosaria, which were too expensive and not within the remit of UNICEF.[11]

At this early point in international anti-leprosy work, "treatment" and "cure" were not self-evidently coincidental because there was no clearly defined endpoint for treatment with the sulphones.[12] At the same time, from a public health point of view there was a calculated and pragmatic trade-off between the long time required to treat the disease and the hypothetical value of reducing infectiousness. It was expressed in this way: treatment "sterilised" the source of infection and therefore "curtail[ed] transmission", albeit very slowly, so that although the hope for a "cure" was attenuated at an individual level, the prospects for "cure" on a public health scale were likely to be enhanced. The UNICEF decision marked the point at which the expectations around a "cure" became nuanced: in public health terms, a "cure" meant an interruption in transmission, whereas, for the individual, a "cure" became increasingly to mean not a permanent remission but a probable lifetime of treatment.

The joint committee decision also marked the departure from the leprosarium as the chief site for leprosy treatment, and the adoption of the mass campaign. The drama associated with this shift from the leprosarium, in which confinement (movement away from the population) was a governing principle, to the campaign in which mobility (movement into the population) was the mode of operation had a direct impact on the staff involved and the people being treated.

From leprosarium to leprosy campaign

The introduction of a new treatment for leprosy ushered in a new set of practices. These were devised in the context of international health, and they were developed and applied as national plans of operation, within the perspective of regional and nationally based public health programmes. They were implemented through district and local networks that were mobile, geographically strategic, and extensive. Instead of tending to and caring for individual sufferers at static sites, mobile teams distributed medication in mass campaigns to thousands. At the beginning of 1958, the WHO Regional Director for Africa, Dr Cambournac, described this extraordinary mobile approach to the disease in terms of the varied modes of transport used by medical auxiliaries:

> There appeared to be at least two million persons affected with leprosy in the [African] Region, sulphone drugs had begun to be used from 1950 onwards, especially in Nigeria and Ghana. New methods for the organization of campaigns were introduced in 1952 and 1953 and campaigns had been still further intensified in 1955 with the help of rural health centers, dispensaries and mobile units. Cars, bicycles, horses, camels and canoes were used for transport, and when none of these could be used, journeys were made on foot. Between 1955 and the end of 1957 the total number of patients receiving regular treatment was 93,000.[13]

A leprosy campaign began in a specific geographical area, and in contrast to isolating people in the leprosarium, campaigns radiated out from local foci or "pilot zones" within chosen endemic districts, as precursors to more extended areas. Then, while trained staff continued to meet ongoing needs for medication, the specialist staff would move the campaign on to the next designated area, gradually spreading their influence outwards, so that the territory within which the campaign operated changed as the activities within it went through several phases. There was an "attack phase", a "consolidation phase" and an "integration phase".[14] The attack phase moved from mass examination of the whole population to house-to-house case finding, to tracing people who had been in contact with individuals with leprosy and examining especially selected sections of the population. The consolidation phase was based on the understanding that "leprosy is a chronic disease and patients need to be treated for years", so it focused on keeping in contact with people who had begun treatment and ensuring that they persisted with their medication. Mobile circuits, outpatient clinics that were visited by paramedical personnel on fixed days, and travelling skin clinics became the chief ways of doing this. A further phase, "integration", was for later, when general health services had become sufficiently developed.[15] Pilot projects were being deployed for different stages of a campaign and for different purposes: for example, as preliminary to a mass campaign, to evaluate the progress of a mass campaign, or to serve as a focus from which a campaign could begin and then radiate outwards.

People were differentiated in new ways and became subjects for mass treatment. Those with the disease, once they were diagnosed and put under treatment, became "cases" and subjects for "case holding"; similarly, those who had come into close contact with people carrying the more infectious form of leprosy became subjects for "contact tracing". Usually this meant tracing family members, especially children, so that they could be treated as early as possible or even given some sort of prophylaxis (which was in an experimental stage). Therapeutic schedules were designed for mass administration, rather than for individuals.[16] In mass leprosy campaigns, names of people with leprosy were unimportant and specific personal identities disappeared altogether.

The leprosy campaign went amongst the people, into their homes and villages, meeting them in their communities, and distributing medication to last until the next visit. Ideally, patients would swallow their tablets under the eye of the paramedical worker. Sometimes an influential village headman, a midwife, or someone in authority would be tasked with ensuring that everyone in the village in need of the tablets received their allocation. If there were no alternative, patients would be given a quantity of tablets to take at home.[17] While people in the leprosarium had been expected to cooperate in their own cure, in mass leprosy campaigns, people were required to self-administer and monitor their progress. The unfortunate consequence was that they could be blamed for a lack of progress and be labelled as "defaulters" or "non-compliant", whether they had failed to continue to take their medication or whether there was simply a pause in their remission.

Progressively, leprosy became less of "a disease apart" and more of an appropriate public health priority for a country, even though there was great variation in what sort of priority the disease was accorded. UNICEF supported anti-leprosy work in the same way as they provided support to TB and yaws campaigns.[18] The *IJL* applauded this association between leprosy and other infectious diseases as a triumph against the practices of the past. Leprosy was just like any other public health matter, such as tuberculosis, which was "a much more infectious and more often fatal disease", and this would "contribute to the disappearance of the unreasoning horror attached to leprosy".[19]

By 1956, large-scale campaigns were officially part of the "increasing efforts to control leprosy" in the WHO programme presented at the Executive Board.[20] The results seemed to indicate that it was indeed possible to organise, detect, treat, and record new cases on a large scale. From this point on, delegates at the World Health Assemblies expressed a degree of optimism that the disease could be swiftly brought to heel. A resolution on leprosy control programmes was passed "to provide program and budget estimates for furnishing assistance to Member States" at their request.[21] Countries such as Thailand, India, and WHO regions such as the African Region Office and the European Regional Office optimistically reported expanded programmes, in spite of the expense.[22] Campaigns were gradually extended over vast territories, treating people in the hundreds of thousands.[23] By 1958, the regional director for the African Region anticipated that in the near future all leprosy cases in the region would be under regular treatment. By then, there were thirteen national leprosy control projects jointly assisted by UNICEF and WHO.[24] The new leprosy services were established within departments of health, with their own personnel. These services were responsible for reporting, gathering statistical information, and evaluating the effectiveness of the newly implemented mass campaigns. Administrators were advised about what was needed for a successful leprosy campaign, how to assess the extent of the disease in their region, and how to evaluate the results of a campaign.

Rehabilitation

The growing tension between the treatment-focused approach to the disease and a rehabilitation-focused approach surfaced at the ILA Congress in Tokyo in 1958. The panel on the social aspects of leprosy compared the "old days" – before effective treatment, when social action for leprosy-affected people had outstripped medical treatment – to the present. The panel suggested that "medical advances" would "yield their full advantages" only when there were "parallel advances in social attitude", emphasising that medical advances brought an increase in social responsibility, rather than a reduction.[25] From this point on, Congresses and expert committees would include rehabilitation in their agendas, although they most often argued that prevention of disability should be the priority, rather than surgical correction.[26] By the Third Expert Committee on Leprosy in 1966, rehabilitation had been expanded to include health education, vocational training, social welfare, simple strategies to prevent disability, surgery, and orthopedics, all of which were to be integrated into leprosy control programmes without diverting funds from field work to reconstructive surgery.[27] Early detection and the prevention of disabilities, rather than correction, became a mantra. And in 1960, a schema for the classification of disabilities was devised, ushering in another layer by which leprosy-affected people could be classified. "Disability" was defined as a "loss of function or earning power" and was "graded" only by the extent to which disability interfered with a person's ability to earn a living or enjoy a normal life.[28]

In the midst of this jostling amongst medical and public health practitioners around the notion of curing people, the people themselves had their own sticking points. As the mass campaigns were intensified, representatives to the WHA from countries in the African and Western Pacific regions mentioned the difficulty they had in discharging people from their leprosy colonies. Originally, people had been driven out of their villages, and now, even though they were being treated and their symptoms were abating, they had no desire to return.[29] The delegate from Liberia, Dr Togba, complained about the difficulty of discharging patients from the leprosy colonies after cure.[30] It was only a small step then to deplore the "professional leper" as one who, even when their disease had been cured and left no permanent sign, still expected to "live indefinitely, comfortably installed in a model leprosarium without making any effort to resume normal social and working life".[31] If the experts were to be believed, it so often seemed that the patients themselves were the least cooperative of all in this whole process of becoming "cured".

Epidemiology and the leprosy campaign

There was still so much that was unknown about the aetiology of the disease and, although various congresses had attempted to standardise the data being collected, there was very little definite knowledge about what actually happened during a leprosy campaign. Changes in data before, during, and after a campaign offered a snapshot of the effect of a campaign, provided all of the data had been gathered using consistent criteria, in the same way, and under the same conditions. Hence, the preliminary epidemiological survey was crucial for establishing a baseline for a leprosy control campaign. UNICEF–WHO required a preliminary survey lasting between three and six months, covering a good sample of the population, and taking the work already done as an initial point of reference.[32] Other surveys would follow based on observations over the period of the campaign in a set area.[33] From these surveys, indices of clinical and bacteriological effectiveness and effectiveness in case finding were devised so a campaign could be evaluated.[34]

The mass campaigns produced uneven results. At the International Leprosy Congress in Tokyo in 1958, Doull called for more careful evaluation of the effectiveness of treatment, especially in mass treatment campaigns.[35] In 1961, Rodriguez, in his capacity as the delegate from the Philippines, asked the Executive Board of the World Health Assembly for a proper evaluation and for statistical proof to demonstrate that the leprosy control programme was as successful as claimed in the Director–General's report. He argued that the results of treatment, the performance of different units, and the trend of the disease needed to be understood.[36]

Possibly in response to the issues raised by Doull and Rodriguez, the Leprosy Unit at WHO set up Leprosy Advisory Teams (LATs) designed to improve the quality of information about leprosy control projects. WHO began random sampling surveys in the Katsina Emirate of Northern Nigeria, in Monrovia, Liberia, and Cameroon, and then in Thailand, Burma, and Indonesia.[37] V. Martínez Domínguez was team leader, and K. M. Patwary acted as statistician.[38] These teams made it possible for Bechelli and Martínez Domínguez to publish research entitled "The Leprosy Problem in the World".[39] The findings of the LAT in Africa (Northern Nigeria; north, central, and south Cameroon) and Asia (the Philippines; Khon Kaen, Thailand; and Myingyan and Shwebo in Burma) showed in random sampling surveys that even in countries with good case detection, 75% of those already registered were new cases. Taking into account the many difficulties in gathering the data – including variations in case-finding processes, as well as variations in the quality of register-keeping, and differing criteria for releasing patients from treatment – Bechelli and Martínez Domínguez attempted to establish "an idea of the magnitude of the problem in the world" and provide "a better approach to the leprosy problem from the epidemiological, human and socioeconomic aspects".[40] They found 2,831,775 registered patients and 10,786,000 estimated cases.[41] An estimated 1,928,000 people were being treated for leprosy, and of the total estimated number of patients in the world, 3,872,000 had disabilities.[42] Five years later, in 1973, it was still unclear if the mass control programmes had achieved a decline in incidence.[43] There had been considerable work on the statistical analysis of data on diagnosed cases of leprosy, but if the goal was to detect people infected with *M. leprae*, there was a great deal of information lacking on individuals, households, and communities associated with the transmission of infection.[44]

The limits of leprosy control

A great deal of energy was invested in the mass leprosy campaigns which had heralded the dawning of a new and exciting era. Over the next fifteen years, the policy and procedures for campaigns were increasingly finetuned, but these new practices of leprosy control reached their limits within two decades. Initially, it looked as if people could be treated in large numbers and then discharged, cured. But as time went by, and in spite of continuously finetuning the leprosy control campaign and exhorting countries to exert their best efforts and extend their budgets, the campaigns became increasingly drawn out. As the lack of progress became apparent, and even before the real difficulties of drug resistance were recognised, many different administrative elements in the campaign came in for blame. And, as always, the person with the disease was represented as the biggest obstacle to their own cure. Even after ten years of treatment, a large proportion of those who had been receiving dapsone still showed signs of *M. leprae* in their skin smears. Additionally, the scale of the programme did not decline: as more people were treated, more appeared for treatment.

In 1951, in the earliest days of the mass campaigns, Wade prophetically editorialised mass campaigns as a "large-scale experiment":

> Here has developed a situation without parallel, the wholesale adoption of a potent but highly toxic drug, in use for a relatively short period and still under active discussion regarding dosage and route of administration, to be used as the standard drug under a wide variety of conditions, mostly where medical supervision cannot be regarded as close and to a great extent in outpatient practice. The outcome will be of great interest to all who are concerned with the treatment of leprosy patients. It is to be hoped that arrangements will be made for the frank reporting of the results of this large-scale experiment, with respect to untoward effects as well as favorable results.[45]

A "large-scale experiment" that could have both "untoward" as well as "favorable results" proceeded using a drug about which very little was known on a disease that was still largely mysterious. Over the next twenty years, the notion of a "cure" would not only be increasingly qualified, but it would become more and more unstable. In spite of the optimism apparent in the reports of the efficacy of the sulphones, a "cure" for leprosy also continued to slip just beyond the grasp of both those subject to its ravages and those who treated them.

While medical professionals who were closely observing the impact of the new drugs in the field were cautious right from the outset, there had been sufficient optimism for Chaussinand, for example, to claim that "leprosy should become a rare disease in the next twenty years provided an enlightened and well-organized anti-leprosy campaign could be put into operation".[46] To do this, a convincing case had been made for the new approach which hinged on the potential for a "cure", the value of the mechanism of the "mass campaign", and the shift of leprosy into the domain of public health. The First Expert Committee on Leprosy unambiguously confirmed the therapeutic potency of various sulphones, including DDS, recommending an optimum dosage of dapsone of up to 600mg a week. Crucially, they recommended that it be introduced initially in small and then in increasing doses over a period of several weeks: a recommendation that sprang from the fear of adverse reactions to the drug.

"Certain limitations" in the use of the sulphones and the need for "more rapidly effective drugs" had been expressed as early as the 6th ILA Congress, held in 1953 in Madrid.[47] By then, the commission had realised that the persistence of bacilli in the body meant that the sulphones were bacteriostatic and not bactericidal, inhibiting multiplication of *M. leprae* rather than killing the bacilli. There were other puzzling effects: the tolerance of different people and different ethnic groups to DDS seemed to vary.[48] Some people, once they began treatment, improved within a period of months: their symptoms abated; their lesions receded; their general health improved; their appetite, body weight, and strength increased; but, frustratingly, their bacteriological improvement was slower: they continued to show the presence of *M. leprae* in their skin smears.[49] All of this meant that the later phases and end results of their treatment varied widely from one individual to the next, and often from one ethnic group to the next. In some places, after lengthy treatment, a high proportion of people were delighted to experience "clinical and bacteriological arrest of the disease" and happily stayed like that for many years. Disappointingly, in other centres, only a small proportion of people experienced this, and, worse still, many "relapsed".[50] There were wide variations in response to the treatment which seemed to indicate vagaries of the disease, and which influenced the "end result of treatment". People in whom the disease had come to a halt became known as "arrested cases"; rarely discharged as "cured"; and still requiring "management" in case their disease became "reactivated" and they suffered a "relapse". The *IJL* told readers: "Recent observations suggest that arrested cases are not completely freed of leprosy bacilli, and that reactivation of the disease is therefore not unlikely." All "arrested" cases had to be kept under observation in case of reactivation.[51]

By 1957, UNICEF claimed that it was "premature to believe that by organizing mass treatment for a few years leprosy could be completely eradicated".[52] The leprosy campaigns were increasingly considered "among the most difficult to organize and continue" because "treatment did not provide immediate and spectacular results".[53] Then reports began to indicate that there seemed to be no end point to the campaigns. In the Congo, a campaign had started in 1954, and at the end of 1960, 15,780 cases had been registered. There were 2,900 arrested cases and 2,700 under observation but not receiving treatment. The intention had been to integrate the campaign into general medical services by 1962, but UNICEF faced having to maintain financial support for years to come.[54]

The duration of treatment depended upon the form of the disease, its severity, and the condition of the lesions, as well as other unlisted and possibly unidentified factors. A cure could be defined only by certain negative clinical signs that were then confirmed by repeated bacteriological and histopathological examinations. In mass campaigns, monitoring the pathology of numerous individuals in order to determine a decline in bacteria was difficult – if not impossible – especially in poorly resourced countries, so the only basis for a conclusive verdict of a cure was to be gathered from observing clinical criteria. Over time, lesions could be compared in terms of their site, aspect, and size. But even this was difficult without clinical assessment by an expert. Usually in a campaign, a nurse would make the diagnosis, but this was not always sufficient to replace the specific and detailed clinical examination a clinician would perform.[55] In spite of this, people continued to enthusiastically present themselves for treatment. More than 1 million leprosy sufferers had been treated in the twenty-six projects assisted by WHO and UNICEF, and medical practitioners and public health professionals were unanimous in agreeing that the public be informed that leprosy could be cured.[56] But, increasingly, the difficulty of arriving at an end point in a leprosy campaign forced a narrowed focus upon the most contagious patients: those diagnosed with lepromatous leprosy.[57]

By 1964, mass campaigns had gone out of favour for reasons that had nothing to do with leprosy, and more to do with the malaria and tuberculosis campaigns. The WHO convened a study group to assess the role of mass campaigns, in general, in the evolution and development of health services.[58] In concert with this disenchantment, reports indicated that the numbers with leprosy were going up, rather than coming down, and although the disease may have been halted in individual instances, some people were actually suffering "relapses". In 1965, the Americas reported that "the numbers of new cases and the total numbers of patients undergoing systematic treatment was on the increase in Latin America".[59] The Director–General told the WHO Executive Board in 1970 that with the resources then available, it would take "at least twenty years of control" before there was any hope of reducing prevalence.[60]

The risk of relapse overshadowed every leprosy patient, even if they had faithfully continued treatment until they had attained bacterial negativity. This was reinforced when Jacobson and Trautman at Carville also reported on a long-term follow-up of Faget's initial patients who had received Promin.[61] Thirty years after they were started on sulphone therapy, ten of the thirteen patients still living continued to have active disease. This meant that "successful control of this disease is possible only if adequate follow-up and treatment are maintained on all lepromatous patients for life".[62]

By 1973, at the tenth ILA Congress in Bergen (where Hansen had identified the bacillus), Bechelli, who had been head of the leprosy unit at WHO from 1961 to 1970, and Hubert Sansarricq, his newly appointed successor, had to confess that the mass campaigns of the 1950s and 1960s were at an impasse. In a summation entitled "Advances in Leprosy Control in the Last One Hundred Years," Bechelli stated quite plainly that "At present, with the drugs available, the prospects of controlling leprosy in a few decades are not favorable for most areas of the world, and these prospects can only be improved by intensifying research."[63] Contrasting the triumph of technology demonstrated in the first moon landing to the lack of basic knowledge about the disease, Professor Michel Lechat, the Belgian epidemiologist, mused that "action" was no substitute for "knowledge":

> We need to know more about the deep mechanisms involved in the life and transmission of the infective organism responsible, the reaction of the human host, and the behavior of the disease in populations. This means increased knowledge in the fields of microbiology, immunology, and epidemiology. Then we shall be able to face leprosy with more powerful weapons.[64]

Leprosy and other campaigns

The use of dapsone (DDS) against leprosy, when placed in the broader international public health context of the 1950s and early 1960s, was typical of the proliferation of WHO-supported national vertical programmes, which were conceived as narrowly focused, technology-driven campaigns targeting specific diseases such as malaria, smallpox, TB, and yaws. Such short-term programmes based on chemotherapy seemed to offer a highly efficient process with easily measurable targets, thereby providing a dramatic solution for communicable diseases.

Efforts against leprosy in Africa encountered some of the same issues as efforts against malaria and tuberculosis, even though the technologies were different.[65] The anti-malaria, anti-tuberculosis, and anti-leprosy campaigns all made use of UNICEF support. All conducted mass campaigns, whether they administered medication or vaccinated people. Efforts against disease in the 1950s and 1960s were dictated by available technologies (DDT and DLD or synthetic drugs in the case of malaria; BCG and antibiotics in the case of tuberculosis; and DDS in the case of leprosy), even though the actions of these technologies were not understood and even though the disease vectors (in the case of malaria) and the disease process, in the case of leprosy – as well as the reactions of the disease to the various technologies – were unknown.

Anne-Emanuelle Birn refers to 1946–70 as a period of bureaucratisation of international health conducted in the shadow of the Cold War and impelled by a development ideology.[66] Webb writes that this was a time of hubris for anti-malaria efforts. McMillen writes that those in tuberculosis control were more cautious, aware of the long-term nature of the problem.[67] All the campaigns were underpinned by the imperative that doing something, using whatever means were available, was preferable to doing nothing. The optimism was founded on the technologies. There was also arrogance: for example, in how the acquired immunity against malaria of African populations was held in little regard. There was arrogance in deploying a biomedical model of disease control without regard to the everyday reality of social and economic conditions within which people lived. As McMillen points out, this is not to say that the researchers in Kenya were unaware of the futility of trying to defeat tuberculosis without making major changes in people's everyday lives, but they worked within the limitations of a biomedical paradigm to produce a biomedical solution.[68]

Was the work against leprosy part of the hubris of the 1950s that envisaged an end to contagious diseases? Those who worked against leprosy were indeed optimistic and eager to join in, but they were very conscious that they were starting from behind, when it came to public health interventions. Leprosy had been barely acknowledged as a concern that would reward efforts. People who worked against leprosy were delighted just to have leprosy included in international disease efforts. They knew very early that there was no end point to treatment, but they calculated that it was worthwhile in public health terms.

Their participation can be justified by the monumental shift in attitudes to leprosy that took place. Leprosy control now belonged to the domain of public health, a notion which would be increasingly refined into the twenty-first century. At the very core of this new approach to leprosy was the expectation for the first time that the disease could be cured. With the discovery of the effect of the sulphones against leprosy, it seemed briefly as if a definite cure had been found, although close examination of the medical response to the sulphones indicated caution and constant calls for more research.[69] That this conservatism was justified became increasingly obvious. The disturbing consequences of what Wade expressed as the "untoward effects" of the vast clinical trial were becoming impossible to ignore, to the extent that it was beginning to look like those working against leprosy might lose the one efficacious drug that they had available to them.

OWNERSHIP OF LEPROSY TREATMENT (1966–73)

International efforts to coordinate the fight against leprosy and introduce large-scale assessment and treatment campaigns did not emerge in virgin territory. The new entrants to the struggle found that they had to modify their expectations and initiatives to take account of certain institutional, financial, and personality issues that were long entrenched. What developed could luridly – but not inaccurately – be termed a struggle for the ownership of leprosy treatment. This chapter examines more closely the benevolent, non-governmental societies working against leprosy, their own attempts to develop efficiencies of scale through federation and specialisation, and their sometimes fraught relations.

The original force in the struggle to control leprosy was a group of benevolent associations, some of whom had been active since the mid-nineteenth century, rising out of the decay of colonial empires, while others had appeared in the wake of World War II. The former had a missionary foundation, mostly Protestant, while the latter were mainly Catholic, taking their point of departure from what was termed Christian social action and forming a counterpart to the rise of the Left. As much as they were about anti-leprosy work, and while they were overtly apolitical, their emergence is inseparable from their political context. Moreover, although the increasing secularisation of these organsations served to distance them from their ideological underpinnings, their identities retained a benevolent character.

There is a view that "With the increasing secularization of leprosy and the changing role of mission societies has come a decline in religious fundraising for leprosy work and a lessening of public attention to leprosy as a dramatic disease."[1] According to this opinion, the missionary societies that worked against leprosy had had their day by the end of the 1980s. But such societies have proved resilient, partly because the popular imagination in the West persisted in entertaining contradictory notions of leprosy: on the one hand that "leprosy had died out" while on the other that it was meritorious to give money for the "poor lepers" in "far-flung lands", wherever they may be.[2]

The extraordinary ability of leprosy to generate charitable donations still allows the anti-leprosy organisations to play an indispensable role, both nationally and internationally, in anti-leprosy work. This strength is paradoxical, for it is based on individual, incremental beneficence, a wellspring that always seems at risk of drying up but never quite does. These micro-donations continue to flow from appeals from the church pulpit, through the media, and at street level through large annual campaigns such as World Leprosy Day. From this cottage funding, these organisations have flourished over the decades while generally good stewardship and judicious investment have resulted in their accruing significant sums of money for work against leprosy.

The father figures and the narratives of origin

Several of these societies take their inspiration from a charismatic founding father around whom stories of personal illumination, dedication, ideals, and personal sacrifice congregate. In most instances, their writings have been preserved and continue to contribute to this process of hagiographic representation. Some have become less visible as the organisations have become more secularised; nonetheless, the values espoused and associated with the "father figure" still permeate the individual organisations and lend them their specific character.

To cite just a couple, Joseph de Veuster, or Father Damien, was a Belgian priest who spent sixteen years on Molokai in Hawaii improving the basic living conditions of the people, building adequate shelter, and representing their needs and fundamental rights to the parsimonious Board of Health. The story of his labours and his battles with the authorities became famous while he was alive. When he noticed the first signs of leprosy on his body in 1876, he famously addressed his congregation in a sermon as "we lepers". When he died in April 1889, at forty-nine years of age, his death seemed to indicate conclusively that leprosy as a germ disease was communicable. Inspired by Damien, Pierre van den Wijngaert formed Les Amis du Père Damien (APD) in 1954, and in 1964, the Damien Foundation amalgamated all the Belgian anti-leprosy societies.[3] This new association developed a well-rounded social mission that focused on prevention, accessible treatment using ambulatory services, rehabilitation through physiotherapy and surgery, and awareness through education in public health programmes.[4] The foundation supported several Belgian researchers in international research programmes, and its efforts impacted particularly on Zaire, Rwanda, Burundi, India, and Korea.[5]

At almost exactly the same time as Damien was beginning his work on Molokai, an inspiring advocate for people with leprosy emerged from the Protestant tradition in India, and, as a result of Wellesley Bailey's inspiration, The Mission to Lepers was founded. The Mission began by providing small amounts of funding to Protestant missionary asylums where leprosy work was being carried out.[6] After several expansions of activity and corresponding name changes, it became the Leprosy Mission International, and it has maintained spiritual and holistic goals: "To minister in the name of Jesus Christ to the physical, mental and spiritual needs of sufferers from leprosy, to assist in their rehabilitation and to work towards the eradication of leprosy."[7] The Leprosy Mission reached into Africa, India, and most of Asia, giving birth to offshoots in Canada and the United States. One of those, the American Leprosy Missions (ALM), has consistently supported key scientific research and training institutions.[8]

Raoul Follereau, who was an indefatigable fundraiser for the Sœurs Notre-Dame des Apôtres and their leprosy settlement of Adzopé, on Île Desirée in Côte d'Ivoire, was inspired by Charles de Foucauld, an ex-army officer who became a Cistercian Trappist and retired to live in the desert as a hermit, like the forefathers of Christianity. In 1946, Follereau founded the Order of Charity which would become the Raoul Follereau Foundation.[9] The practical side of this organisation's work included constructing leprosy centres and clinics and providing transport for ambulatory treatment.[10] However, the organisation also ministered to the wider spiritual and material needs of people, engaging in a battle against broader symbolic "leprosies". Follereau became a pioneer in championing the human rights of leprosy-affected people. In 1952, he petitioned the UN to establish an international convention on the dignity of people with leprosy. In 1954, he initiated the annual World Leprosy Day, on which a coordinated media campaign helped raise funds for the support of those with leprosy.[11] He was also instrumental in setting up the leprosy congress organised by the Order of Malta in Rome in 1956, out of which emerged the Comité Exécutif International de l'Ordre de Malte pour l'Assistance aux Lépreux.

Emmaüs-Suisse was inspired by the famous call made by Abbé Pierre for solidarity with the poor.[12] Like Father Damien in Belgium, Abbé Pierre was (and still is) so admired in France that he was frequently voted France's most outstanding figure. His political position as a Catholic on the left in French politics marks the extreme opposite of that embraced by the young Follereau, who worked to preserve the status quo of the Catholic elite of the old regime, and yet Marcel Farine cites them both as his mentors. Inspired by Abbé Pierre, Farine began Les Amis d'Emmaüs, which was officially convened in Geneva in 1958. He held the post of president for thirty-two years and became the founding president of the European Federation of Anti-Leprosy Organizations (ELEP).[13]

But while many of the societies had inspiring, even legendary, leaders, they became increasingly secularised and bureaucratised. The giant of these organisations, especially in terms of disposable funds, was a twentieth-century arrival. Deutsche Aussätzigen Hilfwerk (DAHW) emerged from war-torn Germany and aspired to be secular in orientation. DAHW's constitution highlighted "medical and social rehabilitation" of leprosy sufferers as a single goal, coupling them and thereby implying that one could not be achieved without the other.[14] Hermann Kober, the founder of DAHW, dedicated over forty years to the organisation as Treasurer, Executive Director, and finally President.

Apart from the American Leprosy Missions, there were two other organisations with a strongly scientific mandate: the British Leprosy Relief Association (LEPRA) and Nederlandse Stichting Voor Leprabestridjding (NSL). Originally the British Empire Leprosy Relief Association (BELRA), LEPRA focused its energies in specific areas such as the Malawi control scheme and work in Sierra Leone and Zambia.[15] Remaining true to its research aspirations, it also supported research in Oxford and at the National Institute for Medical Research.[16]

The Nederlandse Stichting Voor Leprabestridjding, or the Netherlands Leprosy Relief, was equally conscious of its relationship to the former Dutch Empire and the postcolonial intervention it made into the balance of power within the third world. It promoted "the fight against leprosy in the developing countries, regardless of race, politics or religion". Uniquely, the Netherlands Leprosy Relief placed itself squarely within the network of international health and was careful to state that it "maintains close contact with WHO and makes use of the WHO guidelines".[17]

Leprosy carries such a powerful historical legacy, and given how it has been both loaded with meaning and also deprived, for a long time, of medical certainties, it must have been extremely difficult for leaders in this field to avoid the "Christ-like" aura that would coalesce around them. At the same time, these figures were not oblivious to that celebrity. Some tried to avoid or diminish it, and others accepted it but tried to harness it to their cause. At a symbolic level, these father figures stood at the forefront of efforts to "make whole" a fragmented physical body: persons suffering the devastating effects of the disease were to be restored to wholeness, if not physically, then socially, economically, and – most importantly – spiritually. The motif of "making whole" reverberates through the discourses of these societies. The societies believed that they had a responsibility to the "whole person" affected by the disease, and fiercely resisted attempts to see leprosy care as being circumscribed by clinical pathology. In another direction also, it may be that the societies' donor appeal came from a displacement of the public's desire to see a fragmented world restored to wholeness.

These societies, then, while united in the desire to ameliorate the condition of leprosy sufferers, had differing views on what that entailed, and on where emphasis should be placed. Moreover, they were vulnerable to a diminution of interest or goodwill from their donors. While Zachary Gussow believed that these organisations comprised "a coherent collectivity of mutual interests, similar beliefs, and considerable interaction", fuller consideration reveals that here were many grounds for caution, suspicion, and disagreement. Historically, decision-making in this "coherent collectivity" seems to have required considerable will, after prolonged, exhaustive debate. While the positive aspect of this process was that every facet of an opinion would be aired, the negative side was that concerted action could be delayed. There was a fierce anarchy and autonomy at the heart of their federation. Each organisation had its integrity and its historical orientation. They were flexible – and, in the long run, responsive to shifts in international public health policy – but flexible within the limits and at a pace they believed appropriately responsive both to their donors and to their patients. They took it as point of pride to be "in touch" with the people whom they were serving; equally, they were always careful to cultivate and keep faith with their benefactors.[18] They maintained a balancing act between donor, benevolent organisation, and recipient, and were always wary of being thrown off balance by new policies that could bring everything crashing down.

Towards a federation

In 1963, Hermann Kober suggested that the organisations raising funds for anti-leprosy work should get together, but in spite of his best efforts nothing eventuated. Then, in 1965, Pierre van den Wijngaert, in consultation with Raoul Follereau, proposed a "common market" of leprosy organisations.[19] On 2 October 1965, van den Wijngaert convened the first colloquium of nine European anti-leprosy organisations. Together they created COPECIEL

(Commission préparatoire pour l'étude d'une collaboration entre les Institutions européennes de lutte anti-lèpre) which was composed of four of the associations, with Follereau as Chairman and Pierre Kaélin (from Comité Exécutif International de l'Ordre de Malte pour l'Assistance aux Lépreux, Switzerland) as Secretary. They held two preliminary meetings in London, on 15 January and 11 June, and set up the inaugural meeting in Bern in September 1966, at which the European Federation of Anti-Leprosy Organizations (ELEP) officially came into being.[20]

Marcel Farine (of Emmaüs-Suisse) was given the responsibility for forging a compromise between those who wanted to maintain a great degree of autonomy for individual associations and those who preferred a closer, more formalised entity.[21] Eventually, the meeting settled on a minimalist position, at least in the short term, and decided to trial a European Coordinating Bureau and revisit the matter again in two years. The Minutes stated that "The plan of an association with legal statutes was finally given up. The European coordinating committee shall be ruled by simple regulations functioning as statutes to which members keep themselves for two years. ..."[22] Pierre van den Wijngaert was unanimously elected as Secretary–General and was charged with drawing up the simplified statutes with the assistance of Deutsche Aussätzigen Hilfwerk, Fondation Père-Damien, and Comité Exécutif International de l'Ordre de Malte pour l'Assistance aux Lépreux.

The founding organisations, under the titles they held at the time, were as follows:

Aide aux Lépreux Emmaüs-Suisse, Switzerland
Amici dei Lebbrosi (AIFO), Italy
Comité Exécutif International de l'Ordre de Malte pour l'Assistance aux
    Lépreux (CIOMAL), Switzerland
Deutsche Aussätzigen Hilfswerk (DAHW), Germany
Evangelische Leprahilfe, Switzerland
Fondation Père-Damien (FOPERDA), Belgium
Hartdegen Fund, Germany
Les Amis du Père Damien (DFB), Belgium
L'Ordre de la Charité, France (AFRF), France
The Order of Charity, UK
The Leprosy Mission (TLM), UK[23]

The fiercely guarded independence of the organisations would have an impact upon the decision-making process. Eddie Askew, the General Secretary for the Leprosy Mission and its representative at the founding of

ELEP, recalled in his memoirs: "The decision-making process with such a diverse collection of organizations with similar but quite different objectives ensured that decisions were not always easy to arrive at and it was often a struggle to achieve unanimity."[24] They each had different ways of working, different interests, and different visions for the future. Some of the differences were based on religious affiliations: "Some were committed Roman Catholic groups. Others like ourselves were not. Some were secular and not particularly sympathetic to the idea of medical and social work among leprosy sufferers having a Christian motivation. Other groups too were essentially national groups, each raising support in a particular country."[25] To compound these difficulties, cultural and language differences initially provided the most fundamental problems. He vividly remembered the struggles of one of the earliest meetings:

> In 1966 a meeting was arranged in London. Eleven societies met together from France, Germany, Switzerland, Belgium and the UK. It was a disorganised affair. We had much to learn. Newberry Fox took the chair. He spoke only English. I supported him, speaking English, a few words of German and fluent Bengali. The latter might have impressed but was of absolutely no use. Follereau spoke only French. The Germans spoke German and some English. The Swiss understood all three. It wasn't easy but there was goodwill and we soon realised that we could do more together than we could do apart.[26]

One of the most important tasks of the Federation was to delineate the territory for fundraising. Each organisation had limits to the concessions that it was prepared to make, and there were some difficulties. Some were not happy, for example, that the Leprosy Mission drew from an international well of support, and it came under pressure to confine its appeals to the UK.[27] Askew writes, "We argued for tolerance and freedom of choice for people to support whomever they wished." At the same time, he expressed a sentiment that every member organisation clearly endorsed: "We wanted maximum freedom with minimum restriction. Cooperation was good, coercion wasn't."[28]

The organisational structure of the Federation consisted of two parts. The first part was responsible for the management of the Federation. Decision-making and policy were the purview of a General Assembly (GA) of all the member associations which met every two years. Power was delegated to standing committees which drew representatives from five of the member associations. Administrative work was done by the coordinating bureau, "facilitating the process through which its members should coordinate their relationship with each other".[29] This would include organising meetings, setting up coordination structures, and later running the computerised information network. A standing committee composed of the President and five members elected by the General Assembly would act on behalf of the Federation for all urgent matters that arose between assemblies.

The second characteristic of the organisation included the mechanisms for coordinating activities that were "the cornerstone of the Federation". This would enable members "to engage in a free and friendly exchange of workloads and still present a united front in the worldwide fight against leprosy". These working sessions would be a triumph of collaboration on a quid pro quo basis.[30] In these sessions, in one big room, members coordinated the financing and managing of all their projects; they pooled resources with a specific end in mind; they managed ELEP/ILEP grants to researchers and institutions, and nominated project coordinators. They set up working groups to accomplish common strategies, to make recommendations on projects and policies, and to promote specific aspects of the campaign against leprosy. Finally, they appointed coordinators in each country for when projects were formulated and negotiated; for when members made agreements with governments and local authorities; and for supervising and assessing projects in the field.[31]

ELEP established joint projects in which leadership was assigned to one association and supporting funds were contributed by several others. Leadership in a project was determined by consensus, going to the association that was best informed about the centre or country concerned, and had traditionally made the largest commitment in terms of money or activity. Initially, these projects were located in "centers", old-style leprosaria. In 90% of instances, a single association took responsibility for a centre over a long period. A typical arrangement would be for, say, Emmaüs-Suisse to be allocated leadership, and if their organisation needed US$100,000 for a year, Emmaüs-Suisse, Deutsche Aussätzigen Hilfwerk, Les Amis du Père Damien, and Association Française Raoul Follereau would all contribute varying amounts.[32] Adzopé in the Ivory Coast was another joint project. While Deutsche Aussätzigen Hilfwerk contributed US$5,000, Les Amis du Père Damien US$4,000, Comité Exécutif International de l'Ordre de Malte pour l'Assistance aux Lépreux US$6,337, and Aide aux Lépreux Emmaüs-Suisse US$1,900, Association Française Raoul Follereau committed US$50,560 and had already given US$100,000, so it was entrusted with leadership of the organisation.[33]

And so they divided up the leprosy world. In the Congo, for example, in one year, Deutsche Aussätzigen Hilfwerk gave US$5,000 for centres in the eastern province, Les Amis du Père Damien gave US$3,200, the Leprosy Mission gave US$600, and Fondation Père-Damien asked for the leadership. In Ethiopia, Deutsche Aussätzigen Hilfwerk took on leadership. In Uganda, there were ongoing negotiations between the Leprosy Mission and Deutsche Aussätzigen Hilfwerk. Doing this also enabled them to see if there were any overlaps in funding; for example, in Dahomey, they became aware that the centre manager was "requesting money everywhere".[34]

The Medical Commission

As well as the organisational structures of the General Assembly and coordinating bureau, ELEP established a board of experts that it called the Medical Commission, many of whose members belonged to the International Leprosy Association and had been involved in leprosy work from the beginning of the international initiatives. The first members who were elected for a two-year term were Louis-Paul Aujoulat, Franz Hemerijckx, Stanley Browne, and Maurice Gilbert.[35] These experts, who had their own independent professional lives, made their time and expertise freely available to the ELEP associations as voluntary consultants. In 1971, they gave a job description of the Commission:

> Although members of the Commission are busy people, the point is made that they freely offer their services, as far as may be possible, for personal consultation to Member Organizations, for examining by correspondence any Projects that may be submitted … and also for on the spot appraisal of a situation or a Project, and advice on policy or operation. Because of their accumulated knowledge and experience, the members of the Commission represent a reservoir of local data now freely available to the members of ELEP.[36]

All brought firsthand and often prestigious experience in anti-leprosy work to the ELEP Medical Commission, enabling the Medical Commission to play a significant role in steering the activities of the federation. This ensured changes in emphasis in concert with the shifts in the focus of international health initiatives. Initially, it steered members away from ongoing support for fixed-base institutions that used isolation as the prime measure of leprosy control. It also supported mass campaigns against the disease. But before long, and amidst some resistance and debate, the Commission began to encourage the integration of leprosy control into the general medical services of the countries where ELEP members were active. Aujoulat acknowledged that "The crisis in the campaign against leprosy persists, especially at the government level of the French-speaking African countries: the disillusionment is increasing and WHO, as well as UNICEF stress, after 20 years of effort, the lack of sufficient results." In 1971, the Commission produced a statement on the integration of leprosy into general health services, stressing that while "the leprosarium had been taken over by mobile services; these in turn were to give way to integrated services".[37]

But members in the General Assembly raised objections to integration on the grounds of ethical responsibility to their donors. Funds had been raised on the promise of caring for people suffering from leprosy, not for general medical work. Gilbert and Lechat countered that "integration was a technical matter which is more dependent on experts than on public opinion". The Medical Commission was "quite sure that in the future the only valuable method in the campaign against leprosy will be to set up integrated projects". The rest they left to "public relations" tactics. The onus was on members to educate people about "the most effective way of helping leprosy sufferers".[38]

In bridging the gap between old and new ways of conducting leprosy work, the Commission was at pains to be accessible to the members. It encouraged the presence of representatives at Commission meetings so that problems and projects could be discussed and "points of view harmonized in a way and with a speed and clarification not otherwise possible". After 1971, meetings of the Medical Commission were timed to coincide with the principal meeting of ELEP. Annual reports were also submitted to the General Assembly for observations and recommendations.[39] At the same time, the Commission attempted to govern the conduct of different member associations with national governments, recommending "great discretion and correctness" and counselling members to "avoid any suggestion of by-passing the recognized official channels".[40]

An early instance of difficulties in this area reveals how complicated activity in a specific country and relations with a government could become. Deutsche Aussätzigen Hilfwerk had been conducting work in Pakistan with Dr Ruth Pfau, and in 1970 it was planning a more extensive and ambitious project to reach 15,000 patients and spend 260,000DM.[41] Its work was supported by local authorities and regional governments. In view of the ambitious scope of the project, Deutsche Aussätzigen Hilfwerk asked other associations to share the work and funding with them.

The Medical Commission, while praising Dr Pfau's work, felt that it was too dispersed. The core of its reservation was with regard to the role of Deutsche Aussätzigen Hilfwerk in relation to the public authorities. The

Medical Commission questioned Hermann Kober: "Obviously the public authorities should be stimulated. But would it be advisable to replace them, even if they are long in assuring all their obligations?"[42] Kober felt that the Commission was not taking into account the reality of the situation: "He drew attention to the situation *de facto* existing in Pakistan and on all the work that is accomplished there, regardless of the lack of support from the Pakistan government." This began a debate between Browne and Kober in which neither shifted ground. The Minutes reveal that "the Medical Commission is still opposed to the fact that DAHW would replace the government while recognising that private associations must play the role of pioneer". The discussion ended with Kober assuring the Commission that Deutsche Aussätzigen Hilfwerk would make its best effort "to stimulate both Pakistan doctors and the government". But the matter was raised at a subsequent meeting of the Medical Commission, and the debate once again stalled on the same issue. This time the intentions of Deutsche Aussätzigen Hilfwerk were defended with the rationale that "The only method to force the Pakistan Government to do its duty is to make it ashamed." The Medical Commission then conceded that a representative should go and inspect the situation.[43]

Rehabilitation was another difficult issue for the Medical Commission. It refused to make it a priority, instead arguing for balance. Stanley Browne, for example, was adamant that treatment had the first claim on available financial resources, even regarding Paul Brand's pioneering work of surgical reconstruction in Vellore with reservations.[44] But by the 1970s, the Medical Commission was more responsive to the demand to consider the "whole person". Its solution was "a balanced approach", which it explained as "Having one foot firmly based on scientific and medical fundamentals and the other on the oft-neglected social and non-material considerations of the disease" so that "we can appraise and advise, evaluate and recommend, with both scientific detachment and social involvement".[45]

The Medical Commission did not represent the diversity of approaches and convictions of the associations in their entirety. It was impossible for them to speak for members founded in such varied traditions, cultures, and convictions. Additionally, the fundamental similarities of the members made their differences even more important and prone to accentuation. But when it came to dividing up the work, the bilateral and multilateral working groups at which members discussed their aspirations and commitments in various regions and negotiated compromises demonstrated a triumph of collaboration.[46]

There would always be differences in priorities between the highly progressive committee of medical experts who made up the Medical

Commission and the associations, with their time-honoured commitments to their donor base. It would always be much easier to ask for funds to help people with damaged hands and terribly deformed faces than to ask for money for a vaccine that had yet to be developed, or for work the results of which were hard to gauge, especially if it were to be incorporated into a general medical health service. The organisations also had long-standing commitments to, and personal relations with, the small centres that they supported throughout the third world. While the Commission showed the way medically and scientifically, the associations fiercely preserved their own integrity.

ELEP and the WHO

From well before the formation of ELEP, communication with WHO had never been totally satisfactory. The slow release of the official report of the First Expert Committee had caused much frustration to the *International Journal of Leprosy* (*IJL*) editorial board. This compounded the disappointment at the paucity of advice available to various countries from the WHO consultants. The *IJL* explained to the International Leprosy Association members the procedure and protocols:

> Such things are done under a system – for which there are obvious good reasons – that make for difficulties. As we understood it, reports of such experts are confidential to WHO, so that they may express opinions freely; edited versions of them are supplied to the governments concerned; and if and when these governments authorize the release of these reports, they may be made available to others.

Nonetheless, the International Leprosy Association managed to obtain as much information as it could through its diverse network. James Doull's connections were helpful, and Dr de Souza Lima in South America supplied a copy of his preliminary report (but with a warning that it was "restricted"). Yet they were maddened that, while they were kept in the dark, WHO sent out press releases on "simple factual data" – such as leprosy prevalence, control measures, and special institutions – but overlooked responsible medical periodicals such as the *International Journal of Leprosy*.[47] Even more outrageously, one early report had been entirely inaccurate:

> the public information service of WHO, undoubtedly without the knowledge of the technical authorities and certainly in disregard of the restrictions by which we have been bound, broadcast a press release purporting to give

the highlights of the Committee's report. Since that statement was made public we would be perfectly at liberty to print it. We do not do so, however, because it differs so greatly in certain important respects from the spirit of the actual conclusions of the Committee.[48]

As an example of the individual collaborations between WHO and individual organisations, in 1963, the Order of Malta made an offer to WHO to provide support for research and was given a choice between Lara's research into chemoprophylaxis in the Philippines; Khanolkar's research on neuropathology in India; and Spickett's work on genetics and epidemiology at Cambridge as likely recipients.[49] L. M. Bechelli, the Chief Medical Officer, Leprosy, at WHO also told Dr Gilbert of the Order of Malta about the leprosy control project in Burma, which had been going on since 1952, and how the speed of detecting people affected by leprosy there was outrunning the resources available to treat them. He needed between US$30,000 and US$40,000 every year in order to employ more auxiliary staff because the Burmese government did not have the necessary resources. A five-year plan to provide junior leprosy workers in Burma was devised, and all three organisations – the Order of Malta, Deutsche Aussätzigen Hilfwerk, and Emmaüs-Suisse – committed themselves individually to provide US$150,000 in total, over five years, from 1965 to 1969.[50] Emmaüs-Suisse also confirmed their commitment to this (US$10,000 annually) until the end of 1975.[51]

In June 1967, the Leprosy Unit under Bechelli began to intensify efforts to enlist support for research from individual member organisations such as the Order of Malta, specifically for studies into the cultivation and transmission of *M. leprae*, in the hope of developing a vaccine.[52] These collaborations between individual member organisations of ELEP/ILEP and WHO would continue successfully, but WHO would always be conscious of the need in various countries for more money and would look towards the financial resources that ELEP/ILEP had available.

From its earliest meetings, the Medical Commission was conscious of the role of ELEP in relation to WHO.[53] It recommended regular contact with WHO, and subsequently, after the General Assembly, the Medical Commission would visit the WHO Central Leprosy Service in Geneva to report on its activities.[54] As members of the ILA (and coincidently as members of the Medical Commission), Browne and Aujoulat also attended the World Health Assembly and used this as an opportunity to explore possibilities for financial collaboration with countries that would accept voluntary aid.[55]

While WHO keenly appreciated ELEP support, from the point of view of ELEP there were obstacles. In a Medical Commission meeting with WHO in

1972, the ADG, Lucien Bernard, appealed for closer relations between ELEP and WHO, and Pierre van den Wijngaert, in his capacity as the Secretary–General of ELEP, explained that this was not a simply accomplished matter. This led to a discussion of possible collaboration on "the medical level", and the President of the Medical Commission reminded WHO of the "great importance that ELEP attaches to the social problems of leprosy, which did not seem to be the case at WHO". Dr Bernard then outlined how the relationship between WHO and ELEP could be formalised. There were two options: "official relations" (consultative status) and "working relations" (semi-official status). If they were going to come into official relations with WHO, there were various criteria to be satisfied, such as similar goals and also worldwide representation. Optimistically, he suggested that ELEP join the ILA for combined representation. This must have been met with stony silence, because he then started to backtrack by reminding everyone of the successful relationship that already existed.

He noted that, in the meantime, WHO was establishing working relations with several of the member associations on their own behalf, and the presence of a WHO observer at the Medical Commission meetings had already initiated working relations: "These relations which have only a semi-official character, are in practice, more profitable than the official relations and it is always advisable to begin with working relations before thinking of official consultative status." None of this was really having much success, and the rapporteur adds that "since the question of relationship concerns the management of ELEP, the matter was closed". The Secretary–General then went to the Chief Medical Officer, Dr Sansarricq's office, "to examine the conditions of admission, what procedures should be followed, and what privileges are gained by establishing official relations with WHO".[56]

The next General Assembly in Rome, in April 1973, learnt that "since ELEP does not qualify for official status with WHO, its contacts must be limited to working relations which in practice proved more effective".[57] The following Medical Commission meeting plaintively noted,

> It was clear that it was not possible (or desirable) for ELEP to have official relations with WHO, as an NGO. However, contacts should be fostered on an unofficial basis, and information exchanged from time to time as opportunity permitted. On the professional level, there was everything to be gained by maintaining close links with WHO.[58]

Although today the relationship is now a formal one, the reason why, at the time, "it was not possible (or desirable) for ELEP to have official relations with WHO as a NGO" can be found in the "slight" differences between these organisations, which were in fact profound and specific differences that were determined by their respective historical roots, cultural differences, ideological orientations, and espoused priorities. Over time, all of the organisations increasingly "felt" their difference from WHO's international public health strategy, especially as it became more profoundly pragmatic. These differences were experienced in the light of the longstanding vocational dedication of the anti-leprosy organisations to leprosy work. Changes from fixed-base institutional work to ambulatory care, to integration into general medical services and – for what was to come – integration into primary healthcare would all require a readjustment, especially in what the benevolent organisations would communicate to their donors. Different aspects of those shifts were felt by different organisations at different moments, and up until 1973 the changes were like seeds of difference awaiting their moment to spring into a thick, thorny hedge.

Generally, the points of demarcation coalesced into a polar distinction between holistic care for the individual and a chemotherapeutic blitzkrieg across populations. In response to proposals for mass medicine, the anti-leprosy organisations emphasised care of the "whole" person. It is metaphorically consistent for a disease that had a reputation for fragmenting physical bodies that the federation of organisations would contest a public health approach to the disease on the grounds of restoration of and care for the "whole person", albeit a concept that was defined differently by different organisations.

Although there was a broad movement from individual palliative care to chemotherapeutic treatment, and from sanatoria to mobile campaigns, by the time of the ILA Congress in Bergen in 1973, the private, non-governmental organisations that were supporting work against leprosy had not lost ground in the concerted international action against the disease. In fact, in the face of the problems in the leprosy campaign that were by then universally acknowledged, the resources that they could mobilise had never been so important. Through the federation of these organisations, they were able to coordinate both their fundraising and their anti-leprosy activities. Through the Medical Commission, the organisations were constantly challenged to embrace progressive policies and encourage the people that they supported to do the same.

The organisations themselves, however, would remain responsible and therefore vulnerable to their donors, and this would govern the rate of their response to medical and public health innovation. Individual organisations, each with their own specific culture and ideological loyalties, insisted on remaining independent from each other and especially from WHO. By 1974, the crisis in work against leprosy clearly indicated the need for a different approach to the disease, and while the seeds of irrevocable difference were becoming evident between these organisations and WHO at an international level, there were also other seeds already sown amongst this diverse group that would provide the much-needed solution.

After the period covered by this chapter, in 1975 ELEP became international, renaming itself the International Federation of Leprosy Associations (ILEP). At that time, several new organisations joined, including the Sasakawa Memorial Health Foundation (SMHF), adding to the character and changing the balance of the Federation. As will be discussed in Chapter 5, SMHF's source of funds and its way of distributing those funds brought a disturbingly different model of a private benevolent organisation to the Federation. Although each needed the other, the tensions between WHO and ILEP were never far from the surface. We have seen that these came from ideological and bureaucratic differences and different impetuses in the treatment of leprosy cases, and would intensify around what exactly "a cure" in leprosy treatment might mean.

4

OF MICE, *M. LEPRAE*, AND THE LABORATORY

We have seen that the first attempts to develop a systematic campaign to treat leprosy had stalled. Although progress seemed to have been made, with patients getting remission by taking sulphone drugs at dosage levels that could be tolerated, the incidence of relapse when treatment was suspended meant that the "cure" for the disease involved a life sentence of drug taking. With no patient ever able to discontinue the drug regimen, the available treatment resources were soon at capacity, and medical workers had to prioritise patients for treatment. Worse, the alarming appearance of drug-resistant leprosy made it clear that the sulphones were not the (complete) answer.

This chapter explores the response by the anti-leprosy community to this discouraging moment. It was clear that more needed to be known about the disease, so the story now turns to the laboratory. Two major advances were necessary: a method of cultivating the leprosy bacillus in the laboratory to facilitate experimentation on it, and an extension of the range of drugs with which leprosy could be treated. The first of these advances was achieved in 1960, through Charles Shepard's brilliant use of the mouse footpad as a propagating locus, while the second would take more than a decade to solve.

It is difficult to imagine what it was like to have identified a disease-causing entity and for almost 100 years be unable to learn anything really substantial about it. One of the fundamental ways of dealing with a disease caused by a pathogen is to cultivate it in a laboratory and attenuate it into less virulent forms until it becomes possible to produce a vaccine that will render the pathogen innocuous. This had been successfully accomplished for bacterial pathogens discovered after *M. leprae* such as cholera, tetanus, and diphtheria, as well as for diseases caused by viral infection such as measles, mumps, chicken pox, and smallpox. But despite their best efforts, during a period of extraordinary technical, scientific, and medical developments researchers found it was not possible to do this with *M. leprae*.

Many unsuccessful attempts had been made to cultivate the bacillus under laboratory conditions.[1] Mistaken claims of success were not infrequent. Scientists even attempted to inoculate themselves with the bacillus, and many thought that they had successfully cultivated it, only to learn that they had in fact only succeeded in cultivating bacteria that were often associated with *M. leprae*.[2] Frustratingly, this inability to produce *M. leprae in vitro* limited what could be discovered about leprosy. The organism could not be subjected to laboratory tests; it could not be attenuated: a vaccine could not be produced.

Researchers came at the problem from all of the conventional angles and arrived at an impasse. Neither was there any satisfactory evidence that the disease could be transmitted experimentally to animals or to man, despite many attempts.[3] There was, of course, the oft-cited instance of two US Marines from the same town in eastern Michigan who had received tattoos at a shop in Melbourne, Australia, and who, three years later, both developed leprous lesions close to their tattoos.[4] In spite of this rare instance of likely transmission by injection into the skin, there was a sustained history of attempts to understand how the organism was transmitted to human subjects, without success.

Transmitting *M. leprae* to experimental animals was even less successful. Cochrane described how almost every species of animal and every possible route of inoculation had been unsuccessfully investigated.[5] Carpenter and Naylor Foote, writing in 1959, confessed that knowledge had not progressed in the same way as the understanding of other bacterial infections. This was "because the microbiologic problems are greater than those encountered in any other single infectious disease".[6]

In the absence of a laboratory model of leprosy, researchers attempted to unlock its mysteries by examining under the microscope human tissues containing the bacillus; but in 1959 it was still not possible to describe "what a normal healthy leprosy bacillus looks like in the electron microscope".[7] One of the problems was a basic one: were the tiny, straight, or slightly curved, rod-like forms that had been prepared by staining alive or not? While the resemblance between *M. leprae* and *M. tuberculosis* was unmistakable, scientists were not sure if they were viewing viable or non-viable forms of the bacterium, especially when there were variations in the way the bacilli took up the dyes with which they had been stained. Did *M. leprae* react best to staining with a dye when it was alive, or did only the degenerate or dead forms retain the dye?[8] It was possible to see the organisms clumped together in groups which appeared to be both inside ("intracellular") and also outside ("extracellular") "a capsular-like membrane", but the significance of this was difficult to determine.

In the absence of certainties generated in the laboratory, workers were forced to depend upon clinical observations and epidemiological studies, which would raise questions to be tested in the laboratory. Leprosy was, without question, a communicable disease of bacterial origin, but the relationship between the host and the parasite was not well understood. Scientists were unsure about which parts of the body were most favourable to the life of *M. leprae* and why. It was clear that the bacillus lodged itself in the tissues of the body and multiplied there. Bacteria seemed to cluster in nerve tissues, and perhaps this indicated something about the optimal conditions for the bacteria to thrive.[9] It also seemed that the bacteria preferred parts of the body that had a lower temperature, such as the hands and feet.[10] These observations gave rise to studies of *M. leprae* and its relationship to the body tissue, especially the nerve cells. Loss of sensitivity on the surface of the skin indicated that there had been pathological changes of some kind in the skin. It seemed certain that the sensory cutaneous nerves bore "the brunt of damage in all forms of the disease".[11]

Epidemiological observations also raised many questions about individual immunity, early diagnosis of infection, and transmission of the infection. *M. leprae* certainly spread from an infectious to an uninfected individual. People were categorised as either "open or bacteriologically positive cases" or "closed or bacteriologically negative cases".[12] "Open cases" were considered to be the most infectious.[13] But it was unclear if infection occurred through the skin or through the upper respiratory tract or both. There were also many questions about what made some people more susceptible to the disease than others. Why, for example, were many adults in endemic areas resistant to leprosy, and why were some so vulnerable with seemingly very little opportunity for exposure?[14]

Obviously, some people were infected by contact with a member of their household or with infected members of related families. Some people were even infected by contact with non-related associates. Some people who contracted the disease may have had only fleeting contact with infection, and some no apparent contact whatsoever. This led researchers to conclude that "prolonged intimate contact" was not essential for the transmission of leprosy, contradicting something that had been believed ever since the bacillus had been discovered. On the contrary, now it seemed that "repeated intimate contact may be sufficient", and even "one contact, under ideal circumstances" may be enough to produce the disease. At the same time, it appeared likely that the more intimate the contact, the greater the risk of disease, especially in crowded family households of low economic status, where housing was inadequate.[15] It was equally important to avoid drawing hasty conclusions about the source of infection. Just because one case occurred in a family, it did not follow that another case in the same family had occurred as a result of infection from the originally infected family member. Both cases of infection may indeed have occurred from outside the family, particularly in an endemic area.[16]

There were also inexplicable variations in ethnic groups, across gender, within age groups, and between individuals. To begin with, the influence of ethnicity was difficult to explain. Researchers had observed a greater propensity for lepromatous leprosy amongst Europeans and Mongolian groups, than amongst Indian and African groups.[17] Equally puzzling were variations across gender and even between individuals: males seemed to be infected more frequently than females, but this may have been a result of the opportunity for contact.[18] Susceptibility to leprosy did seem to be higher before puberty, but the pattern of those who were demonstrated to be susceptible to leprosy could not be explained. Variations between individuals were even more puzzling. Of two people similarly exposed to infection, one may contract leprosy and another may not. One may exhibit a mild form of the disease and another show a marked response. In one, the disease may appear chiefly to damage the nerves, and in another, mainly to damage the skin. In one, it may "arrest" its course early and remain like that, and in another, the disease process may progress for the lifespan of the person. One person may develop leprosy at the tuberculoid end of the spectrum and the other, inexplicably, at the lepromatous end.

Understanding of the body's response to the bacillus gradually emerged from pathological and clinical findings. The presence of antibodies did not indicate an effective defensive response to the infection; on the contrary, the greater the antibody response, the poorer the resistance to the infection.[19] There were also examples of leprosy being a self-healing disease. Then there was the question of cross-immunity. While leprosy and tuberculosis were both caused by mycobacteria, the clinical relationship between the two diseases was not really understood. One infection did not confer immunity against the other; people could exhibit both diseases, and those with leprosy often died from tuberculosis.[20] Cochrane concluded that "our knowledge of the exact immunological processes in leprosy is indeed slight, and a great deal of work must be done before definite opinions can be expressed as to the exact mechanism by which the body defends itself against *M. leprae*".[21]

The time taken for the disease to incubate was another great unknown.[22] Clinical signs of leprosy generally appeared three to five years after infection, but even here, there was no way of knowing with any accuracy when "the time at which the implanting of the causative agent" occurred. Usually the first symptoms were minor, and, unhappily, people often delayed seeing a doctor until their symptoms became quite pronounced, by which time they had probably suffered irreversible damage. To compound matters, sometimes leprosy would show itself with only minor symptoms and then seem to subside, only to flare up again at a later date.[23]

The time lag between infection and perceptible clinical symptoms made it extremely difficult to bring the disease under control. Individuals may have contracted leprosy several years beforehand, and even if all those with symptoms were successfully treated at any one time, there was no way of knowing how many others had already been infected and, as yet, did not show it. Those silently incubating the disease may have been sources of infection for several years prior to exhibiting symptoms themselves. It was also very likely that in an endemic area many more people became infected than would ever show clinical evidence of the disease.[24]

Researchers longed for a "diagnostic test" which would indicate when someone had become infected. There were expectations that a "lepromin test" may have been a useful indication of exposure to infection. "Lepromin" was made from a suspension of lepromatous tissue containing large numbers of ground-up acid-fast bacilli. There were two different preparations available: the Mitsuda and the Dharmendra antigens, which were thought to be similar in function to tuberculin. But the significance of responses to these preparations was uncertain, so that in the end lepromin tests were useful only in classifying the disease, rather than in diagnosing leprosy.

There was also some hope that BCG vaccinations, which immunised against tuberculosis, could produce an immune response to *M. leprae*, but there was a great deal of debate about this too. BCG made the lepromin test positive and stimulated a tissue defence mechanism, perhaps preventing a person from developing a more severe form of the disease, but even here, researchers had to admit that the evidence was inconclusive. Furthermore, there were no laboratory procedures by which to measure immunity against the causative organism.[25] These many puzzling aspects of the disease gave rise to investigations into immunology and chemotherapy, and at the foundation of all stood the impenetrable puzzle of how *M. leprae* could be cultivated and how it was transmitted.

Investigative centres and colonial peripheries

In 1931, when the key people interested in progress against the disease gathered in Manila, the seeds were sown for British and American research initiatives that would bear fruit in the 1960s.[26] The American influence, with support from the Leonard Wood Memorial, would come under the chairmanship of James Doull and result in the delicate technical mastery of Charles Shepard, finally making it possible to develop an animal model for the disease. Simultaneously, the British research, initially under the inspiration of Robert Cochrane, would lead to the work of Dick Rees at the National Institute for Medical Research in London, where Shepard's work would be further finetuned. Additionally, some of the other attendees were from the major leprosy colonies and leprosaria in South East Asia and the Pacific, such as Culion in the Philippines, Singapore, China, Fiji, Hawaii, in addition to India and Dutch Guiana, thus securing the connection between researchers and those directly involved in administering the former leprosy colonies and their residents.

In the years to follow, some of the British and American researchers would work on assignment in leprosy centres that had once been leprosy colonies and were now postcolonial laboratories. The lines of connection and communication between these far-flung places and the centres of research in the first world were as important as the transatlantic lines of communication between the various national research institutes. The future achievements would not have been possible without the locally born researchers from Malaya, Nigeria, and the Philippines working in collaboration with those British and American researchers. The interconnectedness and continuing dialogue between researchers across national boundaries in this small world of leprosy would fuel the advances to come.

Although leprosy colonies were fading from sight, they would also play an indispensable role in the production of the new scientific knowledge of the 1960s. *M. leprae* could not be cultured *in vitro*, but it could be observed in human tissue, and people in leprosy colonies had always provided the "raw material" for work in experimental leprosy. In the 1960s, the discrete domains of leprosy colony and laboratory increasingly merged. Cochrane wrote in 1959, "Until recently, modern facilities for extensive laboratory research in leprosy have been physically separate from patients and from clinicians familiar with the disease. Eventually, juxtaposition of adequate laboratory facilities, technical skills, and the patient will permit us to solve the problems presented by the disease."[27]

Subsequently, samples were taken from leprosy-affected people in faraway places such as Sungei Buloh, outside Kuala Lumpur in Malaysia, and flown to the National Institute for Medical Research in London, or sent to Oxford for laboratory analysis. Similarly, biopsy and tissue samples containing *M. leprae* were transported from Tala, outside Manila in the Philippines, to Montgomery, Alabama. The Leonard Wood Memorial, the National Institute for Medical Research, and WHO facilitated this transportation. The *IJL* reported that "WHO has developed the necessary machinery for the regular supply of iced human biopsy specimens by air from Rangoon to London, in order to provide material to laboratories interested in the cultivation of the bacillus and transmission of human leprosy to animals."[28]

This submission of bodies in the form of biopsies and tissue samples was fundamental to the success of the research. From the point of view of the people living in leprosy colonies, it was just one more relinquishment in a long line of submissions to experimental endeavours. Ironically, in Culion, two decades later, when it came time to introduce the drugs that would finally break the stranglehold of the disease in their bodies, the people on Culion refused to take part: by then, they had had enough, and the doctor, Artur Cunanan, who knew that he truly had something that would make a difference, had to use all of his powers of persuasion to encourage his sceptical and trial-weary patients to take the drugs.

The American line of research that led to the scientific breakthrough against *M. leprae* can be traced through the Leonard Wood Memorial, which used the Philippines as "a base of operations for field study of the epidemiology of leprosy and methods for its control".[29] This was centred in Cebu, which was one of the most endemic regions for leprosy in the country and the site from where many of the people in the leprosy colony of Culion had originally been taken. The Eversley Childs Treatment Station was built, with a skin clinic in Cebu and a mobile clinic for rural work.[30] Members of the Leonard Wood Memorial Medical Advisory Board and their Advisory Committee came from Harvard and Johns Hopkins, as well as from the US Public Health Service (USPHS), the Rockefeller Foundation, and the Institute for Medical Research (IMR). They were professors of bacteriology, pathology, and medicine from Columbia, George Washington, Vanderbilt, Harvard and Michigan Universities, as well as Surgeons General from the Public Health Service and from the armed forces. James Doull, in his capacity as Professor of Hygiene and Public Health at Western Reserve University, was amongst those drawn into the advisory committee.[31]

Doull strategically made the most of the expansion of the USPHS in the post-war years by making sure that leprosy would be one of the recipients of the grants-in-aid for research and training that were being made available through the National Institutes of Health (NIH).[32] As a result of this stimulation, leprosy research was carried out in the early 1960s in the programme of the PHS at the Federal Leprosarium in Carville, Louisiana; at the Communicable Diseases Centre in Atlanta and Montgomery, Alabama; at the NIH, in Bethesda, Maryland; and in several other universities and institutions. Support for leprosy research was justified as being both in the national interest and also an American international responsibility. "This much activity," the assistant director of the NIH explained, "may be commensurate with the importance of the leprosy problem as it affects American citizens, but greater support of leprosy research will be required if the nation is to assume a larger share of responsibility for the health of its neighbors."[33]

As a result of the interest of USPHS's subcommittee on leprosy research, to which James Doull had been appointed both in his capacity as a US Public Health Service Officer and as the Medical Director of the LWM, Dr Charles C. Shepard was assigned to the Communicable Disease Center of the Public Health Service, in Montgomery, Alabama, to work on the cultivation of *M. leprae*.[34] In 1960, Shepard submitted two important papers: to the *American Journal of Hygiene* (later to be renamed the *American Journal of Epidemiology*) and to the *Journal of Experimental Medicine*. The first was entitled "Acid-Fast Bacilli in Nasal Excretions in Leprosy and Results of Inoculation of Mice," and the second was "The Experimental Disease that Follows the Injection of Human Leprosy Bacilli into Foot-Pads of Mice."[35] In these papers, he recounts the experimental process that led to the multiplication of *M. leprae* in laboratory conditions. Taking his cue from the Australian scientist, Frank Fenner, who had cultivated *Mycobacterium balnei* (later renamed *M. marinum*) and *M. ulcerans* in the mouse footpad, Shepard suspected that he could do the same with *M. leprae*.[36]

He had started his experiments in 1957 with *M. leprae* from the nasal washings of leprosy patients and later also from bacilli collected from skin biopsy specimens. People with lepromatous leprosy, mainly from Carville, Louisiana, but also from Central Luzon Sanatorium at Tala near Manila, provided samples which were shipped to Shepard's laboratory using wet ice refrigeration. Those from Carville had arrived in Montgomery within twenty-four hours. Those from the Philippines had taken 100 hours to make their journey. They came in vacuum bottles which had been re-iced several times on the trip. Happily, they arrived in good condition, so it seemed that specimens could be sent anywhere in the world, provided that they were kept at the right temperature.[37] They had been collected by injecting saline solution into the nostrils of individuals. Using rubber tubing, the solution would flush up one nostril, cross the nasopharynx, and flush down the other nostril and be collected in a flask on the floor. Shepard described how people cooperated: "The patient, seated with his body and head bent forward, breathed through his mouth, and little or no spillage through the mouth resulted if he leaned far enough forward and the BSS [balanced saline solution] did not enter the nose too rapidly."[38]

Working under sterile conditions in his laboratory, Shepard prepared a suspension of *M. leprae* from a skin biopsy specimen by mincing the specimen, trimmed free of fat, with sharp scissors after adding 1 to 2 2-mL saline until lumps of tissue could no longer be detected.[39] The resulting slurry was transferred on the blades of the scissors to the cup of a Mickle tissue disintegrator, to which a number of small glass beads had been added, and vibrated for 2 minutes. After being allowed to settle for 2 minutes, a 10-µl aliquot of the supernatant was placed, carefully spread, and allowed to air-dry on a counting slide (a glass microscope slide on which ceramic circles of known diameter have been fused).[40]

The slide was then subjected to fixation in formalin fumes and stained at room temperature with a standard acid-fast stain. Under optimal microscopic conditions, the acid-fast bacilli (AFB) present in a strip across the diameter of the circle were counted, and the number of organisms in the original suspension was calculated, using the diameter of the circle and the width of the strip (the diameter of one microscope field, which he had measured).[41] Shepard then diluted the suspension so that it contained 5,000 bacilli per 0.03 mL, the volume injected into each right hind footpad of twenty mice. This injection would make the skin balloon, and the inoculum would spread out under the skin. The mice were then kept in a room at 20°C. At monthly intervals beginning 3–4 months after inoculation, one mouse was sacrificed, and the inoculated foot was removed, fixed in formalin, and subjected to decalcification, after which histopathological sections were cut through the foot and examined microscopically. The lesions that resulted from inoculation of *M. leprae* could be seen only under the microscope.

When a significant lesion was observed, mice were sacrificed and *M. leprae* were harvested from the pooled tissue of several footpads. The inoculated feet were washed and dried, and the footpad tissues were cut off with scalpel and forceps and pooled. The pooled tissues were minced with sharp scissors, vibrated in a tissue disintegrator, and allowed to settle. Aliquots of the resulting supernatant were then spread onto the surface of counting slides; the AFB were fixed, stained, and enumerated; and the number of AFB harvested per footpad was calculated. Additional harvests at intervals permitted the construction of the growth curves of *M. leprae*. If the inoculum were appropriately diluted, the *M. leprae* multiplied consistently to the level of 10^6–$10^{6.3}$ per footpad upon passage into the footpads of uninfected mice. If the inocula delivered 5,000–10,000 AFB per footpad, an increase of 50- to 1,000-fold was observed in each passage. That the multiplication reached a maximum appeared to result from an immune response on the part of the mouse. One patient strain of *M. leprae* multiplied 6×10^9-fold in the course of five passages, and seventeen strains increased 10^4- to 10^7-fold in the course of three passages.

In the first paper, Shepard was reluctant to claim definitively that he had cultivated *M. leprae*, but there was no doubt that the passaged material behaved in the same way as the bacillus. Playing his own devil's advocate, he pointed out that isolating an infectious agent from a disease did not establish that the agent was the cause of the disease, yet there was an evident resemblance between the acid-fast bacillus that he had cultivated and the agent that caused human leprosy. This achievement would make it possible to test drugs, study immunity, and even investigate the possibility of a vaccine.

Forty-six years later, Phillip Draper, who had worked at the NIMR on research directly related to Shepard's, assessed the value of the latter's achievement:

> The discovery of the mouse footpad model by Charles Shepard was characteristic of that remarkable man. Many attempts had been made to infect a variety of animals without success, always using a large inoculum. Shepard had the experimental skill and the patience to use minimal inocula and observe the results, and to be sure that the model was reproducible.[42]

Professor Michel Lechat has subsequently commented:

> What is most probably the third major event in the modern history of leprosy occurred in 1960, when Shepard demonstrated that *M. leprae* recovered from skin biopsy specimens could successfully be grown in the footpads of mice. This brilliant achievement – eagerly awaited since the identification of *M. leprae* almost one century earlier – opened the way to a new area of research in leprosy. From this point on, it became possible to test the sensitivity, or resistance, of *M. leprae* to existing drugs, and to screen new therapeutic compounds for activity against the organism. It was also possible to determine the minimal inhibitory concentration of supposedly effective drugs in the blood of mice.[43]

Yet this discovery did not come with the thunderclap that one might have expected. Draper revealed that initially "the model did not immediately convince everyone; some maintained that the mouse infection was quite unlike the human infection"; nonetheless, it became impossible to be sceptical once the "details of the footpad infection were studied".[44] Dick Rees described the period as one of "great activity" in the field of experimental transmission of human leprosy, "when particularly important claims of success were being made by several other workers, particularly Bergel, Chatterjee, Binford, and Convit and his colleagues".

These other claims were made using different animals and in different conditions from those of Shepard: "Furthermore, all the other infections produced more progressive and extensive infections than those obtained in the mouse foot pad." Eventually though, the consensus on these competing claims would be that they needed further investigation and confirmation.[45] At a conference in May 1965, the transmission of *M. leprae* to laboratory animals was spoken of as "not exactly a new breakthrough", but "a long climb over a difficult trail to a new plateau". Yet at the same time, in the same setting, it was also hailed as "the coming of age of research that was accepted by a few at first, then by others, and finally by all of us".[46]

Shepard was characteristically generous in encouraging other researchers to build on his achievement.[47] Dick Rees belonged to a small group of researchers situated at Mill Hill, before the NIMR was officially opened in 1950. These researchers were assembled by Phillip d'Arcy Hart, who had been head of the former Medical Research Council (MRC) TB Research Unit, when it was situated at Hampstead. When interest in tuberculosis research in the UK declined, the scientists there turned their attention to experimental leprosy and towards finding an animal model for the disease.[48] After Hart retired in 1965, the group formed part of the Division of Bacteriology and Virus Research and later became a separate Laboratory for Leprosy and Mycobacterial Research.[49] Over the next decade, they would collaborate with research centres in Malaysia, Ethiopia, Oxford, and London.

Rees confirmed Shepard's observations using passaged material supplied by Shepard and also nine freshly isolated strains of human leprosy bacilli from patients in Burma, East Africa, and Malaya.[50] He understood the potential of the animal model for studying leprosy.[51] Hilary Morgan, who worked with Rees, tells of the "close transatlantic collaboration (notorious among those who controlled the Institute [NIMR] budget for the length of the telephone calls involved)" that developed between the two.[52]

Rees wondered why at least 55% of bacilli recovered from untreated patients were dead. What was it about the host's response to the disease that rendered many bacilli non-viable?[53] This question led him to think about the immunity of the host and to ask himself how to make mice less resistant to the bacilli so that more bacilli could be harvested. Only bacilli from patients with lepromatous-type leprosy had been used so far to establish experimental infections. What would be the differences if bacilli were obtained from patients with other forms of leprosy? This might help to show whether the different manifestations of leprosy or the different clinical forms in man were determined by differences in the bacilli (perhaps with differences in virulence) or, in fact, by different degrees of resistance from the host. What made the difference in response to the disease: the host or the bacilli?

Rees gathered his tissue samples and biopsy material from Malaya, East Africa, and Burma. From 1959 to 1976, a dynamic collaboration took place between the researchers at Sungei Buloh and those at NIMR in London. In this period, "specimens and samples of sera as well as fresh tissues and fixed biopsy material were flown to London almost every week".[54] As a result of this collaboration, by 1962, Rees was able to be sure of the differences between viable and non-viable bacilli when they had been stained with dyes.[55] He was able to say conclusively that the irregularly stained bacilli were degenerate forms of *M. leprae*, and only those that stained uniformly – the so-called "solid forms" – were "likely to be viable." This meant that all the forms of irregularly stained human leprosy bacilli, whether defined as "fragmented" or "granular" or "beaded," were dead organisms.[56]

He could also say that even in untreated people, a large proportion of their *M. leprae* were already dead. Amazingly, these dead bacilli would remain in the tissues for lengthy periods, even when people were treated with dapsone and most of the bacteria were killed quickly. In quantitative terms, once treatment started, bacilli were killed so rapidly that after six months of treatment there were only 4% viable bacilli left, and yet the actual bacterial population seemed unchanged if the bacterial index that counted all the bacteria visible was used as a measure. So while bacilli could be killed rapidly, the body could only very slowly dispose of them. Perhaps this explained why patients with lepromatous leprosy took several years to become smear negative? Perhaps the presence of dead bacilli in the body explained why lesions took such a long time to clear up when a patient was being treated? It might also explain some of the complications that occurred, often long after treatment.[57] Rees also discovered that they were dealing with a single species of *M. leprae*, in spite of its myriad clinical manifestations.[58] Different types of leprosy arose from differences in the response of the host, and not "differences in the parasite".[59] After such a long time of knowing very little, these were conclusions with much potential.

Drug-resistant M. Leprae

Another puzzle increasingly troubled both clinicians and researchers. Patients were starting to relapse even after they had experienced several years of improvement from continuous treatment with dapsone. Researchers suspected that the relapses occurred because drug-resistant *M. leprae* had emerged. The phenomenon of drug resistance occurs when drug-resistant, mutant individuals, which are already present in the bacterial population even before exposure to the drug, are "selected" by the drug. In a bacterial population, the drug-susceptible mycobacteria – that is, the great majority of "naïve" populations – are killed by the drug or inhibited from multiplying, while the resistant mycobacteria are able to multiply as if no drug were present. In time, these resistant individual organisms come to form the great bulk of the bacterial population and represent a resistant strain.[60]

It had not been possible before the mouse footpad laboratory model to test for the presence of drug-resistant organisms because *M. leprae* could not be cultivated, and the response of the bacterial organisms to the drug could not be quantified. Now for the first time, it was possible to determine whether relapses were due to drug-resistant *M. leprae*. To do this, Rees studied the viability of bacilli in patients who had been treated with dapsone for more than a year, and by 1964 he was able to show conclusively that patients who were not responding to treatment with dapsone carried organisms that were in fact resistant to it. This was the first irrefutable experimental evidence for the existence of DDS-resistant strains of *M. leprae*.[61] This meant that resistant bacilli were being selected to the extent that DDS was in danger of eventually becoming powerless.

While tiny amounts of dapsone were effective against *M. leprae*, dapsone selected resistant bacteria. Not only were the numbers of people resistant to dapsone growing, those infected with already-resistant *M. leprae* were also threatening to increase. A person with lepromatous leprosy, with a bacillary index of 4+, would have about 100 billion *M. leprae* in their body, of which as many as 10% were viable. After they had received their medication, their viable bacilli and the total bacilli in their bodies decreased very gradually, as can be seen from the table below. The decrease of the bacillary index indicated the elimination of bacilli from the body. The rate at which this happened had nothing to do with the anti-leprosy drug that was being used and everything to do with the immune response of the person. It seemed that if the patients stopped treatment, even if they showed negative results from the mouse footpad tests, they would eventually suffer a relapse of the disease, for they continued to harbour viable bacilli.[62]

Table 2: BI and Viable *M. leprae* by Length of Treatment

Treatment	BI	Footpad test	Total M. leprae	Viable M. leprae (fewer than)
	4+		100,000,000,000	10,000,000,000
Three months	4+	-ve	100,000,000,000	100,000,000
One year	3+	-ve	10,000,000,000	10,000,000
Two years	2+	-ve	1,000,000,000	1,000,000
...	0	-ve	10,000,000 or fewer	

To demonstrate the emergence of drug-resistant bacilli, Rees collaborated with Dr J. H. S. Pettit at the Research Unit in Sungei Buloh, Malaysia. They selected seven patients who had been treated for thirteen to fifteen years with sulphone therapy and who still showed signs of the disease. Their pathology revealed a high bacteriological index and a high proportion of solidly staining bacilli. Their bacilli were inoculated into the mouse footpad. They were also given twice weekly injections of 300mg DDS for six months and regular bacteriological and clinical examinations. Four responded well, but three showed no improvement. The bacilli of those who had not responded at all to the six months of intensive treatment had bacilli that were unresponsive in the footpad as well. It was clear their failure to respond to DDS was due to the presence of DDS-resistant strains of *M. Leprae*.[63] Thus, the first confirmed cases of dapsone resistance were patients from Malaysia who had been treated under careful supervision with high-dosage dapsone for more than ten years. Before long, it became clear that patients could experience signs of resistance to the drug from five to twenty-four years after they had begun their treatment. Tragically, many had shown negative skin smears for a long time, so that the disease appeared to have been arrested.

Rees and the researchers at Sungei Buloh began a detailed analysis of all the data from Sungei Buloh Leprosarium in order to determine the true incidence of dapsone resistance and whether there was a real increase. He warned that "Preliminary analyses suggest that the increase is significant."[64]

At the same time, thirty biopsies from potentially resistant patients showed that lepromatous patients were relapsing with dapsone-resistant strains of *M. leprae* from the UK, Europe, Tanzania, Ethiopia, Australia, India, and Malaysia. To make matters more alarming, there was a gradually decreasing interval between the initiation of treatment with sulphones and the emergence of resistance. The incidence of resistance may also have been increasing, but more data had to be gathered before this could be verified.[65]

By 1970, another twenty resistant cases were discovered at Sungei Buloh, and by 1973, 120 cases were being investigated.[66] Three out of 135 lepromatous patients treated in Sungei Buloh twice a week with 50mg of dapsone had "developed proven sulphone resistance in under ten years".[67] Then when J. M. H. Pearson, who had been at Sungei Buloh from 1964 to 1972, was seconded to AHRI, in Addis Ababa, he encountered even more frequent drug resistance in Ethiopia.[68]

Persisters

To make matters worse, something else was happening at the microbial level. This became apparent through the research of Doug Russell, who had trained under Robert Cochrane at Chingleput (CLTRI), and who was testing a long-acting sulphone, DADDS, in Papua New Guinea amongst the Karimui people. As exacting as Charles Shepard was with his mice, Russell was clear, logical, and intellectually robust in his applied research. After he administered injections to more than 95% of his patients at regular intervals and was unable to find any viable bacteria in any of them after 750 days of treatment, to his consternation, solid bacteria began to reappear in five of the patients after three to five years. This occurred even though their blood tests showed they had consistently been receiving their drugs. He sent off skin biopsies to Atlanta to be inoculated into mice, and the results came back showing bacteria sensitive to the drug.

This was a surprising and disturbing discovery: a very small selection of people still had viable bacilli that remained sensitive to inhibitory concentrations of drugs such as DDS and DADDS. These surviving bacteria remained "in a latent or resting state, only very slowly metabolising" and therefore "not incorporating the drug into their metabolic products". Only when the bacteria began to metabolise again "did they become sensitive to the drug". Shepard commented:

> It is intriguing that four of these five patients came from one village and the fifth had an epidemiological connection through family contacts. We could

not help but be thankful that this village has been included. Likewise we could not help but speculate what our conclusions about DADDS would have been if the five patients had not been included or if all 28 patients had been like these five.[69]

Doug Russell's scientific records from 1967 reveal a snapshot of three of these people. Number 4010/20, Waida-Tomage, was a 25-year-old with lepromatous leprosy clearly apparent in her facial features. She came from Negabo village in the Daribi. Number 4021/12, Paiyabe-Bungi, whose father's name was Bungi, was ten and weighed a mere 27kg when his treatment started. Number 4010/91, Yomani-Bai'i Kirage, was 14 years old.[70] They all began their treatment at the same time. They all carried bacteria that was neither resistant nor responsive to the drug when it was given at levels that should have been effective. These "latent bacteria" were known as "microbial persisters".[71]

Subsequently, the patients were given a ninety-day course of 600mg of rifampicin, to which their "persisters" responded. This finding was confirmed when Michael Waters (and Dick Rees) also studied twelve lepromatous patients who had completed 10 to 12.5 years of continuous chemotherapy, principally or entirely with dapsone. They found that while all twelve showed a full clinical response to therapy, three remained smear-positive. Then, using the mouse footpad, the researchers discovered that seven of the twelve patients still harboured viable *M. leprae*. Astonishingly, once again three of these strains of *M. leprae* were fully sensitive to dapsone.

As if matters were not difficult enough, Michael Waters also discovered that microbial persistence was a problem after treatment with rifampicin. This discouraging realisation occurred at exactly the same moment as the realisation that the mass campaigns were not working. Lou Levy describes talking to Charles Shepard about this new development at the International Leprosy Congress in Bergen in 1973:

> Walking from the Congress venue to the "Stavkirche", Shepard told me he was depressed by Waters' presentation, and felt that we had to begin again from "square one". If our most effective chemotherapeutic agent was unable to eradicate persisters, the chemotherapy could not prevent relapse of the disease. ... the disease would be expected to relapse in a large proportion of patients with MB leprosy, who are immunologically tolerant to *M leprae*, rendering the chemotherapy incapable of interrupting dissemination of the organism unless it were administered life long, an obvious impossibility.[72]

There was no standard for combined drugs, and trials would take years to come to fruition. Shepard suggested that "Rifampicin and DDS or rifampicin and DADDS" were "the most attractive drugs for the combination", and when the cost of rifampicin was an obstacle, "other effective drugs such as ethionamide or B663 could be used". But this was more easily said than done, for in 1975 a ninety-day course of rifampicin cost US$125.00, a prohibitive cost for most leprosy-endemic third-world countries. Additionally, ethionamide and B663 had side effects and were also costly, especially when everyone expected treatment to continue for several years.[73] In the face of these discouragements, the panel on Experimental Chemotherapy at the Bergen Congress set up a theoretical basis for drug trials. Out of the 200 drugs that had been screened for activity against *M. leprae*, they identified dapsone ("and other sulphones yielding dapsone in the gut or in the tissues"), rifampicin, and clofazimine, the long-acting sulphones, and ethionamide as the drugs with greatest activity against leprosy. They mapped out short-term, long-term, and very long-term clinical trials as part of an indispensable process: "all the steps listed above should be followed in the development of antileprosy drugs".[74]

The leprosy unit in crisis

The Leprosy Unit of WHO (LEP) was at a crisis point in 1973. The WHO executive requested a review of the Unit, and the new Chief Medical Officer, Hubert Sansarricq, found himself making a case against its being disbanded and reabsorbed into the Communicable Diseases section alongside the Tuberculosis Unit (TUB). As Sansarricq tells it:

> When, in April 1972, I took over from Dr Bechelli, as head of the WHO Leprosy Unit, in WHO, Geneva, LEP was a unit relatively modest in size that Dr Bechelli had succeeded in keeping rather prestigious. LEP was spending approximately US$50,000 per year to support a BCG trial in Burma, to provide "token grants" to some 20–30 reference centres and research laboratories spread throughout the world, and to defray a visit by the Chief LEP to one WHO Region every other year.[75]

In addition to the review, "there was an acute conflict going on between Dr Bechelli, on one side, and Dr Rees and Dr Shepard on the other side". This conflict arose because Bechelli questioned both "the value of the mouse foot pad models and the interest of the Ridley/Jopling classification".

Fortunately for the investment made in work against leprosy from 1948 onwards, the Committee decided not to merge LEP with TUB. Yet even after this, in March of the following year, the Headquarters Programme

Committee thoroughly reviewed the leprosy programme in order to decide "whether LEP should be maintained or abolished". Sansarricq recalls that this review lasted more than a week, but, happily, "Together with Dr Walter, we had prepared for the review in a rather convincing manner and, as a result, it was concluded that seventy-five percent of our programme deserved high or sufficient priority: LEP was kept alive."[76] This was a narrow escape, because three other units subjected to the same exercise were all abolished. Of these units, however, less than 26% of programmes were judged worthy of continued funding. Sansarricq then turned towards research to renew the programme.

THE JAPANESE DELEGATION TO THE WORLD HEALTH ORGANIZATION

Twenty-six years after the Indian delegation went to WHO to lobby for leprosy to be included in the communicable diseases programme, another delegation went to Geneva. This group was from Japan, and they espoused a passionate interest in contributing to the work against leprosy. This intervention into international world health and the anti-leprosy campaign could not have come at a better time. The mass campaign was at an impasse. Sulphone resistance was beginning to be recognised as a serious concern. The international leprosy organisations had federated and were presenting a united front by dividing up the work to be done and taking ownership of leprosy work medically, scientifically, and from a humanitarian point of view. Most importantly, the scientific technology had arrived at a point where it finally had a laboratory model and could test the efficacy of drugs against *M. leprae*.

The first approach from the Japanese delegation was made on 30 May 1974, when Dr Masuo Takabe, the Director of the Division of Communicable Diseases at WHO, received a letter from Dr Morizo Ishidate, Chairman of the Sasakawa Memorial Health Foundation (SMHF), expressing the intention of promoting "international cooperation in the field of health and welfare, primarily leprosy, in the countries of South East Asia".[1] The SMHF had only just been established as a leprosy-related non-governmental organisation with a donation of 1 billion yen (equivalent to US$333,000) for the first year. This was a result of discussions between several influential men: Ryoichi Sasakawa, his son Yohei Sasakawa, Professor M. Ishidate, Dr S. Hinohara, and Professor Kenzo Kiikuni. The initiative received support by consent from both the Ministry of Health and the Japanese Leprosy Association.

WHO had not been the first choice as a recipient. Ryoichi Sasakawa had in fact already tried several other organisations, mainly Christian ones, as potential beneficiaries through which to work, but these offers had been declined because the Japanese Shipbuilding Industry Foundation (JSIF) money, from which support was to be drawn, was considered gambling money, as it had been earned from motorboat racing. Kenzo Kiikuni was the one who suggested the WHO as a possible recipient.

The letter from Professor Ishidate to Masuo Takabe carefully expressed the spirit in which the financial support was being offered: "It is our basic understanding that this kind of cooperation should not be given in anyways unwanted, but each country's historical, cultural and economic characteristics must be given due consideration, based on the long-term interest of the countries themselves with all respect for their initiative."[2] A "Prospectus of the Sasakawa Memorial Health Foundation" accompanied the request. It described the remarkable improvement in national health and welfare standards in Japan and the wish to share the benefits with other countries. Leprosy was cited as a "typical example" of a disease that had been "totally or partially eradicated" in Japan but was still present in other countries in the region. The prospectus recounted Ryoichi Sasakawa's wish to "establish a fund" that would draw upon the "advanced medical techniques and expertise" available in Japan "in an attempt to solve the leprosy problems in developing countries". In the interests of international cooperation, the foundation offered to dispatch experts; exchange the results of scholarly research, education, and training of technical personnel; host conferences and seminars; supply required appliances and medicine; conduct public relations activities; and make research grants.[3]

The Sasakawa Memorial Health Foundation (SMHF)

When the international organisations, such as the United Nations and the World Health Organization, were established at the end of World War II, neither Japan nor Germany as the defeated enemy was included. Japan subsequently joined the UN in 1956, and by 1974 the country had fully recovered from the war years to the extent that it was experiencing a period of prosperity as an economic superpower and was even looking for further status by seeking a permanent seat on the UN Security Council. The HQ of the World Health Organization was quite obviously very happy to welcome an approach from members of the newly created Sasakawa Memorial Health Foundation as an opportunity to establish a stronger connection with Japan. Dr Takabe, in his capacity as Director of the Division of Communicable Diseases at the WHO, warmly endorsed the visitor, writing to Dr Bernard, the Assistant Director General, that "a visit from this health foundation would be most welcome, as up to now the Japanese bilateral foreign aid agencies for health have had insufficient contact with WHO/HQ and the Regional Offices".[4]

Ryoichi Sasakawa

In briefing the ADG, Takabe informed him that the Minister for Health and Welfare in Japan had only recently officially approved the Sasakawa Memorial Health Foundation as "a voluntary non-profit making Foundation", and he suggested that he or the Director–General, Dr Mahler, should meet with the Japanese delegates, the Chief of Communicable Diseases and/or the Chief of the Leprosy Unit (LEP). He added that "In this particular case it may well be worthwhile as the Sasakawa Memorial Health Foundation was originated and funded by a behind-the-scene influential political leader of the Liberal-Democratic party now in power."[5] In handwriting on the memo, there is a direction and a question: "Would you kindly prepare a reply for my signature and arrange for the meeting on the 28th" and "What is your advice? Should the DG be asked to see them personally?"

The "behind-the-scene influential political leader" referred to was to Ryoichi Sasakawa. Amongst the men already described in this narrative of international work against leprosy – men such as Damien de Veuster, Wellesley Bailey, Mahatma Gandhi, Robert Cochrane, Ernest Muir, Sir Leonard Rogers, James Doull, Raoul Follereau, Marcel Farine, and Hermann Kober – Ryoichi Sasakawa was by any account a particularly remarkable man amongst remarkable men. As the preface to his biography reminds us, he must be understood in the historical context of Japan: "Born in Kansai in the late years of Japan's great Meiji Era, Ryoichi's long life … spanned almost an entire century of tumultuous change. Any appraisal of his career must take into account the drastic, almost seismic, transformations that befell Japan – and the entire world – within that time."[6]

Ryoichi Sasakawa, the oldest son of a sake brewer, was born in 1899 in Toyokawa Village, in Osaka Prefecture. In 1916, at seventeen years of age, he studied flying and became a pilot. He established a National Volunteer Flying Unit in 1932, opened the Osaka Air Defence Field in 1934, and then presented the airfield to the army. In 1931, he established the Patriotic People's Party, which was one of many small right-wing parties of the time. He was arrested for extortion in 1935 and held without trial for three years, but then discharged. He admired Mussolini and, given to the flamboyant gesture, flew his own airplane to meet him in 1939. He entered the House of Representatives as an opposition-sponsored candidate in 1942, at forty-three years of age, calling for an end to the system under which certain politicians were preferred and others not endorsed by the authorities.[7] He succeeded in wielding considerable political influence throughout his life, whether he belonged to a parliamentary party or not. He became a patron of many. In 1945, he was imprisoned in Sugamo Prison as a Class A war criminal suspect and was released in 1948, at forty-nine years of age, without charge. The Legal Section of the American occupation forces led by Col. Alva C. Carpenter identified Sasakawa as a "nationalist extremist who had previously been involved in public incitation and violence and war-related business in China". And while Carpenter was not confident that charges against Sasakawa would stand, he was reluctant to recommend his release because he believed he "would be a dangerous man" if set free.[8]

As Westerners, our knowledge of the war years is a story of the aggression of Germany and later of Japan. It is inescapably and irrefutably a story of expansionism, territorialism, and concentration camps, torture, and starvation. To the West, the occupation of Manchuria in 1931, the Rape of Nanjing, and the atrocities of World War II across South East Asia suggest a culture of ruthless aggression. From Japan's point of view, the years after World War I are rather a story of American aggression, trade embargoes, and a necessity to expand its territory to feed the populace. Then, when the atom bomb was dropped on Hiroshima and Nagasaki, a whole new dimension of horror was inflicted upon the population. Earlier that year, in March 1945, when the firestorm of bombing was unleashed by the Americans upon Tokyo in an effort to bring the war to a halt, Yohei Sasakawa, son of Ryoichi, was a little boy fleeing in terror with his mother.

By the end of 1945, the elder Sasakawa had been arrested and sent to prison, where he longed to be the hero who would defend his country's actions to the world. In the diary that he kept at the time, he offers both personal and patriotic explanations for his internment. The war diaries provide a picture of a man with both a naïve simplicity and a grandiose sense of self-importance, to the extent that he identified himself with his nation; for example, he wrote letters to General MacArthur "pleading with him to advance my plans for the total abolition of all arms in the world and the redistribution of food, clothing and shelter".[9]

His rationale for the role of Japan in World War II was expressed as a process of cause and effect:

> It takes two to fight. Japan definitely did not wage a war of aggression. Once people are born, they must live. And to live they must eat. And to eat, a

country must import, produce, acquire land, or rely on emigration. The US, however, took away the one way for Japan to gain the foreign currency it needs to pay for these imports by placing tariffs on our exports. The US then blocked emigration. Since the US had threatened our survival, it became necessary, many people argue, for Japan to advance into the continent [China], which was readily open.[10]

He claimed that his hair had gone white in prison "out of my concerns for the future of Japan".[11] And when the Americans announced that they had no intention of abolishing the Japanese imperial system, he described it as "the moment of greatest joy in my forty-eight years of life".[12] His sense of the great loss of life as a result of the war, and the failure of leadership and lack of moral fibre amongst the leading lights in the country, occasioned his anger and grief:

> According to the newspapers, 777,716 soldiers in the army and 397,400 navy men were killed in action, while 330,000 civilians also died. The resulting total death toll amounted to over 1.5 million Japanese. As many as 2.5 million homes were destroyed. Even after these massive losses, the heads of army and navy and top bureaucrats are still refusing to acknowledge responsibility. This can only be described as madness.[13]

The image emerges of a man who tried to control Japan's representation after the war, as his self-identification testifies: "I am not just Sasakawa Ryoichi, but the ambassador of all the venerable war dead who seek to save mankind from the ravages of war for ever."[14] Viewed in this light, his oft-quoted phrase that the world was one family in which "all mankind is made up of brothers and sisters" makes his dedication to fighting leprosy an index of a greater ambition to repair the Japanese body politic, both at home and internationally. As a counter to this image of the ultranationalist is the astute businessman who emerges from prison with an "idea" for motorboat racing that would establish him as one of the wealthiest benefactors in the world.

In 1962, Sasakawa set up the Japan Shipbuilding Industry Foundation (JSIF), the benevolent organisation which is now called the Nippon Foundation (TNF). JSIF, as does TNF today, drew the funds needed for its many projects from revenues generated from motorboat racing. Three percent of the proceeds would go towards JSIF, from which the funds for international health initiatives would be drawn.[15] After decades of philanthropy to many worthy causes, including leprosy, Sasakawa died at ninety-six years of age in 1995.[16]

Morizo Ishidate

Professor Morizo Ishidate was the Chairman of the Sasakawa Memorial Health Foundation Board.[17] This position held its own challenges, one of which was caused by a difference in personality with Ryoichi Sasakawa:

> It was commonly considered that the relationship between Professor Ishidate, an earnest academic, as well as a devout Christian, and Mr Sasakawa, known as a behind-the-scenes-boss of politics and finance of Japan, and at times a quite strongly emotional man, were like oil and water, and a joint project between them was an utter impossibility.

But, contrary to expectations, the two were united in their strong passion to make a difference against leprosy. A moment that was typical of these personality differences occurred at the inauguration of SMHF by Prince Takamatsu, the younger brother of Emperor Hirohito. Apparently, Sasakawa told Ishidate just before he was to speak at the ceremony that he was going to announce the supply of drugs to twenty endemic countries. But Ishidate advised against this, saying, "Please stop saying that. Even if we deliver drugs globally, in most countries there are no systems to actually deliver the drug to the patients and make them take them regularly, thus your goodwill will be wasted." Sasakawa was apparently upset at this response and perhaps its abruptness, but he managed to restrain himself in his speech.[18]

Ishidate's character and disciplinary orientation informed the work of the Foundation.[19] He took care to avoid leprosy work impelled by philanthropy alone without adequate medical knowledge and skills.[20] He also discouraged initiatives structured upon Japanese outreach programmes, and instead oriented the SMHF disbursements to strengthening existing programmes of other nations and their ownership of those programmes. He also emphasised collaboration with international organisations such as the International Federation of Anti-Leprosy Associations (ILEP) and, particularly, WHO.[21] Both Ishidate and Ryoichi Sasakawa believed that the new organisation should learn from both, as well as from those actually running leprosy programmes in endemic countries.[22] This scrupulousness in showing respect to the beneficiary governments and medical workers may indicate a sensitivity to Japan's wartime reputation for brash ruthlessness and a desire to distance the Foundation from any suggestion of dominance or coercion. Nevertheless, the direct approach to foreign governments and the most important international associations inevitably situated the Sasakawa Memorial Health Foundation as a top-tier participant in the benevolent diplomacy associated with international health campaigns, gaining the Foundation a status and an importance that far exceeded those achieved by any of the earlier European-based non-government societies.

The Mikoshi Shrine

The delegation from Japan arrived at WHO on 28 July 1975, presenting the Director–General, Halfdan Mahler, with formal greetings from Ryoichi Sasakawa, who earnestly if portentously described the world as one family in which "all mankind is made up of brothers and sisters". Stressing interdependence amongst nations and peoples, his message was adamant that

> Japan depends on the world for her existence as much as the world depends on this country while my life itself is dependent on others' lives. As I see it, poverty and illness are the greatest enemy of mankind and of all diseases, leprosy is one of the worst. What is vitally important to cope with this disease is the cooperation of all those concerned including not only dedicated doctors, nurses, assistant nurses and patients but also every member of the society. The spirit of cooperation in which people fight this fatal disease reminds me of "MIKOSHI" a Japanese portable shrine which is carried over the shoulders by a great many people on the occasion of festival.[23]

To symbolise the cooperation of people, institutions, and countries working together against leprosy, the delegation presented a portable shrine of the sort to which Ryoichi Sasakawa refers. This was typical Sasakawa flamboyance. No photograph of this presentation is known to survive, but it is likely that the shrine would have taken up to a dozen people to carry. It must have been an extraordinary sight arriving at WHO.

After the visit, Masuo Takabe wrote to Ishidate expressing appreciation on behalf of the Director–General and Assistant Director–General, especially because this was the "first time that a Japanese voluntary organization in health matters and capable of substantial co-operation has done so".[24] The letter was accompanied by some proposals for work that he hoped would be taken into account in their plans for the future.[25] After the meeting in Geneva, the group from Japan then went on to Paris to meet with Pierre van den Wijngaert from the European Federation of Anti-Leprosy Associations (ELEP) to discuss their mutual interests and future collaboration.[26]

The new organisation certainly benefited from the connection with ELEP. It became part of a global network, with entrée to a number of leprosy endemic countries, especially those in East and South East Asia.[27] Yet

Ishidate clearly envisaged a different orientation for the Foundation. As he told Takabe, "We are deeply convinced that the more effective approaches to the leprosy problem at the present stage are not in philanthropic assistance, but in the contribution to the systematic strategy endeavoured by their own government and in target-orientated research works at the same time."[28] Rather than work through the traditional channels taken by anti-leprosy organisations, the Sasakawa Memorial Health Foundation did something quite different by establishing direct connections with ministers of health in national governments. Not having to rely on individual private donations, it had the security of a set budget from year to year, and therefore a flexibility in disbursements not experienced by the other international non-government leprosy organisations.[29]

Other non-governmental anti-leprosy organisations may have been equally sensitive to the countries in which they worked and eager to collaborate with their governments, but no other organisation actually approached governments with the intention of assisting and enhancing their national leprosy programmes. The Swedish Red Cross, for example, was careful when supporting Paul Brand's work to enlist only Indian personnel. They wrote: "All the personnel perhaps with the exception of one Swedish administrator should if possible be Indian."[30] They stressed that their plans needed to be discussed with the Indian Red Cross and "before making any definite decision discussions should also be undertaken with the Health Department of the Indian Government".[31] They aimed to hand the project over progressively to the Indian authorities, but, unlike SMHF, they would not actually hand over funds to the national programme.[32]

Having been to WHO and to ELEP, the Japanese delegation then met with the WHO regional directors for the South East Asian (SEARO) and Western Pacific (WPRO) regions. On 1 July, Dr K. Saikawa told the Regional Director of SEARO that the Sasakawa Memorial Health Foundation was ready to assist the countries of the region in whatever way was judged helpful. He stressed the desire for "full co-operation with WHO" and asked for advice about the best way of giving assistance to specific countries. SMHF was planning to hold a conference at which government officers in charge of leprosy control and leaders of voluntary agencies could come together, for the first time, to discuss their problems. The Regional Director for SEARO concluded that "this co-operation would be very useful" and he was ready to support it.[33]

Two days later, on 3 July, Kenzo Kiikuni and Dr K. Saikawa together also visited the Regional Director for the Western Pacific Region and "expressed their earnest desire that the Foundation should cooperate and collaborate with WHO in its future operations".[34] Saikawa had spent five years in WPRO, so he was on home ground. The delegation told the Regional Director that they intended to "promote international cooperation among South East Asian countries in the field of leprosy control", and to this end there would be US$200,000 a year available from 1974 onwards. This would be for advisory services, exchange of information on leprosy research, training of personnel, conferences, research grants, equipment, and supplies. The Regional Director told the visitors about the status of work against leprosy in Korea, Vietnam, Laos, and the Philippines. He also briefed them on how the WHO Voluntary Fund for Health Promotion worked, and reported excitedly back to WHO HQ.[35]

The birthday present

Complementary to the creation of the Sasakawa Memorial Health Foundation with its own budget, Ryoichi Sasakawa added something that was quite breathtaking. On his seventy-fifth birthday, he decided to mobilise the Japanese Shipping Industry Foundation funds by making a further gift of US$1 million for global health. This was done as a donation to WHO, directly from the JSIF, for its leprosy programme.

As is already apparent from the previous chapters, leprosy was not the highest of WHO's priorities. On the other hand, the global smallpox eradication programme was in its closing stages, but WHO was experiencing a shortfall in funds necessary for this programme; consequently, Director–General Mahler asked that half of the US$1 million that Sasakawa was offering be devoted to the smallpox eradication campaign. Apparently, Mahler then rather reluctantly accepted the remaining half for leprosy. In his own words, "he was not at all confident that WHO could show some positive results with that fund for leprosy, not as readily as for smallpox".[36] The initial grant in 1975 was US$502,000 at a time when the regular WHO budget for leprosy was only around US$300,000.[37] Subsequently, the JSIF contribution increased to US$1 million and eventually to US$4 million.[38]

Thus double-pronged support for global efforts against leprosy began, using both the JSIF/Nippon Foundation and the SMHF as independent, yet connected, funding sources.[39] There were serious questions within TNF about the advisability of having two different organisations operating from the same funding source, but those involved were convinced that it worked better than if the same amount of money had been deployed by a single organisation. For although "WHO, as an established, publicly acknowledged global authority on health matters had ready access both to the health authorities of the developing countries which had large leprosy burdens and to individual leprosy experts", as they were an international organisation, there were formalities to observe and a bureaucracy to appease. In contrast, "SMHF being private, small and smart … had both flexibility and speed of action, and could be quite innovative."[40]

The contribution from JSIF/TNF was initiated when, in July 1975, Dr Sansarricq received a letter from Professor Ishidate officially proposing to donate the US$1 million to the "WHO project of eradication of leprosy and smallpox".[41] Another letter followed in August, formalising the previous one. The donation had been made by the Japan Shipbuilding Industry Foundation, the President of which was Ryoichi Sasakawa, with advice by the Ministry of Health and Welfare and the Sasakawa Memorial Health Foundation. The donation was intended to assist WHO's activities, specifically the smallpox eradication programme and the leprosy control programme. The initial letter also stated that "We have to discuss with you further in details of how to use this fund." And the second letter clarified this: "As mentioned above, this foundation is acting as an advisor. This is the reason why we mentioned in the said letter the necessity of discussing with you as how to use the fund most effectively for leprosy control."[42]

Sansarricq was invited to visit Tokyo to discuss the allocation of the grant.[43] Sasakawa then presented 300 million yen to Francisco J. Dy, the Regional Director for the Western Pacific, in Tokyo. At the 1975 exchange rate, this amounted to US$1,003,600.[44] Half was to go to smallpox; as to the other half, as Mr Sasakawa stated: "we wish to receive WHO's proposal (plan for its allotment for activities in leprosy treatment and control programme.) Upon it, we wish to hold consultation with WHO for its best usage". He added his overall aspiration that WHO, JSIF, and SMHF would cooperate "to apply this fund for the profitable cause to extirpate [the] leprosy disease in this earth".[45]

In 1976, Sasakawa, through JSIF, donated another US$2 million.[46] Mahler responded warmly and proposed that "further correspondence" about the four programmes should take place "at the technical level".[47] Then in 1977, a further US$2,330,000 was donated.[48] Mahler wrote to Sasakawa again in November 1979 thanking him for the donation at the end of that year. The Director–General informed him that WHO had decided to open a special trust account and call it the "Sasakawa Health Trust Fund" so that all the reports sent to the member states would identify the contributions made to the fund as well as the disbursements to respective WHO programmes.

Interest earned on the fund's unspent balances would also be shown in the yearly financial reports.[49]

Thus began a relationship between WHO and JSIF that would be different from that of the previous donors to the voluntary fund for leprosy. The donor was usually kept at arm's length in relation to the use of funds. Their preferences were considered, but usually, following advice from WHO, the donor would agree to the allocation of their funding support according to WHO priorities. In 1976, at the next year's proposal for allocation of funds, the Chief of WHO's Leprosy Unit, Sansarricq, told the Assistant Director–General, in response to Mr Sasakawa's request of August 1975 for consultation on the use of funds, that "we understand that this final and official list implies no further discussion with the donor on the agreed programme activities, but that it is a mere formality only which, in view of the urgent need for programme implementation, we are happy to comply with".[50] This was the official WHO line with donors. A procedure for the process had been outlined: once the foundation agreed to the research agenda offered by WHO, it would then make an official offer to the DG, who would accept their contribution to the WHO Special Account for the Leprosy Programme. In turn, the Foundation would receive annual progress reports and the money would be handled in the same way as that in the regular budget.[51]

In this instance, the participants recount that there was an element of trust and confidence in the arrangements. The TNF contribution covered the major portion of the leprosy budget of WHO in each of the twenty-five years from 1975. There was no exchange of Memorandum of Understanding or any other written agreement underlying these donations. They were based only on a verbal commitment, but remarkably that contribution continued over twenty-five years up to the present, not only without interruption, but also with a steadily increasing amount.[52]

Sasakawa himself had no personal involvement in monitoring the use of the funds. Everything was initially devolved to Professor Ishidate, and, after Ishidate's resignation, to Professor Kenzo Kiikuni for the JSIF/TNF donations and to Dr Yo Yuasa for the SMHF grants. As time went by, possibly because of the size of the donation, the Nippon Foundation became more and more involved in the WHO leprosy programme. The strength of this relationship would underpin the momentum of the programme, something that would increasingly disturb the other stakeholders. The collaboration involved a succession of heads of the Leprosy Unit – Hubert Sansarricq, S. K. Noordeen, and Denis Daumerie – and thus varied a little according to changes in the personality dynamics. It was especially difficult for Sansarricq because he had to find uses for a sudden flood of money before he really had the technical capabilities to achieve the desired results, yet he set in place the technical foundation for what was to follow.

By the time Yuasa and then Noordeen took on the role, both the technical expertise and the infrastructure resources were available to make a real impact on the incidence of leprosy in the world. All they needed to do was to stimulate the political will. Their collaboration with JSIF was based on pragmatics and a passionate engagement to achieve a set goal. The later collaboration with Denis Daumerie, however, was fraught and bruising. This will be discussed in Chapter 9. Personalities aside, by virtue of Sasakawa's "birthday gift", the whole landscape of international health work against leprosy underwent a seismic shift that continues into the twenty-first century. In the process, the "face" of leprosy would change forever.

The Sasakawa Memorial Health Foundation Seminars

The SMHF budget was initially dedicated to holding seminars and workshops to stimulate cooperation in the region.[53] The first seminar was designed to promote more international cooperation in leprosy control. Directors of national leprosy control programmes from the ministries or departments of health, and leprosy specialists from leprosaria and medical institutions from fifteen countries including Laos, Malaysia, the Philippines, Singapore, Vietnam, Thailand, Burma, Khmer, Nepal, Taiwan, Indonesia, Hong Kong, and Korea were invited, along with two representatives from WHO: Dr F. Noussitou and J. C. Tao (WPRO), as well as Pierre van den Wijngaert in his capacity as General Secretary of ELEP.[54] This was the first time that experts from so many countries, as well as representatives from WHO and ELEP, had met at a seminar, exchanged information, and engaged in discussions about leprosy control.[55] The second seminar concentrated upon discovering the major and most urgent problems in the regions in order to target needs and stimulate coherent efforts.[56]

On the basis of these seminars, Yuasa was able to forge working relationships with programme managers from the countries where he felt that SMHF could be of most assistance.[57] Initially he worked with South Korea, Taiwan, the Philippines, Malaysia, Thailand, Indonesia, Myanmar, and Nepal. Later, he worked with unified Vietnam and Micronesia, and from 1984 with China.[58] The value of his contacts with these national programme managers was two-fold. He was able, through them, to meet high-ranking people in the ministries of health who had influence. This also served to enhance the role of the programme managers who were able to draw the attention of their superiors to what was happening in leprosy in their country.[59]

ILEP and SMHF

Despite having initially restricted its membership to European-based associations, in 1975 ELEP admitted two new organisations from outside Europe: the American Leprosy Missions (ALM) and the Sasakawa Memorial Health Foundation (SMHF). At the same General Assembly, it changed its name from "European" (ELEP) to "International" (ILEP). With annual budgets of over a million dollars between them, the new ILEP members significantly bolstered the resources and prestige of the Federation, although not without reawakening the old parochial fears among some members. The representative from the Order of Malta was cautious, if not outright suspicious, of the wealthy *arrivistes*: "If our Federation intends to safeguard its family feeling, it will have to make the necessary steps, even within the constitution, to prevent it from the tyranny of the richest, to avoid temptation of prestige, in a word to keep on the tradition of its founders."[60]

But the SMHF was not going to alienate anyone by overassertiveness, and within a very short time had succeeded in gaining a level of acceptance from the two most important anti-leprosy networks, WHO and ILEP. As in many other cases, professional and vocational collegiality overcame political suspicion and ideological paranoia. Yo Yuasa's first task when he was appointed to the position of Medical Director at SMHF was to attend the ILEP General Assembly meetings in Paris.[61] Far from excluding or regarding him with suspicion, the network of leprosy experts came to his assistance when the discussions took place in French, and Stanley Browne or Michel Lechat translated for him.[62]

The Japan Shipbuilding Industry Foundation Financial Support

While the Sasakawa Memorial Health Foundation's budget was initially devoted directly to seminars in the South East Asian and Western Pacific Regions, the JSIF money was being allocated through WHO according to the latter's priorities. The first US$501,800 was allocated to three regions – AFRO (African), SEARO (South-East Asia), and WPRO (Western Pacific) – with a portion of the money retained by HQ.[63] There was some difficulty in making use of the money straight away, and it would take some time before WHO would be able to set up the structures to do so, as can be seen from the disbursements over this period.[64] At the end of 1976, only US$141,028 had been committed, and by 30 June 1977, the uncommitted balance approached US$2 million:

Table 3: Leprosy Programme (VL): Contributions From JSIF (USD)[65]

	Received	Adjustments	Disbursements	Unexpended Balance
1975	501,800			501,800
1976	670,000		128,088	541,912
1977	900,000	(13,680)	226,074	660,246
Totals	**2,071,800**	**(13,680)**	**354,162**	**1,703,958**

In December 1977, Sancarricq met with JSIF representatives to discuss the use of the funds and report to the donors. He had to explain why things were taking so long to organise. Quite obviously, some regions were simply not ready to make leprosy a priority. For the African region, for example, where there were 1.7 million people known to have the disease, and although the activities had been slow in starting, "a remarkable effort has been made during 1978 to establish a coordinated effort". By 1978, the African region had received US$294,093, and on 1 January 1977 they still had US$87,099 available for allocation from the funds provided in 1975. In 1976, an amount of US$16,560 had been spent in the Central African Republic, and US$14,604 for further epidemiological studies in Upper Volta, but no further requests had been received for the funds allocated to the region in 1977.

On the positive side, the African region had prepared a programme profile and a plan of work for 1978–81.[66] At least half the countries in the region planned to review their leprosy services and support prevalence surveys in at least ten of these.[67] The region would also identify five training centres in the Anglophone and Francophone countries.[68] To start all of this off, the region had awarded fellowships to twenty-seven people in twenty-three countries and selected consultants to review the national programmes of ten countries.[69] The report therefore expected "a handsome return ... from JSIF contributions for the countries of the African Region".[70]

Most significantly, the funds ushered in a new era. The money (accumulated balances) made it possible to develop long-term training and control activities.[71] Most of the regional offices had developed either leprosy programme profiles (AFRO, SEARO, WPRO), medium-term programmes (SEARO), or with AMRO "a document providing background information and a proposed budget" for 1979–81.[72] The report looked forward to evaluating the operations that were just beginning and then following that up with an epidemiological assessment within two years.[73] While disbursing the funds continued to be a slow process, the foundations were being laid for the future. Describing the impact of the TNF and SMHF money, Sansarricq comments:

> Before 1974, WHO was (with few exceptions) offering only advice and recommendations to endemic countries, and governments were left with the problem of securing their own funds for the implementation of WHO's advice. With the availability of extra budgetary funding, notably Sasakawa funds, it was possible for WHO to offer not only the appropriate advice, but also provide the financial support required to apply it.[74]

So when the work against leprosy was at its lowest ebb, as a result of a second momentous delegation to WHO twenty-five years after the first, international anti-leprosy efforts received a much-needed impetus. The upshot of this support was that SMHF became increasingly involved in the direction of the leprosy programme. At the same time, it ensured field research that would culminate in an unexpectedly efficacious treatment.

were in.[10] These trials were designed to find out if combinations of existing drugs could diminish their populations of persisting *M. leprae*. Ciba-Geigy and Lepetit donated the 60,000 capsules of 300mg rifampicin for the first two years of trials. Researchers were able to monitor different combinations of drugs and the effects of different regimens in 300 patients. They were looking for "a general recommendation for relatively short-term treatment, for infectious forms of leprosy".[11] The steering committee of THELEP then planned trials of different drug regimens in Chingleput in South India and Bamako in Mali. This would determine the effects of chemotherapy on the incidence of leprosy. It would also arrive at a standard protocol for chemotherapy trials for lepromatous leprosy.

The Central Leprosy Teaching and Research Institute at Chingleput in South India and the Institut Marchoux in Bamako in Mali had been places of refuge for leprosy-affected people and then centres from which leprosy campaigns were launched and coordinated. Now in new incarnations, they became sites for internationally coordinated clinical trials.[12] The working group set up a list of eighteen multidrug protocols from which they selected three regimens each for Chingleput and Bamako.[13] By 1978, the working group had drawn up a complete programme covering the African, South East Asian, Western Pacific, and European (Malta) regions. The trials eventually demonstrated several important findings: the strength of the regimen was not linked to the eradication of persisters; people tolerated the regimens; and on average, after three months of treatment, their viable organisms fell to one hundred thousandth of their pre-treatment levels.[14]

While the trials were progressing, there was a policy vacuum around the use of combined therapies. Part of the reason for this was that the Leprosy Unit was still suffering from a sense that it was not really viable, and that it should work with the TB Unit. In 1976, this uncertain status resulted in a fifth Expert Committee compiled of a diverse collection of experts from anti-leprosy work and anti-tuberculosis work.[15] The resulting recommendations on drug resistance were buried in a myriad of other issues, and the guidelines for regimens were far too complicated for those in field conditions and in general health services. Sansarricq judged that "The recommendations were difficult or impossible to apply in practice and consequently were applied in very few instances."[16] On behalf of WHO, he urgently needed a public display of authoritative consensus that would serve as a *fait accompli* in order to arrive at "simple, effective and practicable recommendations".[17] To achieve this, he summoned a meeting of experts, both from the field and the laboratory to forge a consensus on combined chemotherapy.[18] He describes the situation:

The greatest concern was rifampicin being given as a single drug to lepromatous patients by fieldworkers either because they were unaware of the risk of rifampicin resistance or because the drug(s) to be combined with rifampicin had not been delivered in time. Faced with this pattern of rifampicin use, WHO – and many scientists and voluntary agencies – feared the emergence and spread of rifampicin resistance, which would compromise the potential of this potent antibiotic for improving leprosy control at a time which the development of new antibiotics highly active against *M. leprae* was not foreseen.[19]

There were also political reasons for calling the workshop together, as Sansarricq pointed out to his superiors.[20] The voluntary agencies were increasingly purchasing drugs, including rifampicin, and the Damien Foundation and the Sasakawa Memorial Health Foundation were supplying drugs, both at the request of WHO and directly in response to requests from endemic countries.[21] Both the Sasakawa Memorial Health Foundation and the International Federation of Leprosy Organizations (ILEP), through the British Leprosy Relief Association (LEPRA), had produced policies on combinations and dosages of drugs based on the available science. The Sasakawa Memorial Health Foundation had begun chemotherapy trials in Korea, the Philippines, and Thailand. In the same year, LEPRA gathered together experts at Heathrow, outside London, and recommended standard combinations. Additionally, two recent regional meetings had made recommendations for drug regimens.[22] Sansarricq needed to review these proposals and maintain WHO technical leadership.[23] To this end, he gathered together the experts who were best placed to make a decision.

The Study Group on Chemotherapy

The experts had to decide on what drugs should be used, how many simultaneously, and in what combination and dosage to arrive at a regimen that was both cheap and effective. To begin with, all had to agree on what actually constituted "combined chemotherapy". Lou Levy explained that "combined chemotherapy" required treatment with a combination of two or more chemotherapeutic agents that acted on the organism by different means.[24] So if someone whose organisms were resistant to dapsone was being treated with combined drugs and one of those was dapsone, they would not be treated by "combined chemotherapy". Neither would a combination of two drugs that acted in the same way (such as dapsone and a long-acting sulphonamide) be suitable.[25] By this logic, individuals with drug resistance had to be treated with at least two drugs other than dapsone. Levy advised choosing a regimen of at least three drugs, including dapsone, for "a general purpose regimen" suitable for all patients.[26]

Next, they had to choose the most suitable drugs and their dosage. They knew that dapsone was safe, if given in standard doses. They recognised the toxic effect of rifampicin, but the toxic potential of clofazamine had not been clinically assessed.[27] They therefore considered intermittent rifampicin in order to "reduce dosage as much as possible without compromising the efficacy of the regimen". They did not know if using drugs in combination increased their potential for toxicity. Gordon Ellard prepared the paper on "Available drugs for the treatment of leprosy." His criteria for suitable drugs were their inherent potency, their acceptability to patients, and their cost. As a pharmacologist, he pointed out the importance of considering the minimal inhibitory combination (MIC) of the available drugs, for it was crucial to maintain an effective concentration in the blood stream.[28] He also compared costs:

Table 4: Cost to WHO of Drugs for Leprosy Control (17 July 1981)[29]

Drug	Dose (mg)	Cost per dose (USD)
Dapsone	100	$0.003
Acedapsone	225	$1.40
Clofazimine	100	$0.12
Ethionamide	500	$0.27
Prothionamide	500	$0.40
Rifampicin	600	$0.68

Ultimately, the Study Group decided that the standard regimen for multibacillary leprosy should be:

Rifampicin:	600mg once monthly, supervised
Dapsone:	100mg daily, self-administered
Clofazimine:	300mg once monthly, supervised, and 50mg daily, self-administered[30]

While the workshop arrived at definitive recommendations, the truth was that, as stated by Michael Waters and Claire Vellut, "the whole approach to multi-drug therapy of fixed duration is of itself a subject for research". The recommendations were in fact the result of an extraordinary exercise in political brinkmanship. In an account of the events published subsequently, Hubert Sansarricq claimed it crucial "to issue recommendations for MDT regimens *for immediate use*", for it would take "several years of preparation at all levels before any patient would start to benefit".[31] WHO would have required clinical trials before the proposed MDT regimens could have been recommended in the field, and this could have taken up to nine years.[32] Michel Lechat also supported the pre-emptive declaration of a recommended regimen without full testing, on the grounds that drug resistance was increasing at an apparently alarming rate:

> While field data were lacking and unlikely to become available for several years, leprosy control was faced with the rapidly increasing prevalence of dapsone-resistant *M. leprae* strains which jeopardized more than 30 years of efforts to control the disease by dapsone monotherapy. After much debate, the Group opted for MDT – a momentous decision …[33]

Sansarricq had pursued a deft and subtle strategy. The regimen recommended by the Study Group was not very different from that designed by the Chemotherapy of Leprosy Project (THELEP) for its 1979 field trials and was really the result of discussions in the Project's Scientific Working Group and the Steering Committee.[34] He did not try to convince his superiors in advance about what he hoped the Study Group would recommend. He recalls that "LEP could have tried to convince its senior management that the risks inherent in the growing anarchic use of rifampicin justified WHO's designing MDT regimens which, *in all likelihood*, would be effective and safe and recommending them for immediate implementation".[35] But he didn't. As he states, "it was thought that such an approach would be refused, probably on the basis that experience with the monthly administration of rifampicin was too limited". Alternatively, if the Chemotherapy of Leprosy Project had tried to recommend a regimen, this would also have been "judged to be outside its terms of reference".

So the Study Group was convened with the conviction that "the experimental THELEP regimen for MB patients, designed in 1979, was likely to respond to the needs". The aim was to have the recommended regimens ready for immediate implementation by the Chemotherapy of Leprosy Project (THELEP) panel and the leprosy control experts, and have them approved by the Executive Board of WHO. To do this he had to be direct, but not provocative: "It seemed that the best way to have the expected recommendation approved by the WHO decision-making level for immediate implementation was to mention this requirement clearly but with great discretion." And this is why neither the proposal for the Study Group, nor Vellut's and Water's discussion paper, nor even the final report of the Study Group, trumpet the recommendations.

There are different views about what took place at this moment. Some would say that it was all about finding a way of dealing with drug resistance, and the efficacy of the drug regimen that was agreed upon exceeded all expectations. Others would say that it was always only ever about a "cure". The meetings that preceded the 1981 workshop on chemotherapy all attempted to arrive at clear-cut, simple, and effective regimens that could be used in the field. That the multidrug regimen emerging from these prolonged deliberations had to be "managed" in such a way that the institution could "approve of it" without actually having something new to approve is mildly shocking. The long-sought-after "cure" for leprosy was in fact "slipped past the gates" with a view to urgency, in order to avoid a disaster of catastrophic proportions. Arriving at this consensus was a momentous step, because now field workers had a specific chemotherapy procedure with which to proceed. But what was utterly unanticipated was how immediately effective the multidrug treatment would turn out to be.

The WHO determination was not, however, the end of the story. For the recommendations of the Study Group to be implemented, governments and voluntary organisations had to endorse them, patients had to accept them, workers had to find them feasible to implement in the field, and there needed to be adequate (increased) financial support.[36] Marshalling those components would take considerable effort and would not come without a great degree of heart-searching and conflict.

7

WHO, MDT, AND PRIMARY HEALTHCARE

The World Health Organization had adopted a drug regimen which, despite what even then was considered inadequate trialling, would quickly prove efficacious. The other element of the treatment was a delivery system which would enable the provision and distribution of the medication in a reliable and acceptable way. This chapter deals with that system, or rather with the ideological matrix in which individual systems were developed, and their implementation in four countries: the Philippines, China, India, and Brazil.

In 1978, an important conference at Alma Ata in Kazakhstan had issued a declaration calling for countries to develop healthcare systems founded on equity of access to treatment and on a holistic sense of health as a human right. Its slogan was "Health for All by the Year 2000". We have seen that over the decades, leprosy treatment moved from the benevolent, palliative model of the nineteenth-century religious societies to the epidemiological approach of the mass campaigns. The WHO Director–General, Halfdan Mahler, promoted a vision emanating from the community and empowering people to take responsibility for their own well-being.[1] This vision marked a radical shift from vertical programmes against communicable diseases, turning for inspiration to the village programmes of rural India and the "barefoot doctors" of China.[2] Essential healthcare had to be available to everyone in their own community, using universally accessible technologies. Communities shared "political, economic, social and cultural characteristics, as well as interests and aspirations, including health" and ranged from clusters of isolated homesteads to more organised villages, towns, and city districts.[3]

This aspiration changed the site from which medical care would take place. It also shifted the burden of responsibility. WHO had always defined health as something positive: "a state of complete physical, mental and social well-being and not merely the absence of disease or infirmity".[4] The Alma Ata declaration finessed that positive notion of health to include also "a spirit of self-reliance and self-determination".[5] The role of "healer" had been placed squarely at the doorstep of the people who needed to be cured – a counter-intuitive notion to many working in medical care.

Primary healthcare located in the village was both fundamental and integral to national health. It was the "first level of contact of individuals, the family, and community with the national health system", and it carried the responsibility for "bringing health care as close as possible to where people live and work". As such, it was "the first element of a continuing health care process" and a new space, both nebulous and specific.[6] And within this new and idealistic paradigm, leprosy control became a great opportunity to address inequity through "multi-sectoral coordination". The wide-ranging social and economic needs of the poorest people in the community would become apparent and could be communicated to the sectors that could best address those problems.[7]

Following the principles of the Alma Ata declaration, leprosy control and the implementation of multidrug therapy were to undergo a process of translation so that healing became the individual's personal responsibility at each stage from diagnosis, through careful observation of the chemotherapy regime, to assessment and completion. This new approach depended upon individual self-reliance or self-governance and upon community participation. It engaged people to improve their own health rather than passively relying on others to do it for them. The focus of this approach was the family unit, which would be educated to recognise the early signs and symptoms of leprosy and to, by their own initiative, seek out confirmation of the diagnosis and a treatment regimen at the appropriate local health facility. Family members would then ensure that the individual with the disease complied with treatment.

For this to happen, a wholly new process of enlistment and co-option needed to take place. People in the community would be educated about leprosy in a way that was tailored to their ways of understanding. The gap between the public health message and the people it concerned would be bridged by mobilising the structures of authority in the community. This was expressed as a delicate matter of enlisting "community participation" rather than "community control". It was particularly sensitive in view of the stigma traditionally associated with leprosy. Workers were told that

There is far more to motivation than informing and instructing people. It is a matter of mutual human relations requiring an understanding of the patient's nonmedical problems, his way of life, work, religion, wants, fears and attitudes towards traditional and modern medicine. Motivation requires a person who speaks the "patient's language" and is capable of bridging intellectual and social distances, removing cultural barriers and changing attitudes and habits. This can best be achieved by individual family members and the village council or village health committee which has an all-pervading influence in tradition-bound societies.[8]

Leprosy control was to be shaped around the life patterns of the people rather than through structures of authority like those in the vertical leprosy control programme or indeed in the leprosarium.

Anne-Emmanuelle Birn compares the approach used in the successful smallpox eradication programme and the primary healthcare aspirations of the Alma Ata declaration as encapsulating strongly contrasting models of healing. The smallpox campaign was vertical, technical, centrally driven, disease-based, and doctor-centred, while the new primary-healthcare approach to leprosy would be horizontal, social, locally defined, health-based, individual-focused, and community-centred.[9] I argue that in international anti-leprosy efforts both models of healing have been deployed selectively throughout the long history of encounters with the disease.

Before the sulphones, leprosy had always been separate from general health services and was barely recognised by general health practitioners. In the early days of the mass campaigns, when it seemed that dapsone (DDS) offered a solution, an eventual handover to local medical services was always part of the plan, but this was never comprehensively realised because of fears of growing drug resistance. Once the regimen for multidrug therapy was arrived at, the Leprosy Unit recognised that they needed the resources available through primary healthcare, but they were reluctant to trust the populace, the general practitioner, or the general medical staff with all the tasks necessary to successfully implement multidrug therapy, hence the parallel service delivery programmes and progressive integration that depended on the sophistication of the already existing infrastructure and on what was available in medical services in the most marginalised and isolated villages.

Approaches to malaria, tuberculosis, and leprosy differed with the introduction of primary healthcare. Webb declares bluntly that primary healthcare was the nail in the coffin for anti-malaria control.[10] Workers could not envisage an approach other than the vertical campaigns that relied on spraying mosquito breeding grounds. Attempts to issue people with their drugs in mass campaigns were ineffective without continued supervision.[11] This was true also in tuberculosis programs where the patients were lost to follow-up and the state of case holding was lamentable.[12] Although in various locales, anti-tuberculosis experts were quickly cognisant of the importance of communication with the community and of adjusting their programmes to local conditions, as when the vertical programmes were transitioned into primary healthcare, with a consequent reduction in allocated funds, efforts against tuberculosis lost momentum.[13] In contrast, primary healthcare was strategically deployed by leprosy workers taking account of the infrastructure of the local health systems (as in some states in India where the vertical programme persisted but integration into primary healthcare was carefully staged) and the resources at the periphery.

Once the WHO Study Group standardised chemotherapeutic regimens for leprosy, the notion of primary healthcare must have seemed an unwelcome distraction for the Leprosy Unit at WHO. The new regimen of combined drug treatment (multidrug therapy, or MDT) was initially designed not to "cure" leprosy, but to combat the growing problem of drug resistance; that it would also be extremely effective in halting the disease in infected patients was unanticipated.[14] There were only a few drugs available to fight the disease, knowledge of which had been laboriously accrued. Many people in different parts of the world who had been treated with dapsone for years harboured *M. leprae*, which was resistant to that drug, while other patients had been newly infected with a dapsone-resistant strain of *M. leprae*.[15] In addition, there were indications that resistance was developing to the new, more effective drug, rifampicin.[16]

These problems produced a sense of urgency. Once the multidrug therapy regimen had been devised, WHO was anxious to distribute the combined drugs to as many people as possible before resistant bacteria infected more people and leprosy control lost the few effective drugs in its armoury. Making the new regimen available to everyone who needed it was an enormous task. No fewer than 4 million leprosy sufferers in the world were registered, suggesting that there could be as many as 10.5 million people with the disease. All of these people needed to receive multidrug therapy quickly.

While this was the imperative, the push to primary healthcare could not be ignored, although the Leprosy Unit dragged its collective feet. It offered lip service. It saw problems. It made adaptations. Gradually, it adopted the transition out of necessity and pragmatism. The five-year plan proposed a compromise between primary healthcare and a vertical approach to leprosy control. To start with, vertical programmes still existed in many countries because of the "peculiar difficulties caused by the stigma attached to the disease". Many countries had already made a "rapid and ill-prepared attempt" to transfer responsibility for leprosy services to general medical staff, with disastrous results for patients. Despite these experiences, the report commented optimistically that in the future patients would find their contact with primary healthcare "rewarding".

To smooth the devolution process, the Leprosy Unit suggested that "a leprosy service which can develop *pari passu* with an expanding primary health service" would offer "a more reasonable alternative to specialized programs".[17] The community had yet to be convinced that leprosy was just like any other disease and should be managed in the same rational way. Public education would, of course, overcome this problem, particularly if volunteers educated leprosy-affected communities. Village health workers would need to be enlisted and trained to detect and manage new cases, and, if they encountered problems outside their expertise, should refer people on to other levels of medical care as necessary.[18] In this way, leprosy control was to be gradually "integrated" into primary health care so that "use can be made of community participation at the village level".[19]

In this "equal footing" compromise, leprosy control activities were reorganised for the more complex administration of multidrug therapy. Combined therapy was more potent, potentially more toxic, and considerably more expensive than dapsone alone, so patients needed more supervision and workers more training. Leprosy programmes that were already stretched financially and with limited and overburdened staff would find it extremely difficult to take on the added complications of multidrug therapy.[20] The pressure to step up detection, make accurate diagnoses, and initiate appropriate drug regimens would add to that burden. The drug regimen had to be administered "under direct supervision" of a leprosy worker to be sure that people actually took their medication. If people missed their scheduled visits, workers had to find them and, if they suffered from complications or side effects, refer them to general and specialised hospitals. Individual progress had to be monitored regularly. People also needed comprehensive care for all their medical needs, especially physiotherapy, corrective surgery, and rehabilitation. Then, once they had completed treatment, patients needed regular monitoring in case they suffered a relapse. Everyone in the community, including health professionals and patients, had to understand and accept the new regimens, so health education using all available resources, including the media, was a necessity. Most importantly, a continuous supply of drugs and equipment, especially motor vehicles, was imperative. Finally, independent teams would need periodically to evaluate activities and measure progress against their targets.[21] This was a momentous undertaking.

By 1983, the sense of direction of the medium-term plan had changed, with much more emphasis on equipping all the leprosy-endemic countries to plan, put into action, and evaluate their leprosy control programmes through the primary healthcare system, most particularly through community participation. While around 1–1.5 million people had been treated and released from control in the previous ten years, there were now 5.3 million registered cases in the world and an estimated total of ten to 11 million existing cases. Resistance to dapsone had increased dramatically (100-fold in Malaysia). It was now mandatory to use multidrug therapy, including intermittent rifampicin, for all cases of leprosy.[22] As the plan put it, "Multidrug therapy for leprosy control should be implemented as soon, as widely and as accurately as possible" before the leprosy problem became unmanageable.[23]

Adaptations to and difficulties with primary healthcare came from below. Dr N. H. Antia, from India, described a field project covering a rural population of 30,000 in north Alibag, near Bombay in Maharashtra, in which local women had been trained as part-time village health workers to undertake all forms of healthcare, with an emphasis on treating women and children. These women workers had successfully diagnosed many cases of leprosy, even lepromatous cases, at an early stage, thereby preventing nerve damage from developing. They increased compliance with multidrug therapy from 50% to 90%. Their success relied on their belonging to the community within which they worked. They mixed freely with their patients, inviting them into their own homes, and dispelling the fear of leprosy. They did not suffer discrimination as a result. As Antia commented, "The stigma of leprosy does not get attached to such a local worker who looks after all health activities of the village and her word often carries more weight within her community than that of an outsider."[24]

In contrast, the idea of educating the community to look after its own health problems had not been acceptable either to the medical profession or the paramedical workers, for they perceived the community health workers as a threat, both to their practices and also to existing norms of accountability.[25] The biggest obstacles to the change to primary healthcare in this situation were both the dedicated leprosy workers and the general medical health staff, who saw their positions of authority challenged and feared their livelihoods would be imperilled.

Other stakeholders were both critical of and cautiously optimistic about primary healthcare. In a special issue devoted to the topic, the editorial of *Leprosy Review* noted that very few leprosy projects throughout the world were operating through primary healthcare, but suggested that "the PHC concept may go far to providing a solution, better than any which has so far been proposed, to the problems of drug compliance and attendance, which are inseparable from the use of both self-administered and supervised medication".[26] However, in the same issue, the Dutch anthropologist I. Bijleveld struck a cautionary note when he drew attention to the danger of romanticising the "community", which was so often fraught with micro-political struggles, factions, and monopolies:

> The community is made up of different groups with different interests, values and expectations. Every new action, every proposal, is likely to contain the seeds of conflict. If one talks of community participation, this may in fact turn out to be no more than the concerted effort of one group which hopes to strengthen its own position by monopolizing the innovation at hand.[27]

For example, the "felt needs" of the "community" did not necessarily correspond to the aspirations of the public health administrator if, for argument's sake, a village wanted to rid itself of people with leprosy rather than treat them. Ultimately, the unresolved problems of staff compliance in vertical leprosy programmes would be replicated by voluntary healthcare workers or village health workers: "PHC depends upon the goodwill and devotion of the village health worker … Who can assure us that the job performance of an unpaid PHC village worker will be any improvement upon that of a salaried health center nurse?"[28] However, in spite of these reservations, much of the international medical debate focused on the tasks that could reasonably be assigned to a village health worker and the training that would be necessary.[29]

Early examples of implementation of multidrug therapy show some success, some difficulties, and some compromises. The Sasakawa Memorial Health Foundation fathering of the multidrug therapy pilot study in the Philippines relied on midwives and community support. In 1982, the Philippine government had requested the services of a short-term leprosy consultant in order to assess the state of leprosy control in the country and gauge the feasibility of introducing multidrug therapy, as recommended by WHO.[30] The existing programme was a vertical one, run by specially trained staff and separate from the general health services. The WHO consultant, Dr Yo Yuasa, found that the leprosy register was so outdated that it was "almost impossible" to make a fair estimate of the number of people with the disease. People who had been treated had not been followed up with on an annual basis, and control activities had not been properly supervised, monitored, or evaluated. Yuasa recommended that the Department of Health consider three specific areas, using the existing general healthcare system in order to explore practical ways of adopting multidrug therapy as a model for the whole country, and totally integrate the national leprosy control programme into primary healthcare.[31]

The provinces of Ilocos Norte and Cebu were chosen as appropriate areas for pilot studies. People had suffered from leprosy in the Ilocos Region and the islands of Cebu, Mindanao, and Iloilo from before the Spanish period. They were key trading centres, and in spite of all the leprosy control measures conducted throughout the twentieth century, including isolation in leprosy colonies, these areas remained endemic for leprosy. In Ilocos Norte – situated in the rugged, most northern portion of Luzon Island, where 2,069 people were registered in 1983 (a prevalence of 4.52 per 1,000) – people earned their living by growing rice, garlic, and tobacco. There were four health districts, each with a hospital, twenty-five rural health units (RHU), 702 Barangay Health Stations (BHS), and a skin clinic for people with leprosy.

In the province of Cebu, on an island south of Manila, people worked in light industry, crafts, and furniture making. The soil was not good for sustained rice growing, but they managed to grow corn, coconuts, and fruit. This was a densely populated area with forty-eight municipalities, four cities, and 961 barangays. 1.33 million people lived in eleven of the twelve districts in the province, and they were all included in the study, except for those in the city of Cebu. The province had a sanatorium and a skin clinic, fourteen district hospitals, fifty-eight main health centres (RHU/MHC), and 340 BHSs.[32]

The Philippine Leprosy Mission (PLM) played a crucial role in organising and running the project.[33] They began the massive tasks of training general medical workers and updating the registers. Key leaders addressed the community by showing a documentary film, and they engaged in community discussions in the municipalities. Radio, television, and print media were briefed and school principals co-opted. District by district, those in need of medication gathered at the main health centre. There they received pre-treatment education, were assigned to their local health unit, and swallowed their first supervised dose of multidrug therapy. They signed a pledge to complete their treatment, and their local health professional recorded and reported this. Paucibacillary patients left with six doses and multibacillary patients left with twenty-four doses to take home.

This was the first time that blister packs had been used to provide the regular doses of drugs.[34] The brain-child of Yuasa, they were designed in collaboration with Ciba-Geigy in the Philippines. (The packaging – that is, the PVC blisters with aluminium foil backs – was produced in Switzerland, and the filling and sealing were done locally.) A brilliant innovation, this packaging ensured that the potentially toxic rifampicin was delivered safely, while it made central stock control and local storage and dosage easier and more efficient. Some of the community treated the packs as prized possessions and stored them in their clothes cabinets and empty cooking pots. Many followed the suggestion of hanging the packs from the ceiling or wrapping them in plastic bags to keep them safe from rats and insects. The supervised doses, including rifampicin, were administered at the local health units. Health workers, who were generally the local midwives, made unannounced visits to the homes of the patients to check that people were keeping up with their medication. As in India, these local health workers commanded a great deal of respect in their villages, for they knew their families from birth to burial.[35]

Originating from both Cebu and Ilocos Norte, 2,336 people were treated with multidrug therapy, and more than 92% completed their treatment. From the study, it was clear that a strong cadre of well-trained health workers, given opportunities to retrain at intervals, was vital, as were knowledgeable and encouraging supervisors. The community had to be well prepared at the start of the programme and patients themselves educated about the process. The study also revealed new cases amongst those under fourteen years of age, suggesting that the transmission of the infection was ongoing. Clearly, *M. leprae* was well entrenched in these ancient locations in the Philippines.

Now that it was clear that multidrug therapy could be successfully administered by health workers with no previous experience of leprosy, the next step was to create a national plan. The opportunity for this occurred unexpectedly, when in 1986, in the midst of the pilot study, the EDSA or People Power Revolution erupted and the Marcos regime was overthrown.[36] Yuasa happened to be in the Philippines during the coup, and, with the assistance of the Philippine Leprosy Mission, he met with the new Secretary of Health, Dr Alfredo Bengson. Bengson readily agreed to nationalise the pilot programme, and he instructed the Director of Communicable Disease Services, Dr Jesus Abella, to make sure the project was expanded nationwide.[37] A National Leprosy Control Program therefore began in 1987, aiming to put 35,966 people on multidrug therapy for two years.[38]

China

Primary healthcare was based on the model of the barefoot doctors in China, yet the Chinese nationwide anti-leprosy campaign was a vertical programme under the authority of the Ministry of Health.[39] It reached down into provincial, prefecture, county, and commune levels, and included a network of leprosy villages where people were isolated and treated with dapsone. In 1949 there were 500,000 cases of leprosy in China, and by 1982 this had reduced to approximately 200,000.[40] There were still 1,143 leprosy villages and a cadre of leprosy workers trained to participate in mass campaigns. These latter were the barefoot doctors who would detect cases, treat with dapsone, provide prophylactic treatment to family members, and follow up contacts.

In a new era of political and economic reforms and the opening of China to the international community, after the Twelfth International Leprosy Congress held in Delhi in January 1984, six Chinese delegates were invited to visit Nepal, Thailand, and both Agra in Uttar Pradesh and various sites in Tamil Nadu in India.[41] None had been abroad before. The Chinese delegation visited Nepal first in order to observe the national leprosy programme, particularly how it retrained leprosy workers, and to observe the phenomenon of dapsone resistance, the implementation of multidrug therapy, and the activities of mobile leprosy teams. In south India, they witnessed rehabilitation and reconstructive surgery in Karagiri. In Agra, they discussed research at the Central JALMA Institute for Leprosy (JALMA).[42] In Thailand, they visited the WHO Khon Kaen project and observed a primary healthcare centre.[43]

This medical diplomacy was effective, for on Christmas Eve of that same year, Dr Andrea A. Galvez, Western Pacific Regional Office adviser on chronic diseases, received a formal request from Dr Wang Jian, the Director of the Bureau of Preventative Medicine, and Dr Li Huan-Ying, from the Beijing Tropical Medicine Research Institute, to say that the Directors of the Provincial Skin Disease Control Institutes of Yunnan, Guizhou, and Sichu hoped that with further technical guidance and material aid from WHO they could modernise and speed up leprosy control activities in the southwestern part of China.[44] The government wanted to modernise the existing leprosy control programme in these three provinces in order to reduce the prevalence of the disease to less than 1 in 100,000 initially, and to attain a prevalence of less than 1 in 500,000 by the year 2000. They planned to start implementing multidrug therapy in seven areas of the three provinces, then cover the whole of each of the three provinces, and also integrate leprosy control into the primary healthcare system.[45]

The three provinces were quite varied, but in each there were villages that could be reached only by bicycle, foot, or horseback because of the extremely difficult terrain.[46] Yunnan had a population of 32,553,317 people with 129 counties and six municipalities. There were six leprosaria in the

Kunming counties; twenty-seven in Wenshan Zhuang; and thirteen in the Xishuanbanna Dai Autonomous Region. Registrations had been reduced from 20,830 in 1962 to 13,395 in 1983, but every year about 1,000 new cases were detected. Guizhou province (population 28,552,007) was a very mountainous region with cloudy and rainy weather most of the year. Leprosy had been documented here as far back as 1783 when American and French missionaries established hospitals in the region.[47] The Han, Miao, Yi, and Hui peoples, who lived in Bijie in the northwest, would be the first in this province to receive multidrug therapy. Sichuan Province, with by far the largest population (99,713,310), was crossed by precipitous mountains, deep gorges, and swiftly running rivers. There were Han, Yi, Zang (from Tibet), Hui (Muslims), and Mon (from Mongolia) peoples here, amongst others.[48] In 1960, 32,450 people were registered as suffering from leprosy, but by 1983, this number had dropped to 13,008.

Leprosy field workers, laboratory technicians, and doctors attended training courses, starting with a workshop on multidrug therapy in Xichang beside a volcanic lake surrounded by villages in which there were many people with the disease.[49] A team of health educators visited the villages to show specially produced popular movies and educational films, and to discourage stigma.[50] In the first phase, workers reviewed the old case histories, and those who were still clinically active had their histopathology confirmed. All the multibacillary patients, both new and those who had relapsed – as well as any who had received less than five years of dapsone and rifampicin, and any who had received more than five years of treatment and were still smear-positive – were given multidrug therapy.[51] The primary healthcare worker or the leprosy worker delivered the drugs by motorbike.[52]

In September 1985, Dr Andres Galvez from the WHO observed the progress and recommended that they expand outside the designated areas.[53] Finally, they extended multidrug therapy to all the counties of the three provinces. This primary healthcare approach was then evaluated and subsequently adopted as a model for the other counties, and training was extended to the whole of the three provinces.[54] After November 1987, the committee planned to extend the programme and introduce multidrug therapy to all the other provinces of China in order to eradicate leprosy by the year 2000. The goal was to attain an incidence of less than 0.5 per 100,000 and a prevalence of less than 0.01 per 1,000.[55] By 1990, multidrug coverage in the whole of China was between 90% and 95%. What happened next would be critical because of the long incubation period of leprosy. In 1991, evaluation teams found that multibacillary cases were being treated for too long (up to five or six years), but it looked as if China had a chance of eliminating leprosy by the year 2000.[56]

India

The anti-leprosy programme in India was a vertical programme, and efforts to implement multidrug therapy through primary healthcare were hampered by weak or nonexistent health services at the periphery, a problem that was typified in several states. Dr S. K. Noordeen, the new Chief Medical Officer of the WHO Leprosy Unit, visited and reviewed the Indian national programme at least once every year. In July 1986, he visited districts, projects, control units, drug delivery points, hospitals, and training centres. He examined and interviewed several hundred patients. He also spoke to community members in order to assess the strengths and weaknesses of the Indian programme.[57] Again in 1990, he visited districts in the states of Madhya Pradesh, Orissa, Maharashtra, Karnataka, and Tamil Nadu where multidrug therapy was being implemented.[58] He found that the Indian programme had built up a large infrastructure over the preceding three decades, and while it was not operating at its optimum level of efficiency it was quite capable of being activated and revitalised in order to realise its potential (as was well demonstrated in several of the already existing multidrug therapy projects).

He reported positively that the programme was backed by strong political commitment, working towards specific targets with a sense of direction at all levels that ensured administrative flexibility, optimism, and a sense of urgency. The government had taken responsibility for the bulk of activities with very good coordination between the central and state levels of health administration. There was excellent leadership at the centre, state, and district levels. Health workers were enthusiastic about multidrug therapy, particularly those at the periphery. They were seeing substantial changes in the clinical symptoms of the disease, and were also influenced by the positive responses from patients and the community. Even without health education, communities were enthusiastic about the combined regimens, and this was having a very positive impact on stigma. Patients were readily attending for their treatment, and large numbers of new cases were presenting themselves – a big change from the days of dapsone monotherapy. Patient compliance had also improved. Serious side effects were quite rare, and minor side effects were acceptable to patients. The frequency of reactions also appeared to be less. However, he cautioned, the most critical test for the regimens would be the occurrence of relapse after treatment had been stopped, but so far this was rare.

On the less positive side, the training was inadequate at different levels. Technicians needed to be retrained in order to ensure that the skin smears were collected, stained, and read properly. While positive smear results were often checked, the negative results, which were sometimes more important to check, were insufficiently verified. The medical officers experienced genuine difficulties in classifying cases that been treated previously, particularly when the patient's earlier records had not been well maintained. Many medical officers did not understand the concept that clearing skin lesions and a decrease in bacillary index were not directly proportional to bacterial killing. Neither did many understand how multidrug therapy worked in concert with the natural response of the host.

Additionally, the guidelines issued by the Indian programme aimed to classify cases conservatively, particularly amongst treated cases with multiple lesions. These would be classified as multibacillary irrespective of their bacterial index, but this unduly cautious approach added to the workload and wasted drugs. On the other hand, patients with paucibacillary leprosy did not want their doctors to end their treatment after six months of multidrug therapy, and although the guidelines permitted patients to be treated for a further six months if they had fresh lesions, in some places, treatment was unnecessarily prolonged when there were persisting lesions. Some projects also appeared to neglect important medical needs such as treating reactions, preventing ulcers, and dealing with other illnesses, and this had a flow-on effect, for if the services were unable to meet all the medical needs of their patients, the popularity of multidrug therapy would suffer.[59]

In 1988, the national plan for the elimination of leprosy (NLEP) reviewed various states in India and found many shortcomings consistent with Noordeen's observations. Monotherapy was still being used. Many patients had their treatment unnecessarily prolonged, and some arrested cases were still being treated. In one instance, two patients had been treated for twenty years. There were also many unfilled posts and untrained workers, and some reported reluctance of medical workers to treat patients. In Andhra Pradesh, twenty posts of medical officers and 100 posts of nonmedical assistants were vacant. There was a shortage of drugs, and some stocks were close to their expiry dates. States were late sanctioning their physical targets, and stiff letters were written to Bengal and Bihar from Vineeta Rai, Joint Secretary, Health and Family Welfare, India, as follows:

It is unfortunate that no serious action is being taken by your State for the implementation of the program for which 100% central assistance is available. I shall be grateful if the above deficiencies are removed and the endemic districts already approved for introduction of MDT prepared and district leprosy societies formed at an early date. This Ministry may please be informed of the action taken on the above points at an early date. I shall be grateful if you could bring with you the latest up to date position regarding the points mentioned above at the forthcoming meeting of the Health Secretaries to be held on the 27 and 28 October 1988.[60]

The Regional Director for South East Asia received a report from the Indian ministry indicating that

Implementation of the National Leprosy Eradication Program in some of the states namely Bihar, West Bengal, Uttar Pradesh, Madhya Pradesh and Kerala has been slow. The Government of Uttar Pradesh and Madhya Pradesh have been requested at the Health Secretary level to develop infrastructure in their states for taking more and more districts under multidrug therapy particularly when the program is included in 20 Point Program of Government of India and implemented as 100% central sponsored scheme. The Consultants have also been requested to pursue the matter vigorously with the officials of the State Government at various levels and bring the specific difficulties to the notice of this Directorate for taking up the matter at the appropriate level.

Out of the 196 districts identified as endemic with prevalence rate 5+/1000, 70 districts have already been covered under MDT. Sanction for the release of funds to another 28 districts has already been issued on 22.11.88 and the remaining districts are proposed to be taken up under MDT during 1992.[61]

India's leprosy vertical programme would be integrated into primary healthcare only when the leprosy prevalence rate was reduced to two or fewer per 1,000.[62] And even then not all specialised aspects of the leprosy control programme would disappear. In 1990, C. K. Rao was asked to develop a detailed plan for integration of the leprosy programme into the primary healthcare system in leprosy-endemic districts that had been under multidrug therapy for over seven years in the Indian National Leprosy Program.[63] He outlined the broad organisation of the primary healthcare system as compared to the national plan at all the different levels of responsibility:

Table 5: Broad Organisation of Primary Healthcare System Compared to National Plan

Level	PHC	NLEP
National	Rural health division DGHS	Leprosy Division, DGHS
State	PHC Bureau	Leprosy Bureau
District	CMO/DMO	District Leprosy Officer
Taluka	Community Health Centre (1:120,000 pop.)	Leprosy Control Unit (1:400,000)
Sub-taluka	Health Centre (1:30,000)	Non-medical supervisor – 1 (1:120,000)
Sub-centre	Health Workers – 2 (1 male and 1 female) (1:5,000)	PMW (1:25,000)
Village	Health Guide	None

Leprosy Control Units	719
Urban Leprosy Centres	894
SET Centres	6,097
District Leprosy Units	224
VOs	250
Sample-Survey-cum-Assessment Units	36
Consultant Leprologists	32
NLEP Consultants	13
Independent Evaluations	1986, 1987, 1989

Rao considered that it was appropriate to hand over leprosy programme activities to the primary healthcare system staff when multidrug therapy had been in operation for seven years or more and the prevalence rate was 1.5 per 1,000 or less. There were five districts that were eligible for handing over in 1990–1, "after ensuring the feasibility, practicability and the willingness of the systems".[64]

While moves were being made to integrate leprosy into the primary healthcare system in India and all 201 highly endemic districts were using multidrug therapy, sixty-six of the 201 highly endemic districts lacked "a full leprosy infrastructure".[65] At the same time, there was pushback. As C. K. Rao put it, "Despite the simplification of diagnosis, classification, treatment regimens, drug delivery, and reporting, leprosy program activities could not be successfully integrated into general health services: there was opposition from leprosy staff and reluctance among general health staff to assume the responsibilities."[66] Professional boundaries were threatened by the notion and reality of primary healthcare. At the same time, the prejudice against leprosy was still present amongst the general medical staff.

Brazil

Brazil was another instance where weak infrastructure combined with the interests of stakeholders, in this case dermatologists, to delay implementation of multidrug therapy and resist primary healthcare. When Lopez Bravo visited the Americas in 1984, he found that implementation of multidrug therapy was in its most preliminary stage. Even though governments had decided to integrate anti-leprosy measures into the general health services of their countries, this had not yet happened; and yet, they had cut the funds for the vertical programme without a corresponding increase of funds for the general health services. Cases were widely dispersed, and the specialised approach to leprosy made the cost per patient high. In the whole region, only 10% of those who needed it were receiving multidrug therapy.[67]

In Brazil, the vertical leprosy control service had been traditionally run by dermatologists, but the new programme was designed to employ auxiliary workers. This change threatened professional boundaries with consequences that would hold back treatment for many leprosy-affected people.[68] Brazilian leprologists refused to endorse multidrug therapy, claiming that the existing studies were inconclusive. These doctors were dermatologists who had considerable status in their own country. Some had also occupied positions of influence in advising WHO. One had belonged to the 1981 "WHO Study Group on the Chemotherapy of Leprosy for Control Programmes", but, to the consternation of his colleagues in Geneva, had done an about-face once he returned to Brazil and opposed his own previous recommendations.[69]

Lopez Bravo spent several days in Brazil in 1984, in discussion with the self-styled "National Advisory Committee on Alternative Therapeutic Regimens for Leprosy". This committee, formed in August 1983, insisted on clinical trials to assess the WHO-recommended regimens because they felt that the existing studies were either preliminary or inconclusive. They reasoned that rifampicin was unnecessary for tuberculoid patients, "as they would eventually be cured without any treatment". Furthermore, the committee argued that it was unethical to treat patients with regimens such as those recommended by WHO because their efficacy had not been studied anywhere else.[70] They maintained that, although there were a number of dapsone-resistant cases being treated with clofazamine, the magnitude of the drug-resistance problem was unknown, as dapsone resistance had never been surveyed.

There was also a problem with the acceptability of clofazamine because it caused skin discolouration. Lopez Bravo left the meeting hoping that they might at least cooperate in a feasibility study, but he feared that the regimens recommended by the committee would produce resistance to rifampicin.[71] Two days later, Lopez Bravo met with the committee again, and Dr Diltor Vladimir Araújo Opromolla identified two centres where the studies would be conducted, asking if WHO would assist.[72] Taking a firm stance, Lopez Bravo informed him that WHO would be involved only if the studies followed WHO's recommendations.[73] He left optimistic that there was a chance that multidrug therapy would be introduced into certain areas in Brazil, with WHO's cooperation.

A year later, in December 1984, Noordeen visited the Brazilian leprologists, who in the face of the increasing problem of drug resistance, continued to insist that the WHO regimens had not been sufficiently tested.[74] He explained the recommendations of the Study Group, but left less optimistic than Lopez Bravo. Noordeen concluded, "At the end of the discussions there was no clear indication that the Brazilian policy towards multidrug therapy will change in the immediate future." He recommended persistence.[75] Within two years, the National Division of Sanitary Dermatology did indeed support the national leprosy control programme and promote the use of multidrug therapy, but the state health departments were tardy as well. It all resulted in "frustratingly low coverage of MDT in Brazil".[76] In order to speed things up, Noordeen planned to visit Brazil again in 1988 and 1989.[77]

While the opposition of the Brazilian leprologists hampered the impact of multidrug therapy in Brazil, a lack of political will in the region – both towards leprosy and towards building the infrastructure for primary healthcare – also combined to hold back its introduction. Inadequate infrastructure for supervised treatment, insufficient personnel trained to administer and carry out activities, lack of resources for buying specific drugs, the low priority given to leprosy control, and the refusal by leprologists to adopt the therapeutic scheme recommended by the WHO Study Group combined to deprive people infected with the disease of treatment that could have made a significant improvement to their lives.[78]

Conclusion

In spite of all the institutional motivation, integration of leprosy control into primary healthcare was frustratingly slow and uneven, and intersectoral cooperation was halting, where it existed at all.[79] Issues of stigma in the community and amongst health workers and the reluctance of specialised staff to lose their monopoly on roles, as well as the reluctance of peripheral workers to take up leprosy work, were responsible for this lamentable state of affairs.[80] Against all fears and expectations, multidrug therapy was proving to be effective and acceptable to both patients and workers, but its implementation was glacial.[81] Even more troubling was the fear that leprosy work could be given low priority and simply disappear amongst a welter of other equally pressing health concerns.[82] Inadequate public health infrastructure, inadequate functioning of referral levels, scarcity of laboratory services, weak management of the primary healthcare system, and lack of manpower all persisted.

Sometimes communities did not give priority to healthcare. On the other hand, leprosy patients did not have confidence in the multipurpose staff at the primary healthcare centre, and people with disabilities were not tolerated by medical workers. The idea persisted amongst patients, workers, administrators, politicians, and the community that leprosy was a disease apart, deserving of special treatment and services. Workers were unclear on their roles in leprosy control, particularly if some components of a vertical programme were still operating.[83] By November 1986, registered cases had increased in the preceding twenty years from 2,831,775 to 5,340,895. In sixty-five countries, only 9% of the registered cases – that is, 468,222 people – were receiving multidrug therapy, and 93,216 had completed their medication.[84]

Table 6: Distribution of Registered Leprosy Cases by
WHO Region 1986[85]

WHO Region	Estimated population (000s)	No. registered cases	Prevalence per 1,000	% of total
Africa	421,782	886,465	2.10	16.6
Americas	654,958	320,536	0.49	6.0
E. Mediterranean	310,697	74,384	0.24	1.4
Europe	613,418	12,775	0.02	0.2

WHO Region	Estimated population (000s)	No. registered cases	Prevalence per 1,000	% of total
South East Asia	1,130,606	3,801,343	3.36	71.2
Western Pacific	1,359,562	245,392	0.18	4.6
Total	**4,491,022**	**5,340,895**	**1.19**	**100**

There was a desperate need for coordination between governments, WHO, other international, multilateral and bilateral organisations, and voluntary agencies at both the regional and the global levels. The aspirations were there, but the follow-through was lacking.[86] Equally, further political commitment was urgently needed.[87] Letters between Yuasa and Noordeen indicate the desire for a more effective approach to the implementation of WHO multidrug therapy. Yuasa believed there could be an 80–90% reduction in the caseload in the world, and he wrote to Noordeen, "Our clear duty is to reach every case as soon as possible and give every patient a chance of cure by providing basic MDT." Nearly twelve months later, Noordeen pointed out that multidrug therapy was reaching most endemic areas where the health infrastructure was good, where vertical structures existed for leprosy, and where political commitment was strong. Where conditions were not so advantageous, he felt strongly that "it [was] quite unacceptable to wait for the most favorable conditions to develop … before we could think of introducing MDT". He added that "something needs to be done in these countries to increase the awareness on MDT, to make people know of the opportunities that exist for envisaging the end of leprosy in their countries".[88]

In 1988, geographical coverage of multidrug therapy was only 33%, with 1,604,927 people on it and nearly 627,919 who had completed treatment.[89] For the first time, the statistics showed a decline in the total number of patients registered worldwide, but leprosy was not being afforded priority. And by the end of the decade, multidrug therapy coverage was only just over 50%.[90]

Table 7: Leprosy Cases Compared to Treatment and Coverage of MDT

End of year	No. registered cases	No. new cases	No. patients treated with MDT	Cumulative total cured with MDT	Geographical MDT coverage (%)
1985	5,368,202	550,224	78,752	9,425	1
1986	5,341,000	573,790	468,222	93,216	9

End of year	No. registered cases	No. new cases	No. patients treated with MDT	Cumulative total cured with MDT	Geographical MDT coverage (%)
1987	5,078,000	594,145	1,318,964	515,144	26
1988	4,908,000	553,597	1,604,927	627,919	33
1989	3,866,000	550,743	1,751,903	853,706	45
1990	3,737,000	571,792	2,080,998	1,204,821	56
1991	3,087,788	584,412	1,295,640	2,870,944	42

As is apparent from the above exchange, those involved discussed their activities in terms of "duty" and what was universally "unacceptable". These value-laden terms were used in the context of what people needed to know "of the opportunities that exist for envisaging the end of leprosy in their countries."This sense of moral imperative would culminate in a World Health resolution that aspired to bring an end to leprosy even closer.

8

ELIMINATION, THE IDEA

"Nothing will ever be attempted if all possible objections must be first overcome."
— Samuel Johnson

While the Leprosy Unit at WHO was disappointed at the slowness with which multidrug therapy was being taken up in many of the endemic countries, it was optimistic – even visionary – about its potential to bring about a substantial reduction in the number of active cases worldwide. The Unit believed that the total number of registered cases could be reduced by up to 90% within ten years, provided nations made a political commitment and international NGOs coordinated their work and resources. Yet many countries were simply unable to give priority to the disease.[1] As a result, millions of people would inevitably suffer from leprosy's debilitating social and economic consequences, let alone the physical disabilities that were so common, but so avoidable.[2] By WHO's figuring, geographical coverage was only half what it should be, and this seemed utterly unjustified, given the funds available to the programme. An idea of the significant WHO funding available can be gained from the following examples in Table 8 below.[3]

Table 8: WHO Funding, 1988–9 Compared to 1990–1 (USD)

	1988–9	*1990–1*
Regular budget	2,447,600	2,588,100
Research budget (IMMLEP and THELEP)	5,224,000	6,200,000
Other sources	6,073,600	6,345,700
Total	**13,745,200**	**15,133,800**

Getting a resolution before the World Health Assembly seemed the best way of marshalling the necessary political will to allow these funds to be deployed effectively. A resolution for the elimination of leprosy was introduced in January 1991, at the 87th Session of the Executive Board of the same year, by Professor O. Ransome-Kuti, the Minister of Health, from Lagos, Nigeria. As a result, the campaign began to eliminate leprosy as a public health problem by 2000.[4]

If the devil is in the details, he is equally in the definitions. The elimination campaign was fraught with difficulties surrounding both its goals and the ways to measure them. Distinctions between control, elimination, and eradication of leprosy had to be clarified. Issues to do with incidence and prevalence of leprosy were also inherently complicated and gave rise to prolonged debate. The discussion at the Executive Board questioned how realistic the goal was and how reliable the numbers were of cases on which the campaign was to be launched. While the WHO had reasonable confidence in its registers of infected cases which were compiled by field workers and national-level bureaucrats, it had to admit that a proportion of leprosy cases remained undetected and unreported, since a scientifically accurate sample would be "prohibitively expensive", not least because the disease was widely and unevenly scattered.

In the discussion at the Executive Board, three amendments were proposed. These had the effect of emphasising that multidrug therapy was one amongst many leprosy control measures, of producing a numerical notion of elimination, and of including "social and economic rehabilitation" as a goal of the programme.[5] The concept of "cure" therefore became quite expansive, embracing not only the disappearance of clinical signs of the disease but also the restoration of patients to satisfactory social and economic relations. And in an attempt to make the reduction target rigorous in a disciplinary sense, the "elimination" of leprosy was defined as reduction to "less than 1/10,000", even though the population group concerned – "global" or "national" – was left deliberately ambiguous. This residual ambiguity around the notion of "elimination" would make it a target for debate between epidemiologists and specialists with a public health focus.

Resolution WHA 44.9 for the elimination of leprosy was presented two years before the "International Task Force for Disease Eradication", which considered more than eighty infectious diseases and judged six to be eradicable. The Task Force defined elimination as the cessation of transmission of a disease in a single country, continent, or other limited geographic area (e.g., polio in the Americas), as opposed to "global eradication". They considered it to be theoretically possible to "eliminate" a disease in humans when the microbe remained at large (e.g., neonatal tetanus). For although a disease itself may remain, a particularly undesirable clinical manifestation of it may be prevented entirely (e.g., blindness from trachoma) or new transmission interrupted (e.g., infectious yaws). They also included a notion of control of a disease "to a level that it is no longer considered 'a public health problem'". This "level" was as an arbitrarily defined qualitative (e.g., onchocerciasis in West Africa) or quantitative (e.g., leprosy incidence below one case per 10,000 population) level of disease control."[6] It is worth noting that this definition refers to "leprosy incidence", not "prevalence".[7]

The WHA 44.9 resolution on leprosy clearly did not refer to "eradication" and neither did it refer to "control". It was a resolution to reduce the prevalence of leprosy to less than one in 10,000, rather than the incidence. To compound matters, when the goal for the elimination of leprosy was set, with its inherent tensions clustered around the notion of a "cure", indicators of incidence and prevalence had already been established as complex compromises. Prevalence was defined as "the number of cases of a particular disease in a defined population at a specified time".[8] But prevalence statistics were often calculated from the number of registered cases by subtracting cases who had been cured, those who had moved away from the population in question, and those who had died. Thus, their accuracy depended upon how well the registers were maintained. Incidence was defined as the number of new cases of a particular disease that occurred in a defined population during a specific period. This was expressed as a proportion or rate of the population in which the new cases had been discovered. Incidence was valuable in determining the effectiveness of a control programme, but new cases might take many years to be recognised. Accurate figures were difficult to obtain, so the number of new registered cases was frequently used to estimate incidence, however approximately.[9]

Because the date of onset of the disease was notoriously difficult to determine, the new case detection rate depended upon the nature and intensity of case detection, so it was considered feasible for most leprosy control programmes to "provide estimates of incidence in the form of case-detection rates". The source of the denominator had to be clearly stated. If active case detection was employed, the denominator was the number of people actually examined. If passive case detection was employed, the denominator was an estimate of the population from which the cases were derived.

Although causal interpretation of trends was a problem for a number of reasons in determining the possible decline in leprosy in an area, leprosy trends in a population would be able to be monitored by analysing prevalence and incidence statistics that had been collected over a number of years. This would indicate the progress made by a leprosy control programme in interrupting transmission until the disease no longer represented a public health problem, and in treating people so that they were cured and did not develop deformities.[10] The degree of disability from which a newly diagnosed person suffered also served as an indicator of how long the person had been infected before diagnosis.[11]

Operational indicators had been devised to assist in practical managerial tasks such as planning a leprosy control programme, operating from day to day, and evaluating the programme's effectiveness. These were particularly important in determining the appearance of, and increase in, drug resistance, and in gauging the impact of the switch from dapsone to multidrug therapy. The ratio of the known cases to the estimated cases was considered a good measure of the progress and efficiency of case detection, but both numerator and denominator were problematic. Accurately determining known cases was complicated by diagnostic errors, out-of-date registers, and people lost to follow-up.[12] Most countries had working estimates which were drawn from a variety of historical and current sources, and although actual case numbers could be obtained only from specially designed population-based surveys, these estimations were useful provided they were challenged and continually revised with experience and improved data. The number of cases registered each year was the most widely used statistic, and the simplest to obtain, although it revealed little about the case finding in the programme. A fall might mean one of several things (e.g., a fall in incidence, or a fall in the backlog effect, or a decline in case detection activities).[13] Information about the cases actually detected, such as age, clinical type, and disability, as well as information about the type of case detection that was being carried out, would also be crucial aids in determining the progress of a campaign.

For Noordeen, the "concept of elimination" was entirely distinct from the idea of eradication. On the basis of his professional understanding, "eradication" of a disease was "completely removing a disease from a community" if the epidemiological situation, the technology, the possibility of applying the technology in the community, and the resources were all optimal. This not only meant "the absence of disease in the community, but also complete stoppage of transmission as well as the removal of the disease agent from the community".[14] This would happen "throughout the world so that there is no possibility of reappearance of the disease or its agent anywhere". The first and only example of this was the eradication of smallpox. On the other hand, "elimination" was a concept that did not have the same clear-cut meaning as either "eradication" or "control":

> This in-between situation between control and eradication came to be referred to as 'disease elimination'. While in some situations disease elimination meant eradication limited to certain geographic areas, in others it referred to steep reductions in disease occurrence to levels so low that it could be in the realm of acceptability from the public health point of view.

So, in Noordeen's words, "elimination" meant "a reduction in the size of the problem to extremely low levels".

When the idea of the "elimination of leprosy" was conceived, Noordeen recognised that "it would envisage an arbitrary definition" and require the qualification, "elimination as a public health problem". "Prevalence" would be used as a marker, and the level of prevalence to be attained was also arbitrarily set at 1/10,000, as was the goal of the year 2000. Apparently, the notion that the goal be reached at the "global level" "was mentioned in the early documents", but "it was assumed that elimination should be attained in each endemic country at the national level". He explained that

> As far as WHO was concerned, the use of the term elimination varied with different diseases and as long as it was clearly defined as in the case of leprosy it did not worry too much about the Dahlem definition. In this I got very good support from my ADG, Dr Ralph Henderson. Even at the time, I knew that the resolution and the goal was going to make a big push for leprosy, notwithstanding the reservations of some who thought that leprosy would go the way of malaria and fail.[15]

The rationale behind the initiative was clear at the outset for Noordeen. It was vital to seize the opportunity presented by the success of multidrug therapy and break the "lethargy" amongst those who were prepared to accept the disease as a "perennial problem". (He was surprised when he joined WHO that leprosy was considered so intractable, and he set about looking for opportunities to solve this problem.)[16] He also believed that there was "a very good epidemiological opportunity in most endemic countries irrespective of the inability to reach zero disease and zero transmission".[17] For him, it all hinged on the "technological breakthrough" and the necessary political support.

An elimination initiative had been started earlier in the Western Pacific Region in 1989, when the newly elected Regional Director of WPRO, Dr S.T. Han, was looking around for some achievement to mark his legacy and saw the leprosy programme as a possibility. Capitalising on Han's request, Dr Lee Jong Wok, a Korean doctor who would subsequently become the Director–General of WHO and who was the regional officer in charge of leprosy at the time, and Yo Yuasa spent time before the Manila Regional Leprosy Conference appraising the leprosy situation in the region and discussing what could be achieved.[18] They were convinced that the countries in the region could bring down their prevalence rate to around 1/10,000, or roughly one-tenth of the existing rate.

They had a budget of US$20 million, so they cast around for a name that would ensure the programme was accepted by the health authority of each member country. They were joined by Dr Robert Jacobson from Carville, who had with him "a small pamphlet published by the US Public Health Department entitled *Elimination of TB in the USA by 2010*". This plan carried a quotation from Samuel Johnson: "Nothing will ever be attempted if all possible objections must be first overcome." Yuasa describes what followed:

> Taking a hint from this, reducing leprosy prevalence rate to less than 1/10,000 was named the 'elimination of leprosy as a major public health problem.' Although the program was not officially presented at the regional committee, the members at the conference adopted the initiative and took it back to their own Ministries of Health.[19]

Noordeen maintained that the WHO's decision to go ahead with the elimination initiative was not primarily influenced by the Western Pacific initiative:

> It was certainly one of the factors contributing to the decision, but more important was the need to take a strong initiative in the light of the great opportunity with MDT. With the resolution and subsequent drug donations, we were able to make sure that leprosy was squarely in the public health domain and countries had to respond to the opportunity.[20]

Noordeen's retrospective recounting of the thought and motivation behind the resolution indicates a degree of flexibility in the "spirit" of the decision. His concern was consistently for what could be achieved to reduce the disease in real terms.[21] Sansarricq has admitted that "It may have been felt that a technical meeting was likely to express some reservations about the elimination concept, whereas a WHA resolution proposing a relatively simple objective could be readily adopted and would also have a greater impact on governments and other interested parties."[22]

Policy decisions and recommendations that came from the WHO were negotiated at the Executive Board and at the World Health Assembly so that they could be issued as the consensus of the member nations. The technical recommendations that emerged through the specialised units, such as the WHO Leprosy Unit, were hammered out and issued as Expert Committee Reports, drawn from lengthy consultation with independent experts from the Regions who were acknowledged to be the best in the world. These technical experts wore many different institutional hats and juggled different institutional affiliations and allegiances. The direction that work against leprosy took rested on their professional and scientific integrity which, as is apparent from previous chapters, they considered to be not only professional but vocational.

At the heart of the debate of responsibility for international policy, particularly the elimination resolution, is a fallacy about the agency of WHO. While the power and authority of WHO comes from the consensus of nations and the authority of its expert consultants, the priorities of the organisation may be influenced by the priorities and pressures of substantial donors. The WHO can be steered by outside influences, as it has been throughout its history. Hence the lobbying by Robert Cochrane, the International Leprosy Association, and the Indian delegation in 1949 that enabled leprosy to be included in the WHO programme of works.

In many ways, it can be said that the structure of WHO has been designed for this sort of pressure, as it is dependent on funding from either member nations or independent donors. As Brown, Cueto, and Fee show, the United States exercised considerable influence during the Cold War years: "when the Soviet Union and other communist countries walked out of the UN system and therefore out of WHO in 1949, the United States and its allies were easily able to exert a dominating influence."[23] However, East–West cooperation was still possible. The smallpox eradication campaign initiated by the Soviet Union and Cuba in 1959 was supported by the United States government in 1965 when "Lyndon Johnson instructed the US delegation to the World Health Assembly to pledge American support for an international program to eradicate smallpox from the earth," enabling the "Intensified Smallpox Eradication Program" to be launched in 1967.[24]

As Dr Yo Yuasa described it: "The working relationship [between SMHF and WHO] became much closer in 1982 in terms of actual collaboration ... after the publication of the *Report of the Chemotherapy Study Group on MDT*, because SMHF's support to leprosy endemic countries became concentrated around MDT implementation in these countries."[25] The Sasakawa Memorial Health Foundation and Nippon Foundation were influential in setting the course for WHO's work against leprosy over the next decade. And much of the negativity towards the leprosy elimination programme was not only a criticism of the technical aspects of the decision to set an "elimination goal", but also a veiled criticism of the Japanese intervention in this area and a suspicion of their agenda. Interestingly, the World Bank also played a considerable role in supporting the leprosy programme in India, yet did not receive the same resentment.[26]

This realignment was not peculiar to leprosy. The growing reliance of WHO on extra-budgetary funding "coming from donations by multilateral agencies or 'donor' nations" shifted the balance of power within the organisation: "By the period 1986–87, extra-budgetary funds of $437 million had almost caught up with the regular budget of $543 million. By the beginning of the 1990s, extra-budgetary funding had overtaken the regular budget by $21 million, contributing 54% of WHO's overall budget." Brown, Cueto, and Fee describe the problem that this created for the organisation: "Wealthy donor nations and multilateral agencies like the World Bank could largely call the shots on the use of the extra-budgetary funds they contributed. Thus, they created, in effect, a series of 'vertical' programs more or less independent of the rest of WHO's programs and decision making structure."[27]

Refashioning leprosy

Following on from the resolution, to the consternation of many, the clinical descriptions of the disease and its management were "re-fashioned" so that recommended field operations became increasingly simplified and streamlined. There were changes to definitions of a case of leprosy and its cure, the classification of the clinical symptoms, the procedures for diagnosis and treatment, post-treatment surveillance, and the duration of standardised treatment. These changes were viewed suspiciously as a means of hastening the elimination initiative, but the WHO Leprosy Unit and its expert advisers argued that simplification was necessary in order to implement multidrug therapy successfully, and advisable in light of the increasingly obvious success of the new chemotherapy.

One change in the process of refashioning leprosy that actually preceded the elimination resolution was a more restricted definition of a "case" of leprosy. Until the Sixth Expert Committee met in November 1987, people who were defined as a "case" of leprosy were quite a heterogeneous group.[28] They included those who needed to be treated, those who were undergoing treatment, and those who had completed treatment but were still under surveillance. Additionally, people with residual deformities or disabilities who needed care were also kept on the leprosy register as a "case of leprosy". This "lack of distinction between these categories" was judged to be "a source of error in computing and comparing prevalence and other statistics necessary for planning and organizing leprosy control programs".[29]

The new definition of a "case of leprosy" was "a person showing clinical signs of leprosy, with or without bacteriological confirmation of the diagnosis, and requiring chemotherapy".[30] This redefinition necessitated setting up two other registers: one for those who had completed their treatment but required (or were under) surveillance, and one for those with deformities or disabilities "due to past leprosy". Computations of the prevalence of leprosy were based on the first category of patients, those requiring chemotherapy, although this did not mean that responsibility towards the patient ceased with the completion of chemotherapy.[31]

Consultants for various NGOs were sensitive to the potential problem. Colin McDougall, for example, a member of the LEPRA Medical Board and editor of *Leprosy Review*, understood that many of the difficulties of determining prevalence derived from ambiguity in what was meant by a case of leprosy. At the same time, he flagged the potential for misunderstanding:

> On first reading, this implies that such patients are no longer part of the leprosy control program (once chemotherapy is completed), but … I see that this is not necessarily intended. To me, the section here on community-based rehabilitation is of outstanding importance; surely one of the 'new concepts' to be fully discussed by the Expert Committee.[32]

With a case of leprosy defined as one requiring multidrug therapy, this excluded people with residual disabilities who required ongoing care. Yet once people were removed from the leprosy register, they were at risk of being denied access to the precious financial investment made for work against the disease.

On the other hand, medical administrators such as Adeleye, the Director of Health Services in Nigeria, had no problem with the changed definition of a case of leprosy. He observed that "as much as 50% of cases on registers need not be there. Many of them are the mutilated, disabled persons needing no leprosy drugs who are still kept on the register".[33] He believed that a standard definition of a leprosy case was very important "because of the variables applied in various areas and by various workers, apart from the observers' variations that make data from various places difficult to compare".[34] He made comparisons between other diseases that produced disfigurement and deformities, such as smallpox, polio, and tuberculosis of the spine, reasoning that "I believe that *sequaelae* of leprosy should not necessarily keep the patient on the treatment register for ever after they are 'cured'. Such should no longer be considered as leprosy patients but should be transferred to the general rehabilitation program where this is available."[35]

In contrast, John Hargraves, a microsurgeon, whose field experience was amongst the indigenous people in the Northern Territory of Australia, pointed out that in his experience, if people with disabilities were not treated as part of a leprosy programme, he would not be able to get the others to take their medication: "where no effort is made to correct deformity, patients have regarded medication as useless." He found that the shift in the definition of a case of leprosy was therefore "counter-productive to the overall control of leprosy."[36]

Then, almost before the debates had subsided, the next Study Group on Chemotherapy (1993) standardised the duration of the regimen for multibacillary patients at two years, dropping the caveat "or until smear negative". The Study Group also recommended that post-multidrug therapy annual surveillance of patients be discontinued, along with a relaxation of the requirements for bacteriological surveillance and supervision of monthly doses of rifampicin. Two years later, the Seventh Report of the Expert Committee on Leprosy redefined categories of patients from a clinical point of view on the basis of their skin lesions. Patients with a single skin lesion were distinguished from those with two to five lesions. Patients with more than five lesions were to be classed as multibacillary cases. Drug regimens would depend upon the category of "cases". In what was almost unimaginable to some and to others an entirely logical development, those who were categorised as "single lesion PB patients" were to be given a single dose of chemotherapy. Those with five lesions or more, the multibacillary group, needed to be treated for only twelve months. Additionally, health professionals were instructed to send people off with more than a month's supply of their drugs, if necessary.[37]

The implementation of multidrug therapy on an increasing scale, together with the changes to the definition of cases, categories of patient, and length of regimens, precipitated changes to the prevalence of the disease. As Lechat so pithily put it: the "introduction of MDT had or will have the effect of reducing prevalence drastically, since patients will be discharged after a relatively short course of treatment. In other words, MDT could reduce prevalence much more quickly than incidence."[38] Multidrug therapy promised to push the whole epidemiology of leprosy, which was already a matter of many different determinants, into completely uncharted waters. To many, this seemed like a *fait accompli.* Then there was an added complication in determining what was actually happening, for in spite of the dramatic drop in prevalence, the "new case detection rate" remained virtually static, as it had for a decade.

This, of course, could mean any one of a number of things. It could mean that the implementation of multidrug therapy was so effective that many previously hidden cases were presenting themselves for treatment. It could mean that there was a huge backlog of cases still to be treated. Or it might mean that transmission of the infection continued and multidrug therapy was not getting to people early enough before they infected others. A further possible explanation was that there was a non-human reservoir of *M. leprae*, as yet undiscovered. No one knew, and all of this would cause a great deal of consternation that would intensify as the deadline for elimination drew closer. Working Groups on Leprosy Control, held on a yearly basis from 1991 to 1994, kept the goal of elimination uppermost in everyone's minds – planning country, regional, and global strategies – with the full participation of all the actors involved, including the NGOs.[39] No one was doctrinaire about delivering multidrug therapy by either vertical or integrated leprosy services, instead relying on whatever system was the most appropriate in the local situation.[40]

Meanwhile, the pressure on the elimination strategy surfaced at the Third Meeting of the Working Group on Leprosy Control. By WHO reckoning, there were still 6.5 million cases to treat before 2000, at a cost of US$420 million. Representatives of the International Federation of Anti-Leprosy Associations expressed concern about the negative impact of the elimination rhetoric and media attention on their fundraising activities.[41] They expressed "the potential negative impact on donors of loose use of the 'elimination term'", and they asked WHO to put the targets expressed in press releases into the context of the unchanged level of newly detected cases in areas where it would be difficult to implement multidrug therapy.

They also asked for publicity about the continuing needs of patients with disabilities.[42] They were concerned that people would think that the problem of leprosy had been solved.[43] Funds were becoming more difficult to obtain because of the recession and competition from other charities.[44] The representative for the Damien Foundation, Dr L. Janssens, added that "The organization felt uneasy with the definition of elimination as it was a purely arbitrary one, depending on the duration of treatment and the definition of leprosy." The group concluded that while much had been achieved with the elimination resolution of WHO, "successes scored should not be overstated nor the challenges ahead understated". In short, the International Federation of Anti-Leprosy Associations was asking WHO to tone down its publicity.

In 1991 and 1992, Noordeen produced two strategic papers. The first clearly and brilliantly explained the value and importance of multidrug therapy (MDT).[45] The second revised the global estimates of leprosy. This was the first major publication since Bechelli's estimates in 1966.[46] Noordeen reasoned that the introduction of MDT had reduced the prevalence of the disease so that a reassessment was necessary. He estimated that there were 5.5 million leprosy cases in the world and between 2–3 million people, now cured, with residual deformities.[47] This was half the number estimated throughout the 1960s, 1970s, and 1980s.

Many had already been cured through treatment with MDT. With the new definition of a "case", many people had been eliminated from the registers. There were possible longer-term effects of dapsone therapy that had to be taken into account in some areas. Some countries had better and more efficient leprosy control activities because of the introduction of multidrug therapy. Finally, there was a natural decline in some parts of Africa.[48] This revision would provide another point of contention, for it seemed to some that Noordeen was making the problem disappear, that is "eliminating leprosy" by means of arbitrary redefinitions and guesstimates.

The response to the resolution on elimination

The International Federation of Anti-Leprosy Associations' Medical Commission responded positively to the WHA 44.9 resolution at their meeting in June 1992 in Bern, with the proviso that "patients who need care after cure" be considered. They also thought that they should start post-elimination planning immediately.[49] But the elimination target was not universally hailed as desirable, as was evident from the response of Paul Fine, an epidemiologist at the London School of Hygiene and Tropical Medicine and consultant to the British Leprosy Relief Association (LEPRA). Fine's response would encapsulate, justify, and fuel much of the growing unease.[50] He criticised the change in case definitions, which he summarised as taking place merely for the purposes of "diagnostic criteria, classification criteria and administrative criteria". These were changes with implications for research and control.[51] The diagnostic criteria were in his view "dogmatically" expressed by WHO, even though diagnosis was not always straightforward. As he rightly pointed out: "An appreciable proportion of registered leprosy cases in the world are never seen by a medical officer, let alone biopsied. We must appreciate the implications of the diagnostic difficulties under such circumstances."[52] He argued too that classification had been confused by shifting criteria, and he pointed to long-standing and well-known uncertainties to do with classification, some of which stemmed from unreliable laboratory procedures: "the routine smear services upon which the classification dichotomy is based are often not of sufficient standard to give reliable results".[53]

But for Fine, the most significant problem had been created by changes in administrative criteria for defining a "case". These changes had produced "an artefact": "a massive discharge of patients from registers" and a consequent "dramatic decline in numbers of registered patients".[54] Fine conceded that "a large proportion of patients" who had been "discharged in the 1980s as a consequence of the new short duration treatment policies had already been effectively cured and were on registers only because there had been no appropriate discharge policy beforehand".[55] But this artefact concealed, in his view, a glaring inaccuracy. It represented "a fall in administrative burden but not necessarily a fall in morbidity incidence – or indeed true morbidity prevalence – in leprosy-endemic populations". On the contrary, "Long-term progress in leprosy control should be reflected in declining incidence of disease." Fine justifiably stated that "Unless incidence is reduced, all the problems of case finding, diagnosis, and registration remain unchanged."[56] He also rightly claimed that "We have no evidence that MDT has or will have any appreciable impact on incidence at all."

Fine had been in large part responsible for the comprehensive *Epidemiology of Leprosy in Relation to Control* report, referred to earlier. In this, the difficulties of obtaining figures for incidence and prevalence were clearly spelled out, and case-detection figures and prevalence indicators were arrived at in all their compromised figuration. It is therefore interesting to note that at this point Fine makes an argument for a decrease in incidence that is natural and quite independent of the implementation of multidrug therapy. His argument shifts from suggesting preferred measures of incidence as a substitute for the "deeply flawed" measures of prevalence to claims about dramatic declines in leprosy incidence (or "case-detection rates") that "have been documented in many countries of the world for more than a decade".[57] He cites natural declines in the incidence of leprosy in Norway, Japan, Portugal, China, Thailand, Mexico, and Venezuela, well before the advent of multidrug therapy. He hypothesises that a combination of "improving socio-economic standards" and BCG anti-tuberculosis vaccination may have been responsible.[58]

With his characteristic rigor, Fine criticises the elimination initiative for two weaknesses. The first is that the application of the term "prevalence" is vague. What does it refer to? He assumes that it refers to persons "having clinical signs of leprosy … and requiring chemotherapy". The second object of criticism is the numerical goal of 1/10,000 population, with Fine asking, "what population is implied?" If it means the total global population of those with leprosy, then that would be approximately 7/10,000. Did global elimination therefore mean that the prevalence of the disease should be reduced sevenfold? And if it did, "would a sevenfold decrease in India mean elimination from that country?"[59]

In retrospect, Fine justifiably complained that the administrative changes made the job of the epidemiologist extremely difficult: "Such changes pose considerable problems for efforts to compare disease types or treatment effects between populations or over time," so that "the change in statistical criteria had made it difficult to see if it [leprosy] is even dying, let alone to measure the speed of its demise".[60] But he was also quite sarcastic, referring to the discharge of cured people from the registers as "a fall in administrative burden". The elimination campaign was, in his view, a "political" initiative with "a strong lobby" that exhibited "crusading zeal" in support of multidrug therapy. He predicted that there would be "much number-dancing over the next decade, as different people try to interpret the target and as different organizations twist it in various ways in order to suit their own publicity needs".[61] In conclusion, he emphasised the evidence indicating that socioeconomic improvement and BCG had had an impact on the incidence of leprosy, adding: "We should not forget this, since it opens up a variety of approaches to leprosy control beyond case finding and treatment alone. If elimination is to be achieved, it will not be by MDT alone."[62]

Response of the International Federation of Anti-Leprosy Associations

S. K. Noordeen made every effort to marshal the resources of the NGOs to the leprosy elimination initiative. During his time in office, he attended International Federation of Anti-Leprosy Associations meetings and also met separately with members. As has already been indicated in Chapter 3, ILEP and its member associations were by no means homogenous in any respect, especially in their attitude to WHO's objectives. When Jean Loiselle became President of ILEP in 1990, he stressed in his speech that "Exchanges with the World Health Organization, with the International Leprosy Association and with the ILU [International Leprosy Union] and with all those involved in the fight against leprosy are essential in my view and we should continue to further them, respecting each other's identity and objectives."[63]

Yet the record shows that from the International Federation of Anti-Leprosy Associations' (ILEP's) point of view, WHO needed to be more consultative, and from WHO's point of view, ILEP needed to collaborate more with governments. WHO kept pointing ILEP towards national programmes, and ILEP kept asking for more international input. For example, when Noordeen suggested various ways in which WHO and ILEP could collaborate in the Leprosy Unit's Program for 1991, he suggested that members of the associations meet with leaders of the national leprosy control programmes in the countries where they were active. He also suggested that WHO could collaborate at a technical level "through participation at Medical Commission meetings and contacts with its members". But both the President and the General Secretary of ILEP expressed a desire for "more open and flexible cooperation with the Leprosy Unit" at the "level of global initiatives". They complained that "too often, useful activities or meetings occur without ILEP being informed well in advance". They suggested that "closer cooperation could lead to better identification, planning, coordination and practical follow-through of initiatives". They clearly felt the need for more reciprocal contact at the highest level and refused to be redirected to make more contact at the national level.[64]

To its credit, ILEP was actively pursuing its own agenda, and its Medical Commission was equally productive, developing numerous technical advisory documents such as those making recommendations on the use of blister packs, improving skin smears, and reading the bacterial index.[65] The Medical Commission was reorganised with expert groups that appointed temporary subgroups; for example, in 1991, the Expert Group on Leprosy Control had temporary subgroups on disability prevention, integration of leprosy control activities, extending the coverage of multidrug therapy, an editorial team for issuing guidelines, and one on ILEP indicators for monitoring leprosy control programmes.[66] The Expert Discipline for Therapy also had a temporary expert group on the treatment of reversal reactions.[67]

Member Associations were earnest in their desire to implement multidrug therapy in all of their programmes which they regularly evaluated, but the bureaucratic processes were quite lengthy and risked robbing the initiatives of their momentum. In June 1991, as part of the process of self-evaluation of the goal of "MDT for All, by the year 2000", the International Federation of Anti-Leprosy Associations' "Leprosy Control Expert Discipline, Expert Group on Extending the Coverage of MDT" reported to the coordinating bureau that they had identified fifteen countries that accounted for 86% of the known cases of leprosy. They were slightly shocked to discover that in ten of these countries "either no ILEP national coordinator had been appointed or co-ordination was in some way exceptional", which meant that "it appears not to be easy to apply ILEP coordination procedures to those countries or Indian states with particularly large numbers of leprosy patients". They also pointed out that in three of the four Indian states which accounted for 25% of the world total of registered cases, "LEP supported projects are treating 7% or less of the state total of patients".[68] They planned therefore to hand these findings over to the "Expert Discipline on Leprosy Control" so that it could prepare to be more involved in those key endemic areas.

Eighteen months later, they admitted that nothing much had changed in addressing this shortcoming: "Conscious that they had committed themselves eighteen months ago to increased activity in the priority States [in India] but that relatively little has so far happened, Members determined to take the important step of appointing ILEP coordinators for states in India."[69] At the same time, the fourth interface meeting on "achieving MDT for all by the year 2000" analysed the leprosy situation in five major countries or areas in order to set up temporary partnerships at the next working session so that members for each area would be able "to share their interests and co-ordinate their plans for the future".[70]

In light of this glacial pace, Noordeen's criticism in the same year appears a valid one. When he attended the ILEP Medical Commission meeting, on 3 June 1992, he complained that in spite of initiatives by ILEP members to increase multidrug therapy coverage, to study reversal reactions, and to initiate health education, there was continued reluctance to work closely with WHO and coordinate activities. He felt that the multilateral discussion revealed "ILEP's lack of interest in working with governments" and their predilection for planning in the abstract.[71] On a more encouraging note, he reported that "The bilateral discussions on Myanmar revealed ILEP members' continued interest in supplying drugs to the Myanmar programme through WHO."[72] Happily too, Trevor Durston's reminiscences indicate that ILEP coverage in India did improve:

Although ILEP had been established over 25 years before this time, it is interesting that only a few ILEP members (notably The Leprosy Mission as a lead player) were operational in India where about two thirds of all people affected by leprosy (whether new cases or people with disabilities) are living. ILEP started to challenge itself on these issues, and in 1994 agreed to be more proactive by allocating an ILEP member to be the lead (or coordinator) in each of the 6 priority states in India. Over the following years other ILEP members also joined forces to give more resources to the fight against leprosy in India.[73]

As a counter to the public health policies that underpinned the elimination goal, the International Federation of Anti-Leprosy Associations began to formalise its focus on care of the whole person by setting up a working group on the social aspects of anti-leprosy work. This was designed to "promote normalization of the life of persons with Hansen's disease within his/her community by non-medical means". (Normalisation meant both physical and social rehabilitation.)[74] To this end also, in 1996, the Medical Commission became the Medico-Social Commission.[75]

In its proliferation of committees and subcommittees, the International Federation of Anti-Leprosy Associations was in danger of becoming top-heavy and overly bureaucratic. André Récipon cautioned against what he called the "temptation of bureaucracy, commissions and numerous meetings", in his speech as outgoing president. He urged the member associations to:

> Avoid Parkinson's law, characterized by a sprawling administration, devouring time, money and human resources and, furthermore, totally inefficient. I am afraid that I see the beginnings of this temptation in the regular increase in the number of members attending different ILEP events. I am also afraid to see the lengthening of the meetings and the fact that the meetings are now held in the middle of the week and in places so far from the headquarters of ILEP which progressively excludes volunteers, as indeed does the increase in the number of meetings.[76]

Coordination between WHO and the International Federation of Anti-Leprosy Associations took place more successfully at regional and country level. For example, in 1991, the meeting on leprosy control strategy for the Americas was held between representatives of WHO, its American Regional office (AMRO), and ILEP in order to brief members on leprosy in the Americas and the initiatives being taken by AMRO on elimination.[77] There representatives of the member associations of ILEP reported on their work in the respective countries of the region.[78] There was activity in more than twenty countries, from Mexico and the Caribbean to Argentina. As well as the international agencies like WHO and its American regional office, there were benevolent associations based in Italy, the UK, Germany, Switzerland, Denmark, and the United States. Most either ran institutions or oversaw drug therapy programmes, while the Sasakawa Memorial Health Foundation supplied medications to Brazil and funded training for fieldworkers in Mexico, and LEPRA supplied vehicles for American Leprosy Missions projects in Mexico, Brazil, and Paraguay. Attendees agreed on the uncontroversial proposal that they should improve communication and coordination with each other, and they promised to develop ways of doing this at subsequent meetings.

Conclusion

The elimination campaign changed the definition of leprosy and its cure. Many felt that the emphasis had shifted from a "cure" in a diagnostic sense to a manipulated "cure" in a quantitative sense, and the grounds for contestation became the statistics. Two worlds of value were at odds here. The International Federation of Anti-Leprosy Associations' notion of a "cure" for leprosy was not the same as the WHO's notion of a "cure". In 1994, the General Secretary for ILEP, Paul Sommerfeld, described the differences between these two world views. The voluntary donor agencies had "the traditional vision of not-for-profit charitable organizations in liberal democracies". This was "to seek support for the needy, and to fill the gaps in provision".[79] Their vision was based on assumptions "antithetical to a purely public health approach". NGOs were ill at ease with the public health approach, if it meant that "the greatest good for the greatest number is achieved at the detriment of particular individuals".[80] He described the International Federation of Anti-Leprosy Associations' mantra of "MDT for All by the Year 2000" as "reflecting the hesitation of autonomous associations to be formally committed to common action" so that "it is more a statement of determined intent than a fully fleshed-out coordination strategy".

In contrast, the World Health Resolution for the Elimination was more managerial, with a measureable target; it was more political, in that it offered governments a dramatic achievement within a relatively short space of time; and it was less ambitious because it limited the horizon to leprosy as a public health problem, defining it at an arbitrary level which, although not easy, was "a practical possibility". The WHA resolution had an underlying assumption, which Sommerfield described as "difficult for the traditional humanitarian to accept". This was "that there will still be people whose problems either need not be seen as significant or who must be left to a later stage and further targets". For the International Federation of Anti-Leprosy Associations, this was the assumption inherent in the new definition of a "case of leprosy". For while the ILEP associations had "long accepted the opportunities offered by MDT – to reduce drastically the bacteriological load and thus the pool of transmission, and to prevent disabilities by early cure", they recognised that even with the most optimistic view of the success to be achieved with multidrug therapy, it must be assumed that at least the present generation of patients so affected will require some care throughout their lifetime. That in turn means maybe a further thirty to forty years of significant demand on health services.[81]

Sommerfeld finished his interpretation of the NGO position with a declaration on behalf of the member associations of "a lasting commitment to leprosy": "it is probably fair to say that there will be voluntary agencies active in support of people with leprosy long after the governmental bodies such as WHO have moved on to other organizational and political priorities".[82] For "With their humanitarian origins and purpose, however, they do not forget that at the end of the day it is the stigma of deformity, not the bacterium, which is the human tragedy of leprosy."

9

ELIMINATION, THE REALITY

It is astonishing to realise from the evidence of the documentary record that the whole process of distributing drugs to national programmes with enormous benefit for hundreds of thousands of people was up until then totally reliant upon the personal requests, placatory apologies, and expressions of thanks of Noordeen. The Chief of the Leprosy Unit of WHO was at the mercy of the benevolent organisations when it came to marshalling the necessary resources for the treatment of the world's leprosy patients. He had to mediate between the cash-strapped third-world governments and the NGOs on a case-by-case basis and often in circumstances of crisis. This is not to imply that the NGOs were not eager to supply the drugs. It is quite evident that the Damien Foundation, the American Leprosy Missions, and the Sasakawa Memorial Health Foundation, for example, were making every effort to facilitate these supplies. The logistics were also complex and involved many people, but at the core of the whole project were the will, conviction, and energy of a tiny group of individuals.

For the elimination programme to be successful, a regular and timely supply of multidrug therapy was of paramount importance. When Yohei Sasakawa offered to provide US$50 million for drugs over five years, the elimination campaign received a significant boost. This enabled WHO to assume the role of the major supplier of multidrug therapy, which it was able to distribute free of charge to leprosy-endemic countries.[1]

Following Yohei Sasakawa's announcement, in Hanoi, Kenzo Kiikuni began arrangements with WHO for setting up the leprosy drug fund on 16 August 1994.[2] This was to be a special fund, known as the Sasakawa Leprosy Elimination Trust Fund (SLEP-FUND), independent of the general budget and the already existing Sasakawa Health Trust Fund, and with separate accounting. It was exclusively to be put towards buying drugs for the global leprosy elimination programme for five years, starting 1 April 1994 and finishing 31 March 1999.[3] This made it possible for the Leprosy Unit to purchase and distribute multidrug therapy in blister packs to the twenty endemic countries with the highest prevalence of leprosy, from 1994 onwards.[4] The packs were prepared with doses appropriate to multibacillary or paucibacillary adult and child patients, and distributed to project workers in Asia, Africa, and South America.

The intervention of the Leprosy Unit into the distribution of the multidrug therapy supplies caused some precautionary anxiety among project workers. Wim H. van Brakel, the Project Director in the International Nepal Fellowship Leprosy Control Project in Pokhara, Nepal, expressed his concerns to Noordeen when he placed his order with the Chief of Leprosy Services in Nepal:

> Could you please inform us of the procedure of drugs supply? Will the drugs be sent directly to the project as before, or will they also be processed through His Majesty's Government Ministry of Health? If the latter is the case, this could lead to serious delays in the drug supply, which would need to be anticipated well in advance by ensuring a sufficient buffer stock of drugs.[5]

However, with an assured supply of chemotherapy from the Leprosy Unit, governments and voluntary organisations were able to reallocate funds to other aspects of leprosy control.

By 1997, forty countries were requesting blister packs,[6] with 7.5 million blister packs delivered the previous year to treat 920,000 people. From 1995 to 1997, 1.5 million people had been treated annually and about 700,000 cured every year. By then, WHO was supplying all of the drugs needed in twenty-two out of forty countries.[7] In the following year, this increased to fifty-four countries, in order "to cure over 2.35 million patients".[8] The blister packs were available in all the endemic countries without charge, in sufficient quantity to allow buffer stocks to be built up.[9] This was very reassuring for the local project workers whose access to the medications had often been precarious, and it made a huge difference to the efficacy and morale of the campaign.

In addition to the standard control efforts, very specific dedicated Leprosy Elimination Campaigns (LECs) and the Special Action Projects for the Elimination of Leprosy (SAPELs) were created. The Leprosy Elimination Campaigns were designed to find cases, reachable but for some reason not yet reached, while the Special Action Projects were designed to reach those who were unreachable by existing routine or health services.[10] SAPELs were based on the principle of equity, which ensured access to multidrug therapy by every leprosy patient, no matter how inaccessible their home. These special approaches were devised for difficult-to-access locales, but also served to heighten awareness of leprosy amongst those in general medical services and in community health services. In effect, they were vertical programmes executed with community participation.[11]

In looking back, Noordeen appraises these extremely creative initiatives with mixed feelings:

> LEC and SAPEL were initiatives to push further towards elimination. SAPEL was comparatively a smaller endeavor with varying results. On the other hand, LECs involved big funding running into millions of dollars. While the LECs produced excellent results in terms of awareness creation and detection of hidden cases it also had its negative features such as over-detection. As with any campaign, questions were also raised on its undermining general health services and also its cost effectiveness.[12]

Randall Packard was correct when he argued in 1997 that "Verticality remains a central organizational principle within WHO-sponsored programs despite years of post-Alma Alta rhetoric about the need for horizontal programs, infrastructural development, primary health care, and popular participation."[13] This was especially true if leprosy control in India is taken into account. However, as I have already argued, the Leprosy Unit was pragmatic on the question of whether or not to mobilise the resources of primary healthcare. If the implementation of multidrug therapy could be furthered by community involvement, then so be it. If a specialised vertical programme would make a difference, the Unit did not hesitate to institute it. If a large and populous country with poor infrastructure at the village level had a vertical programme for leprosy, then the transition to primary healthcare was deliberate and measured. At the same time, when running a quasi-vertical programme, administrators mobilised volunteers and the whole community, from its most influential members to villagers.

To implement the drug regimes, they drew on primary healthcare principles to entrust multidrug therapy to people for self-administration. Similarly, they simplified chemotherapeutic regimens in keeping with the values and more basic technologies of primary healthcare. They also streamlined administrative procedures in the same way, much to the chagrin of the epidemiologists. Yet special targeting and very local vertical campaigns were deployed as well, in spite of the criticism that this might rob primary healthcare in remote regions of funding and opportunities to develop. In all, there was a pragmatic application of whatever approach was feasible, and, at the same time, a progressive assimilation and integration of medical services across the whole community.

The Leprosy Elimination Campaigns (LECs) operated within the context of there being up to 1 million people with the disease who were as yet undetected.[14] They were innovative approaches that mixed vertical campaigns with community participation that would garner a great deal of publicity for detecting, treating, and informing people about leprosy. The campaigns were very specific events with predetermined end dates. They might be designed to provide training for local health workers, to mobilise volunteers for elimination activities, or to increase community awareness about leprosy, and they were framed within a country's overall programme against leprosy so that health and ministerial staff at the highest level were involved. WHO and other agencies were also to be present with whatever expertise was required. But it would all come down to volunteers and their community leaders.[15]

The LECs started first in areas with a population of around 500,000, but were later modified to cover larger areas and populations. They were carried out in twenty-four countries, identifying more than 450,000 new cases between 1995 and 1998. They were so successful that the LEC became one of the core activities of the Elimination Action Program.[16] The project grants varied considerably in size, as can be inferred from Table 9 below for 1996.

Table 9: Number of LECs Compared to Project Grants by Country

	Number of LECs	*Allocation/project (USD)*
WPRO		
Philippines	6	25,000
Vietnam	6	25,000
Cambodia	5	20,000
PNG	2	25,000
SEARO		
India	17	25,000
Bangladesh	14	20,000
Myanmar	15	15,000
Indonesia	6	35,000
Nepal	6	30,000

	Number of LECs	Allocation/project (USD)
EMRO		
Sudan	6	25,000
AMRO		
Brazil	4	45,000
AFRO		
Nigeria	5	30,000
Zaire	6	25,000
Ethiopia	6	25,000
Mozambique	6	25,000
Mali	3	25,000
Madagascar	3	25,000
Chad	2	25,000
Niger	2	25,000
Guinea	2	25,000

Noordeen then made arrangements to compile a photo library, for he reasoned that the success of the programmes would depend upon the level of community interest and energy generated. To that end, he made plans for developing the resources to create posters that would inform the general public about the disease and treatment.[17]

Fifty-two Special Action Projects for the Elimination of Leprosy had detected 3,396 patients. Ten Leprosy Elimination Campaigns had detected 4,500 new cases, in all. Ninety-three new LECs were expected to detect a further 23,000 cases. The whole south Indian state of Tamil Nadu carried out an LEC amongst a population of 59 million people and detected 12,865 new leprosy patients.[18] Leprosy Elimination Monitoring (LEM) had been carried out in six countries, and eight more were to follow. But while multidrug therapy was clearly making inroads, progress was neither extensive enough nor rapid enough to enable the elimination target to be reached on time. Locating and treating patients in cities, towns, and accessible villages was now almost routine, but did not come near the goal of "reaching every patient in every village".[19] International Conferences on Elimination first in Hanoi and then in Delhi, in October 1996 were held to buttress political commitment for further efforts.[20]

Failing to reach the elimination target

Surprisingly, while the data from twenty-four countries showed a dramatic decrease in prevalence from 1985 to 1995, the rate of newly detected cases remained static.[21] Admittedly overdiagnosis of paucibacillary (PB) patients, especially those with a single lesion, was boosting the newly detected cases. Patients were also being recycled; that is, people who had received an incomplete course of multidrug therapy, even if almost complete, were being re-treated and re-registered as new cases. Happily, though, several countries had achieved the target. In the American region (AMRO), Ecuador, Cuba, the Dominican Republic, Mexico, Uruguay, and the English-speaking Caribbean countries had achieved elimination of leprosy as a public health problem, as had the whole of the Eastern Mediterranean region, with the exception of Sudan and Somalia.[22] In the South East Asian Region (SEARO), Sri Lanka and Thailand had achieved elimination. In the Western Pacific, most of the countries in the region had reached the goal, and the region itself would achieve elimination by 1998. American Samoa, Kiribati, the Lao People's Democratic Republic, the Marshall Islands, Samoa, Singapore, and Vanuatu were expected to reach it within two years.[23] While registered cases had fallen from 5.4 million in 1985 to 888,340 in early 1997, the third Leprosy Elimination Advisory Group (LEAG) meeting learned that the new case detection rate remained about the same as it had for the last ten years.[24]

To the chagrin of many – and *schadenfreude* of others – the numbers of new cases that were being detected annually were still relatively stable. In the twelve most highly endemic countries, there were still 735,000 registered cases and 750,000 new cases, or about 4.5/10,000, just one year before the goal for elimination. Once again, further efforts had to be marshalled against the disease.

In 1997, Angelo Simonazzi, a new General Secretary for the International Federation of Anti-Leprosy Associations, was appointed to replace Paul Sommerfeld. The new president for 1998–2002 was Terry Vasey. The head of the Medico-Social Commission was Cairns Smith.[25] They would take the troubled relationship with WHO and the fight against leprosy into the new millennium. Also in that same year, in a sign of what was to come, Kommer Braber (Netherlands Leprosy Relief Association), expressed deep concern about the continuing publicity associated with the WHO "elimination" programme. In his view, the press releases "implying that the fight against leprosy is almost over" were "having a serious impact on the ability of leprosy associations to persuade potential donors to give funds for the work that we all know will be needed for decades to come". He saw the culprits as being "not so much the Leprosy Unit, as the DG and the press staff of WHO exaggerating a good story". Accordingly, he urged the President "to speak directly with the Director–General", and he called for the International Federation of Anti-Leprosy Associations to mount a counter-campaign.[26]

The Assembly discussed the degree of coverage for WHO press releases in various countries and the impact on donor governments. A "public attack on WHO" was inadvisable. It would be better "to express concerns within the network", to campaign for people affected by leprosy and not to campaign against WHO. Publicity should focus on the total burden of leprosy (social, disability, economic, and psychological, not just chemotherapy). At the end of the discussion, with no sense of irony, the President reminded delegates that the "Action Group on Fundraising" had been asked to consider these issues and advise on how best to counter the impact of "elimination" over the next two to three years.[27] He also indicated that he would ask to see the Director–General early in 1998.

For Noordeen, on the other hand, the world of value from which he was operating held out for a longer-term greater good. As he explains the varying degree of support that the elimination initiative received, he touches upon the different levels of comprehension and interest. He found that "the response to the WHO initiative was overwhelmingly positive". The WHO Regional Offices adopted resolutions at their Regional Committee meetings. The endemic countries also responded very positively, "although in some cases it took some time for them to act".

However, in his view there were problems with some international donor NGOs, "particularly those under the International Federation of Anti-Leprosy Associations (ILEP)". As he put it, "Their main concern was the fear that their donor community will interpret elimination as if leprosy will no longer be a problem after the year 2000." For him, the imperative was also very clear: "In terms of the long-term future, the importance of the public health goal of elimination of leprosy far outstripped the human problems to be faced in the short and medium terms." He drew support from those who shared the same public health aim: "The decision-makers at the ministries of health at the country level well understood the public health purposes of the WHO initiative and strongly supported it."[28] As a counter to this viewpoint, Geoff Warne emphasises that "ILEP member NGOs were out in the community delivering leprosy treatment and rehabilitation, as well as running hospitals, vocational training programs, and IEC activities, etc."[29]

The difference between two worlds of value ran deep and produced a great deal of ill feeling. There were many instances when the gap between the work towards elimination and the work of the NGOs widened. A further attempt to heal this wound would be forged through the formation of a Global Alliance for the Elimination of Leprosy (GAEL), at Abidjan, in Ethiopia, at the Third International Elimination Meeting in 1999.

As the target year of 2000 approached, the WHO's "Action Program for the Elimination of Leprosy" streamlined its name to the "Leprosy Elimination Project" (LEP). If this was in preparation for a triumphal conclusion to the campaign, it was premature. By June 1998, while "virtually every patient was receiving MDT", it was realised there were some countries that would not reach the elimination target by 2000.[30] There were other shadows, too. In the same year, S. K. Noordeen's term as Chief of the WHO Leprosy Unit concluded and he retired, while the great warrior and founder of Deutsche Aussatzigen Hilfwerk / German Leprosy Relief Association, Herman Kober, passed away. With Kober's vetoing influence removed, in the following year the General Assembly of the International Federation of Anti-Leprosy Associations "unanimously approved the request to enter into official relations with WHO". But it was an arrangement that was not to last for long, as the next chapter will reveal.[31]

In spite of the failure of twelve countries to achieve the elimination of leprosy as a public health problem by the year 2000, enormous progress had been made, and the leprosy landscape had changed forever. As early as 1987 Melville Christian had reported extremely encouraging developments: "Where MDT has been implemented in a systematic manner, there has been a dramatic decline in prevalence rates, within two to three years."[32] He was no longer seeing multibacillary cases amongst children. None of the new cases was showing deformities.[33] Most extraordinarily, he could also report a "perceptible decline in the social stigma against the disease".[34] People with the disease were "now being increasingly accepted in the main stream of community life in both towns and villages of the rural hinterlands in all countries in the South-East Asian Region".[35] By 2000, although the rate of new infections did not seem to have abated, Christian's optimistic observations had been replicated in all the endemic countries.

10

THE GLOBAL ALLIANCE FOR THE
ELIMINATION OF LEPROSY

We have seen that the International Federation of Anti-Leprosy Associations (ILEP) renewed its leadership in 1997–8 with Terry Vasey, Angelo Simonazzi, and Cairns Smith being the new incumbents as President, Secretary–General, and Head of the Medico-Social Commission respectively. A comparable change of leadership occurred at WHO, for when Gro Harlem Brundtland became the new Director–General in 1998 she announced that the top staff would be replaced by a completely new team. Brundtland described "the 'new' WHO as having a 'flatter structure, [with] better communication, more transparency, [and] a clearer distribution of responsibilities'".

This organisational change was viewed positively in the medical press. The authoritative *British Medical Journal* (*BMJ*) heralded it as "a radical break with the WHO's tarnished past", and praised the number of non-WHO personnel appointed to the board, their geographical mix, and the radical gender balance:

> Unusual within the United Nations system is the broad spectrum of background and experience that the new leadership brings to bear. Of the 10 holders of the cabinet positions, eight come from outside the WHO, and, remarkably for a traditionally male dominated organization, six (including Dr Brundtland) are women. All of the WHO's six regions are represented, with an even split between north and south.

Continuity, as far as leprosy was concerned, was limited to the reappointment of David Heymann whose task was to combat "new, emerging, and other communicable diseases (CDC), especially in the poorest countries".[1]

This chapter argues that while the organisational change accomplished in this new regime may have been generally good for WHO – and while David Heymann, Maria Neira, Denis Daumerie, and V. K. Pannikar took responsibility at various levels for the leprosy programme – the programme was managed within a consultative "cluster" by which decisions were shared. This had the effect of creating a leadership vacuum, especially after the strong leadership provided by Noordeen. Additionally, a culture gap opened out, for while Daumerie and Pannikar had belonged to the "Action Programme for the Elimination of Leprosy" (LEP) under Noordeen, neither Heymann nor Neira had worked with people in this field before, and its unique culture of single-minded dedication to a cause, as much as dedication to work against a disease, must have come as something of a shock. In short, they were outside the "family", admittedly a dysfunctional one, but still a small group of people who spoke the same specific language.

The international politics of the alliance

The changes at the top level of WHO made Yo Yuasa, of the Sasakawa Memorial Health Foundation, concerned about what was happening in the Leprosy Unit. Maintaining a place for leprosy on the international health agenda, and specifically within WHO, had required a deal of advocacy in 1948 and again in 1973 when Hubert Sansarricq was appointed. Yuasa was uneasy about the momentum of the Elimination movement and was keen to ensure that the Nippon Foundation would continue to be involved. At the end of September 1998, he wrote to David Heymann asking for the Director–General to reassure the Nippon Foundation, both in writing and at a face-to-face meeting with Yohei Sasakawa on 26 October, that WHO expected further financial support "for at least two more years, up to the end of the year 2000, if not longer".[2] David Heymann responded two weeks later reassuring him that the partnership with TNF was fully recognised and highly valued. He also assured Yuasa of the place of leprosy within the structure of the Communicable Diseases Cluster: "following intense discussions last week it has been agreed that leprosy elimination will be undertaken through the establishment of a Special Project, which will be fully responsible for its mandate".[3]

WHO had a new strategy in mind for leprosy: to marshal new partners, in a new configuration, with support from a new donor. In appraising Brundtland's "reinvention" of WHO, Brown and Cueto describe the way in which she strengthened WHO's financial position "largely by organizing 'global partnerships' and 'global funds' to bring together 'stakeholders' – private donors, governments, and bilateral and multilateral agencies – to concentrate on specific targets" such as "Roll Back Malaria" in 1998, the

Global Alliance for Vaccines and Immunization (GAVI) in 1999, and "Stop TB" in 2001.[4] On the downside of this, Brown and Cueto noted "a worrisome bias towards the private sector and, particularly, the seeming favoritism of the pharmaceutical industry in the *Commission on Macroeconomics and Health and the Private Public Partnerships*". Within this readjustment and re-securing of WHO's financial position and the role of donors, the position occupied by the Nippon Foundation was readjusted, specifically as regards its donation of drugs to the WHO leprosy elimination programme.

The drugs that made up multidrug therapy, or WHOMDT, were produced by different companies in a variety of locations. The manufacturers of the MDT blister packs for WHO in 1995–6 were Wolfs (Belgium) and Scanpharm (Denmark), but blister packs were also produced in Brazil, India, and Switzerland. Dapsone was manufactured mainly by Parke-Davis, Wellcome, Roussel UCLAF, and Bengal Chemicals. Clofazamine was mainly made by Ciba-Geigy and Astra India. Rifampicin was manufactured by both Lepetit and Ciba-Geigy. All three drugs were individually off-patent, and MDT, as a combination, had never been patented. The major producer of both clofazimine and rifampicin was now Novartis, which had been created by the 1996 merger of Ciba-Geigy and Sandoz Laboratories, so it was to Novartis that Bruntland turned. At the end of five years of the Nippon Foundation's financial support for anti-leprosy drugs, WHO set about securing another five years' supply directly from Novartis.

In May 1999, Dr Daniel L. Vasella, the President of Novartis International, in Basel, received a letter in the name of the Director–General thanking him for the offer from Novartis to donate multidrug therapy for the elimination of leprosy from 2000 until 2005. The letter explained that the offer was particularly opportune, "as the drug fund that has kindly been provided by the Nippon Foundation" was finishing, and a continued supply was imperative for intensive work in ten countries, for "If, as we project, the overall elimination target is not attained, there can be no question of bringing elimination efforts to a close."[5] Revealingly, the letter concluded by expressing "the need for WHO to reassert its role of leadership and advocacy in this field", and to that end a memorandum of understanding was prepared.

The other dimension of WHO's strategy was to reconfigure the alliance of partners involved in the elimination strategy. Leprosy prevalence in sixteen countries was still almost four times the level at which elimination could be declared, only one year before the target date. Furthermore, in other leprosy-endemic countries, the prevalence rate had levelled off at 1.6 per 10,000, and the new case detection rate was increasing. Clearly, ten countries would not reach the elimination target in time, and at the beginning of 1999, V. K. Pannikar called an informal meeting to review critically the global leprosy situation. Twelve days later, a Leprosy Elimination Advisory Group (LEAG) meeting was held with "potential partners" in order to forge "new and intensified partnerships" at the global, national, and local levels for an effective "Focused Strategy". This was designed to actively promote ownership of the goal, as well as make a place for partners "from other health disciplines" and also "from sectors other than health".[6]

While this made good theoretical sense, it failed to recognise the highly specific body of expertise that had been accumulated in the work against the disease, and more seriously failed to understand the importance of the (admittedly fraught) culture that had grown up amongst those who had a stake in that work. Obviously, it was designed to break the deadlock that Noordeen had experienced in dealing with the International Federation of Anti-Leprosy Associations. Even more obviously, it was an attempt to wrest away the initiative taken by SMHF/The Nippon Foundation. Most of all, it was designed to reassert WHO's leadership and authority. In doing so, it failed to recognise the subtle balance between those long-standing organisations, whose conflicts were paradoxically founded in the passionate conviction of each in the importance of their differing, but ultimately overlapping, goals. This was something that Noordeen appreciated, but not something that Brundtland, Heymann, or Neira grasped as truly significant.

Meanwhile, in a countermove, Yuasa made a separate and strategic approach to the ILEP organisations. That he was able to do this, effectively switching his allegiance from WHO to ILEP, demonstrates how much of a shared culture existed between these long-standing organisations and how closely related were their goals, even if they differed on how to reach them. Yuasa arranged support between the Nippon Foundation and the Raoul Follereau Foundation for the next international gathering on the elimination of leprosy to be held in Africa.

The location had originally been planned for Ethiopia, but its government had been unsupportive. WHO/LEP had then unilaterally approached Tanzania, whereas Yuasa hoped to reorganise the venue in a French-speaking African country that needed to be encouraged towards the elimination goal as a beneficial side effect of the gathering. As he explained it to Ji Baohong, the Medical Consultant for the Follereau Foundation, WHO/LEP had taken the initiative to approach Tanzania "without our prior consent ... but we are assured by WHO/LEP that it is possible to choose some other country within the African region, if our Foundation so desire, and it is also possible to cancel the request to Tanzania without too much difficulty".[7] Then he formally approached André Récipon, President of the Follereau Foundation, to insinuate that the Nippon Foundation would be withdrawing from collaborating with WHO after the year 2000, "at least in monetary terms". He suggested that "the sooner WHO established closer ties with other ILEP members the better". He suggested that the Follereau Foundation's collaboration with WHO/LEP made its sponsorship of the forthcoming conference extremely important.[8] This gathering, the Third International Conference for the Elimination of Leprosy, was eventually held on 15–17 November 1999, in Abidjan, Côte d'Ivoire, co-sponsored by WHO, TNF, and FRF. Here the seeds of dissension would finally sprout their first clearly visible shoots, as the individual trajectories of WHO, the International Federation of Anti-Leprosy Associations, and TNF inevitably collided.

The increasingly poor communication between WHO and ILEP can be illustrated by an informal meeting, held by Maria Neira the month before the planned international conference, during which she presented the conclusions of the supposedly consultative process as if they were a *fait accompli*. She told the invitees that "All partners are convinced that the creation of a Global Alliance will help to solve the remaining problems and will best facilitate the function of coordination."[9] In telling potential members of the Alliance what they were supposedly "convinced" of, she pre-empted what they were being asked to consider. This high-handed mode of discourse would rapidly alienate and in some cases infuriate the Associations. Even allowing for difficulties of cultural interpretation, it is understandable that many interpreted this as condescending.[10] Thus, from its very launch in November 1999, the Global Alliance for the Elimination of Leprosy (GAEL) was hindered by communication difficulties which would rapidly take on a financial dimension.

The new Global Alliance was announced at the Elimination Conference in Abidjan in a press release with the title, "Abidjan – Today." This partnership was designed to complete "the elimination of a disease from which humankind has suffered, physically and psychologically, for thousands of years". The press release stated that each of the partners pledged financial support: The Nippon Foundation pledged US$24 million; Novartis, US$30 million in medications over six years; and the International Federation of Anti-Leprosy Associations, US$19.5 million, from their US$65 million budget. Terry Vasey, the President of ILEP, was quoted as saying, "ILEP members believe that the Global Alliance is an essential part of our wider strategy for the fight against leprosy. We welcome the creation of the Alliance and we look forward to working closely with all the partners in a renewed spirit of collaboration."[11] The press release was embargoed until "11.30 GMT on 15 November 1999".

Four days before the embargo expired on 11 November, ILEP Press Officer, Joyce Massé faxed her counterpart at WHO, "Melinda. I know it is very, very late, but is it possible that you can amend the press release? We would like you to omit the figure of US$19.5 million. Please get in touch a.s.a.p. Thanks, Joyce."[12] The WHO copy of the fax is endorsed for reply: "Sorry – PR already printed and distributed (under embargo)" signed: "G. Hartl INF, WHO". But there is a further unsigned endorsement addressed to Robert Sattele, the Deputy Head Base Business of Novartis, expressing concerned incomprehension: "Robert, This is a mystery. Joyce Massé is apparently the ILEP Press Officer. Will let you know if we have any further information on this." It appeared that ILEP had pulled the plug on its donation to the Global Alliance at the last minute.

Two months later, in February 2000, WHO held discussions on GAEL in Geneva. On behalf of the Director–General, David Heymann expressed support for the private/public partnership typified by GAEL. He drew attention to the Director–General's personal efforts to bring the elimination goal to the attention of various countries. He described GAEL as an "open, transparent partnership that anyone could join or leave as they saw fit (including individual NGOs)" that would "provide a forum for coordinating leprosy elimination activities". It was "a high-level political forum" for leprosy elimination with a mission to facilitate the exchange of ideas and advocacy, to mobilise political support, to ensure a common strategy and approach, and to identify gaps and mobilise resources to fill them. WHO was to act as the "secretariat" for the Alliance and provide technical leadership. A Technical Advisory Group (TAG) would review progress and guide WHO and GAEL. The guiding principles of the Alliance were "complete transparency of the partners with regard to strategies, activities and budgets", "a clear definition of roles and responsibilities of partners", and a focus on field activities rather than "on preparing for committees and meetings".[13] Denis Daumerie outlined the current status of the elimination initiative, pointedly drawing attention to a "critical funding gap" of US$44 million.[14] Contributions from the Nippon Foundation and Novartis were then described by their representatives.

At the meeting, Terry Vasey underscored the fundamental independence of the individual member associations of the ILEP: "At their General Assembly meeting in Delhi in December, most members had endorsed the Alliance and given the President/Standing Committee a mandate to support it." He reiterated that ILEP was made up of individual autonomous member associations. He also clarified the support offered by ILEP to GAEL: "The US$19.5 million that had been promised as ILEP's contribution to the Alliance comprised the individual member associations' activities." His hands were tied, for as he put it, "He was only able to encourage individual associations to be guided by the strategy." To that end, "Bilateral discussions with some members were being held and further discussion was required with other members at country level."

To a large extent, this was a replay of old problems in a new arena. In its effort to streamline and focus the anti-leprosy work, GAEL had come up against the jealously guarded independence of the individual ILEP Federation members and the consequent powerlessness of the ILEP executive. Thus, GAEL partners had to understand that the pledge from ILEP was not new, or even dedicated money, but rather a guesstimate of what its individual members would be spending on their own anti-leprosy programmes in the coming year. This support covered diverse activities and had never, at any stage, been intended to be at the disposal of GAEL.[15]

Additionally, ILEP were concerned with WHO's dissemination of public information, and they issued a veiled criticism of several press releases from Brundtland herself about elimination. Terry Vasey complained that "this provided a false illusion that after leprosy elimination had been achieved, no further resources would be needed for any sort of leprosy activities". Such messages were "totally counterproductive to traditional ILEP activities that dealt with the social aspects of people whose lives have been affected by the consequences of leprosy and for whom, according to ILEP, considerable resources would be required for many years after elimination had been achieved".[16] This again was a replay of an old ILEP anxiety that the WHO approach was broad-brush, overly concerned with media-worthy "results", and neglectful of the ongoing physical and social needs of patients, especially those who had suffered nerve damage and deformity.

The meeting concluded with both sides undertaking to make changes. Vasey agreed to write to those member associations appealing for money for treatment. WHO also "officially requested ILEP to revise its strategy and to actively include leprosy elimination in its activities". ILEP agreed to encourage the members "to ensure that core leprosy elimination activities are implemented in all areas in which member associations were active". In return, WHO "agreed to ensure that in future the media would be adequately briefed on the full meaning of 'elimination' and made to understand that it did not mean that the physical and socioeconomic after-effects of leprosy would have disappeared".[17]

Politically, though, irrevocable damage had been done. Vasey's defence of the "withdrawal" of the ILEP pledge persuaded the GAEL partners that if they wanted to achieve anything with the ILEP members, who actually controlled the resources, they were better off dealing with them individually. After politely but perfunctorily acknowledging that "The role of ILEP is important," GAEL proposed exploring "bilateral agreements directly with individual associations" or "multipartite agreements ... for elimination activities in some major endemic countries".[18]

GAEL was formally inaugurated in Delhi, at the end of January 2001, but instead of forging bonds and alliances between anti-leprosy organisations, it furthered division. At this meeting, the aspirations of the "Delhi Declaration" – the public resolution that the attendees enunciated in support of the elimination initiative – was the final straw for ILEP. In their view, it enshrined assumptions running counter to their *modus operandi*, particularly the promise to consign leprosy to history with a "final push". The declaration announced that "In order to make *The Final Push* to detect and cure all the remaining leprosy cases in the world and thereby eliminate leprosy from every country by the year 2005, a Global Alliance for the Elimination of Leprosy was created in November 1999."[19]

Étienne Declercq, as the chairman of ILEP's Medico-Social Commission, wrote to WHO on 8 October 2001. "I have been asked by Mr Terry Vasey, President of ILEP, to outline the reasons that have pushed the ILEP Medico-Social Commission to advise ILEP to withdraw from the GAEL."[20] The ILEP MSC expressed concern that "the Alliance has become an instrument of WHO to achieve its political agenda to reach the elimination target at any price". They argued that using the "prevalence of registered cases as the single indicator to evaluate whether leprosy has been eliminated from a country or not" had "no sound epidemiological basis". Furthermore, they objected to the message that leprosy will disappear naturally once prevalence is below 1 per 10,000, and they objected even more to WHO's disseminating this through the media. They described the rhetoric of "the final push" as "completely misleading" because it gave the wrong impression that, by the year 2005, "the leprosy problem will not exist anymore". This would then have a long-term detrimental impact on work yet to be done.

The MSC also expressed concern about WHO's technical policies: "Despite strong opposition from ILEP experts and the scientific community, WHO had unilaterally introduced a number of technical policies in the field, with very weak, if any justification at all." Patients were sent off with their whole course of treatment in blister packs, no longer needing to attend the health clinic, which the MSC considered an "absolutely unethical" practice. Slit smear examination was no longer mentioned; lip service only was paid to preventing disabilities. Worse still, the MSC complained that WHO had damaged ILEP's credibility with various countries:

> There is no real partnership within GAEL. It is currently dominated by the WHO. Its operation lacks transparency and democracy. The views of other partners, particularly those of ILEP, are deliberately ignored. What is more, the role of ILEP has been repeatedly minimized by the WHO, including in public meetings. This undermines the position of ILEP, with the result that difficulties are met with some governments. It is felt that WHO, which is in a stronger position than ILEP to influence governments, is instrumental in current attitudes to ILEP. A final example to illustrate the fact that the spirit of partnership has never been developed: representatives of the WHO and the TAG have been invited to attend the last three meetings of the MSC, unfortunately to no avail.

The letter concluded that "In view of the above, we advise ILEP to clearly differentiate itself from the Alliance. To withdraw from the GAEL is probably the only way for ILEP to show its disapproval of these policies."[21]

David Heymann, as Executive Director, Communicable Diseases, emailed Étienne Declercq to announce that the WHO Leprosy Unit was referring the issues to its body of experts (the Technical Advisory Group) and seeking "official permission" to circulate Declercq's letter to members of that Group. "If TAG members agree with your views, that the ILEP position is not compatible with the GAEL principles, WHO will inform other partners in the Alliance."[22] This move had the effect of publicising ILEP's withdrawal threat to non-aligned leprosy experts and crystallising it, so that it would be very difficult to retreat from.

In response, the Technical Advisory Group pointed out that the question of interrupting transmission was an unknown area, and "elimination" had been defined as "lowering [the] disease level to a threshold from where it would disappear in the natural course," but "nobody knows this level of threshold".[23] The TAG did record "reservations regarding [the] projected expected outcome of [the] strategic plan on reducing transmission to [an] insignificant level, for solid evidence to make such a statement was lacking" and "as a result, WHO had modified its strategic plan based on these observations". Regarding the length of multidrug therapy regimens, they noted that "further observations strongly suggest that it should be possible to shorten the period of MDT particularly for MB cases, detected in program situations". It requested studies on accompanied MDT and stated quite strongly and pointedly that "sustainable vertical leprosy programs will be a nonviable proposition" in the future.

Importantly, in their view: "the political will and commitment generated through the goal of leprosy elimination has been tremendous and needs to be sustained". They concluded with a glimmer of evident frustration: "All these issues have been discussed threadbare by the TAG. TAG is of the considered opinion that there is no need to change the present definition of elimination of leprosy." The meeting concluded that the "TAG is therefore entirely satisfied with the very responsible secretariat for leprosy in WHO." Additionally, and rather confrontationally, it added that

> If ILEP thinks otherwise, they may feel free to quit GAEL. Leprosy Elimination programs in different countries need technical inputs from WHO at this decisive stage of the war against leprosy. We therefore encourage WHO to concentrate on these issues, and not to get bogged down with issues like membership of GAEL.

It is one of the ironies of this disputatious situation that the field of international experts was so small that the same figure could appear in opposing camps. Cairns Smith belonged to both the WHO's Technical Advisory Group and ILEP's Medico-Social Commission, and would be a member of the organising committee for ILEP's forthcoming Technical Forum.

Meanwhile, WHO prepared to declare that the disease had been eliminated globally. To this end, Yohei Sasakawa was invited to attend a special event at the WHA at which a select panel reported on the global achievement of elimination to delegates from all concerned member states.[24] It is quite extraordinary that the goal of eliminating leprosy, as declared in the WHA 44.9 resolution, had been achieved, yet the official acknowledgement of this became a non-event in the face of the conflict between the stakeholders.

In WHO's report of activities to the Nippon Foundation for 2002 and their proposal for 2003, this achievement is put into historical perspective. It marked the final phasing out of traditional control programmes carried out by specialised workers and institutions. Responsibility for making a diagnosis of leprosy and treating people with the disease was now integrated into the primary healthcare system. Intensive media campaigns had made communities more aware of the importance of detecting and treating leprosy early so that people had a chance of escaping serious disability. Leprosy could be treated "like any other skin disease". Treatment was free and available in the community. Amidst all of the controversy and passionate debate, this had been a remarkable achievement that WHO felt vindicated the elimination strategy.[25] Yet the objections to the nature of the goal and the means employed to reach it still had to run their course, as the Alliance continued to deteriorate.

Members from WHO and ILEP met on 7 December 2001 in Geneva at the request of the President of ILEP to discuss the recommendation of the ILEP Medico-Social Commission to withdraw from GAEL.[26] Heymann, who in no way was going to allow ILEP to use the threat of its leaving the Alliance as grounds for renegotiating WHO policy, declared: "Two years after the creation of GAEL, it is clear that the time has come to diverge partnerships away from global federations such as ILEP to individual NGOs that were already working closely with member countries at national level, as well as in the field." The meeting therefore accepted "the recommendation for ILEP's withdrawal from GAEL" and decided that "Individual ILEP member associations together with other international, national or local NGOs, who agree to subscribe to the GAEL principles, would be invited to join GAEL as full partners."

Maria Neira of WHO emailed all members of the Alliance and the WHO Regional Offices to inform them that ILEP was no longer a member of GAEL,[27] reinforcing this with a specific instruction to "ensure there is no mention of ILEP as a member of GAEL in any documents, speeches or notes". They were encouraged to invite "only relevant individual national and international NGOs" to meetings "and not ILEP as a Federation". The way ahead was that "from now on GAEL will be open to other partners, including individual NGO members of ILEP and any others who subscribe to GAEL principles".[28]

11

A QUESTIONABLE VICTORY

This period began with the creation of the WHO-inspired Global Alliance for the Elimination of Leprosy (GAEL) to make a "final push" against leprosy. This was followed by a counter action by the International Leprosy Association (ILA) to initiate its own Technical Forum to weigh, reconsider, and revise the technical advice provided by the WHO. Since WHO's Leprosy Unit had been the primary source of technical expertise on leprosy treatment, the ILA was staking a claim to more agency in producing its own recommendations for treatment of leprosy. The period culminated in the specially commissioned independent evaluation of GAEL that attempted to mediate between the former members of the fractured Alliance. The difficulties and disagreements within GAEL eventually enabled the individual member associations of the International Federation of Anti-Leprosy Associations (ILEP) to forge a new alliance with a geographically resituated WHO leprosy unit in New Delhi, and convert the leprosy elimination programme into a sustainable leprosy control programme. Meanwhile, as this disturbing international contest played itself out, ordinary people accomplished the extraordinary task of bringing treatment to the millions suffering from leprosy. Yet in spite of all their efforts, and in spite of all the high-principled contestation of the international bodies about the reliability of the statistics, the numbers of new cases being detected throughout the world showed little, if any, decline.

The ILA Technical Forum

A scientific front in the struggle against the WHO for leadership of leprosy treatment was opened in 2001 by a former WHO staffer who then worked as a research scientist in Paris and served on ILEP's Medico-Social Commission. Dismayed at a decline in new research findings, and intrigued by the technical debates around the elimination strategy, Ji Baohong proposed the establishment of a regular Technical Forum sponsored by various ILEP members.[1]

In preparation for the forum, Ji emphasised that "All the activities should be transparent," and "major decisions will be taken only by consensus".[2] He desired a purely scientific document that would withstand scrutiny and peer review and was authorised by the ILA. He knew that the Forum would not have the status of the WHO Expert Committee, but he hoped that the opinions from the Forum would carry comparable weight. Moreover, the objectives of the Technical Forum had to be clearly defined, well formulated, and achievable.[3]

There were difficulties in trying to review the effectiveness of current technical policies because documentation and reporting were often non-existent. A number of policies had never been formally recorded, or were recorded only in working papers of WHO meetings or non-peer-reviewed journals. Ji was concerned that there was simply not enough solid data "to support some of our arguments". Neither was it possible to collect new data within the coming months.[4] As a solution, Cairns Smith suggested using the criteria established for "evidence based medicine". Each piece of literature could be examined for relevance and then classified according to the weight of evidence it contributed. The best evidence was produced from meta-analysis of several randomised, controlled trials. Expert opinion, unsupported by evidence from clinical trials, had a lower status. "So while there may not have been much 'solid data' to support some of our arguments," he stated, "it would be progress to admit this and identify the gaps in our knowledge rather than making recommendations which are poorly supported." He suggested that "if we systematically searched and critically reviewed the evidence and presented recommendations in this way it would give the document much more credibility".[5]

From 25 to 28 February 2002, the International Leprosy Association Technical Forum was held in Paris.[6] Its findings were published in the *International Journal of Leprosy* and *Leprosy Review*.[7] The report had the status of an authoritative document under the auspices of the ILA, and it was circulated at the ILA's 16th International Leprosy Congress, held in Salvador, Brazil, in 2002. The Technical Forum tested the WHO-recommended policies on diagnosis and classification, treatment, prevention of disability and rehabilitation, epidemiology and control, and finally the organisation of leprosy services. Evidence in each of the areas was assessed in a hierarchy of categories, in accordance with those employed under the rubric of evidence-based medicine.[8] The conclusions and recommendations of the report were graded so that evidence-based recommendations were designated as "EB". Those conclusions for which evidence was found to be lacking were designated as "best practice" (BP), and those requiring further research were designated (R).[9]

The underlying impulse in the ILA Technical Forum report was a desire to wrest back control for administering MDT on scientific grounds. Under the WHO policy, control of diagnosis and treatment had been progressively relegated to quasi-primary healthcare/general medical services since the 1970s. The scientists of the Forum made a case for better monitoring by the experts who could keep ongoing records for scientific and epidemiological purposes. This underlying impulse is evidence of the ongoing conflict between the public health model of healthcare based on primary healthcare, which gave responsibility back to people at the periphery, and the leprosy control model that took medical and scientific responsibility for "cases", with the long-term aim of being able to measure the success of the treatment.

The report stressed the importance of integration into general health services (a process that had been going on for over thirty years), as something that should be well-planned and implemented methodically. There was little faith in the notion that people could take responsibility for their own health, and even less faith in the quality of general medical services in third-world countries and in their readiness to care for people with leprosy. People were absorbed into the larger healthcare system, and after they had been treated were no longer considered "cases". They were not followed up and their records were discarded, so their progress after treatment was not monitored.[10] In short, the broad success of multidrug treatment in the community militated against monitoring the success or otherwise of individual cases.

The rhetoric of leprosy control for scientific purposes permeated the Forum. The policy of handing out multidrug therapy to patients for self-administration drew strong reservations because less frequent contact between patients and health workers raised issues about their compliance with treatment, especially since monitoring successfully completed treatment was necessary to evaluate the success of a programme.[11] The Forum outlined "best practice" as opposed to the profound pragmatism of the simplified public health approaches evolved by LEP, along primary healthcare principles. The Forum emphasised the need for more research, the need for more evidence about the optimal duration of regimens, and generally a return to greater surveillance of the patient. This ran counter to the impetus towards integration into general medical services and the emphasis on primary healthcare which handed responsibility back to the community and the patient. The Forum, in contrast, mourned the "loss" of the patient as "evidence" for the way in which the programme was developing. The "success" of the devolution and democratisation of treatment made it difficult to measure its success empirically and scientifically.

The report concluded that actual prevalence was likely to differ significantly from the available figures, which were based on the patients registered for treatment. To that could be added the large number of people living with the consequences of leprosy. Importantly, "despite a dramatic reduction of the number of registered cases, the global new-case detection-rate has not declined. Furthermore, there is no evidence that, once a predefined level of prevalence rate was reached, leprosy will necessarily die out". Significant numbers of new patients would continue to present themselves for many years to come so that it was essential to sustain leprosy control activities, even in countries or areas that had officially reached the elimination target.

These findings provided a foundation for the discussion and debates that took place at the ILA Congress in Salvador, Brazil, in 2002, where everyone was encouraged to "review their recommendations and guidelines for leprosy related activities in the light of the [ILA Technical Forum] report".

The evaluation of GAEL

By the end of 2002, the drama in GAEL occasioned a WHO-commissioned independent "Evaluation of the Global Alliance for the Elimination of Leprosy", whose report was handed down in June 2003.[12] The evaluation attempted to draw all the collaborators into a balance that respected their various areas of expertise and rebuilt respect for the "entire spectrum" of activities against the disease by addressing the Manichean divide between a public health approach and what it termed a "clinical approach" or a "patient-centred approach".[13] While the evaluation applauded the smooth collaboration between partners in various countries, it observed that the relations between some of the collaborators at the international level were very bad, to the extent that the Global Alliance was "not adding the value that it could and this poses threats to country leprosy programs and to the reputations of collaborators on leprosy work".[14] It recommended that the Alliance be "rebuilt and refined immediately".[15]

Problems had sprung from several areas:

> The evaluation team believes that the clinical *vs.* the public health approach may drive some of these differences of view. Some may be driven by

personality differences. Some may be driven by the desire of organizations that work on leprosy to maintain the base of their constituents and their programs. Some may be driven by honest and well-founded concerns.[16]

While difficulties and misunderstandings were inevitable, those that had arisen had not been dealt with at all well.[17] At the outset, understanding of the nature of GAEL, the roles that individual members would play, and how the Alliance was to be governed had not been clear.[18] People perceived that the Alliance had been too embedded in the WHO, and it was not sufficiently open and consultative.[19] Specifically, there were technical issues that had not been sufficiently discussed to the satisfaction of all the participants.[20] The new team at the WHO was perceived to be target-driven at the expense of other important aspects of the work against leprosy.[21]

To counter this, the evaluation recommended that the collaborators learn "appropriate lessons from the Alliance's work to date and its breakdowns in trust and communications". This they must do, the evaluation stated, "with humility and a spirit of give-and-take".[22] It recommended that the NGOs and the Foundations convene a Collaborator's Forum at which issues could be openly discussed and debated.[23] It recommended that collaborators complement each other by working through country-led task forces. The WHO was to focus on technical advice to country programmes, and coordinate evaluation and monitoring by appointing an independent panel of experts.[24]

It is disturbing to find, in light of the evidence provided already, that the evaluation mentioned several times that ILEP had been expelled from the Alliance.[25] This seems to indicate that the whole chain of events described earlier had not been made available to the evaluation team. More importantly, no one recognised that the problems in GAEL had been brewing in the anti-leprosy community for a very long time and had only been brought to a head by the creation of the GAEL. WHO's representation of its achievements had been a matter of concern for the ILA from the very earliest days, when the 1st Expert Committee on Leprosy met. The policies on shortened regimes and the changes to the definition of a case and the shifts in classification occurred before the Alliance had been formed.

Many of these simplified approaches to treatment had developed out of WHO's focus on primary healthcare. Some of the blame for the complete breakdown in communication may actually be traced to the structural changes within WHO in which the authority for decision-making and communication took place amongst those who simply did not appreciate the culture of the participants. At the same time, ILEP was not straightforward in bringing all of its objections against WHO to bear on the technical changes. ILEP's very existence was threatened by the elimination programme. Noordeen had managed to handle this because he understood that in spite of the problems between the different groups, they all shared the same goal. But he was no longer there to mediate in the way in which he had previously. Denis Daumerie had a different, less compromising, approach. He saw the voluntary organisations as having too much influence, and he confronted them, whereas Noordeen had delighted in "reasoning" with opposing opinions. And behind it all, Yuasa, who had been humiliated by WHO's rejection of TNF donations for medication, attempted to wrestle back influence. The evaluation told the truth in the most diplomatic way possible, but as a result of this enquiry WHO's Leprosy Unit seemed to lose a great deal of confidence and direction.

People power in India

In sharp contrast to what was happening in the international politics of leprosy, in the nations of the world, people at every level of society were willingly being marshalled as volunteers to find and treat those infected with leprosy. In one of the major achievements of the elimination initiative, the programmes that mobilised whole populations in dynamic and creative ways did so with a view to handing over responsibility for their health to the people.

In the second half of February 1997, the whole of the vast state of Tamil Nadu in South India conducted a Modified Leprosy Elimination Campaign (MLEC) designed to find hidden cases of leprosy "of consequence". This involved directing volunteers and the entire health infrastructure of the State to uncover any "substantial hidden caseload" of MB leprosy.[26] Guidelines for the campaign were produced by the Director of the Medical Services with the State Leprosy Officer. All of those involved were instructed according to the standardised format prepared at the state headquarters to understand and identify the disease, to encourage people to diagnose symptoms themselves and report to their health centre, to minimise stigma, and to improve the multidrug therapy services.[27]

Initially, the media were saturated with information about leprosy, especially about reducing stigma and encouraging people to go to a health centre if there were any suspicious physical signs of the disease. While the messages were prepared in the state ministry, using Information, Education and Communication (IEC) experts, the district leprosy officers were given the freedom to adapt the messages so that they would be appropriate in their localities. Much of this media time was donated. C. K. Rao reported that

> Doordarshan had contributed its time liberally free of cost on all its channels to convey the message and appeal by high political and administrative functionaries and so had the All India Radio. Several donors/NGOs paid for the time on private TV channels to convey messages on leprosy relevant to the campaign involving public/popular film personalities.[28]

This succeeded in creating "a wave of awareness" in preparation for the leprosy campaign. Messages "reached all communities including the highest social and economic strata of society".

The district leprosy officers then planned with the primary healthcare centres how to go about the house-to-house and village-to-village searches for anyone with the disease. The national leprosy programme was still a vertical one in Tamil Nadu, so that this was the first time many primary healthcare workers were engaging with leprosy. There was a primary health centre for every 30,000 people in the state, and the Director of Public Health and Preventive Medicine thoroughly endorsed the involvement of medical officers and the staff of the centres. The medical officers themselves were also positively disposed and did not feel that their involvement in coordinating the campaign in their area took away from their routine tasks.

Members of these centres were assigned to teams with one or two others, to act as searchers for groups of 2,000 or 3,000 people for eight days. People were drawn from such health services as the "Tamil Nadu Noon-Meal Programme", the "Nutrition Programme, the Integrated Child Development Service". Additionally, numerous volunteers – students from paramedical schools, high schools, and colleges – were recruited as searchers and helpers in their communities.[29] Various members of the community also contributed to the campaign in a spirit of generosity and with a sense of collective endeavour. C. K. Rao comments in an astonishing admission, in light of the history of stigma associated with leprosy throughout the world, let alone India, that

> It was heartening to observe that posh localities in corporations/districts considered it a privilege to receive the searchers and co-operate with them. Some of the experienced NGOs have reported that they were pleasantly surprised to see the unprecedented awareness in the communities on leprosy elimination. They considered that this campaign has achieved a lot more than what was possible with the health education activities under the program during its last 40 years of operation.[30]

After the eight-day campaign came to a close, several of the medical officers and staff in the primary healthcare centres continued to seek out new cases amongst their outpatients and also during field visits, and so continued their role in treating leprosy. As a result of the campaign, some defaulters returned to treatment, and C. K. Rao observed that having primary healthcare doctors involved helped persuade people to undergo treatment once more.[31] Similarly, those drawn from allied health services enjoyed their tasks and were well received in the community. Even after the close of the campaign, health workers continued to be aware of the possibility of leprosy and were prepared to refer suspected cases for confirmation of their diagnosis.[32]

The district leprosy officers oversaw the campaign daily. Medical officers coordinated the campaigns in their areas and worked with the specialised leprosy staff to review and confirm the diagnoses of people who had been found by the searchers. The enthusiasm of the searchers produced many false positives. There were only 12,556 cases confirmed from among 228,724 suspected cases. Those who had missed the examinations were given the opportunity to present themselves for examination, and out of another 116,859 who reported to the primary health centres 705 people were diagnosed with leprosy. In addition, most of the staff were also examined, and 12,868 were confirmed as having leprosy.[33]

The funding for the campaign came from the National Program, the World Bank, and the Danish Assisted Leprosy Eradication Program (DANLEP). Most of the money was spent on the IEC materials, training, and mass media. The searchers received Rs 25 a day.[34] Rao stated that "The program did not seek the funds from ILEP member participating agencies as the resources mobilized met the needs of the campaign." Nonetheless, "All the NGOs participated in subsequent Modified Leprosy Elimination Campaigns (MLEC) in their area."[35]

Of those diagnosed with leprosy, only 8% of the 12,556 new cases suffered from MB leprosy, and of those less than half showed positive skin smear tests. Between 80% to 90% of the PB cases had only a single lesion. Rao concluded that "the assumption that considerable hidden cases exist in the State has not been supported by the results of the campaign". A large proportion of these single lesion cases would have healed spontaneously. Happily, only 2% of the new cases had a disability of grade II, which meant that most of the newly detected cases were recent and early.[36] Nonetheless, in the two months following the campaign, the number of people presenting themselves voluntarily for diagnosis and treatment increased.[37] The community was now aware of leprosy, and people were volunteering for treatment at the merest suspicion of the disease. The age-old fear of leprosy was disappearing.

C. K. Rao wholeheartedly endorsed the responses to the campaign from all levels of politics. He commented that "Despite the declining number of leprosy cases during the last ten years in the State, it is heartening to note that the political will displayed towards this MLEC was unparalleled and perhaps comparable to [the] successful pulse polio campaign undertaken recently."[38] The Chief Minister and the Health Minister directed the MPs, the Members of the Legislative Assembly (MLAs), and the mayors to give the campaign the highest priority so that it would be successful. This response filtered down to the local leaders in the districts, blocks, and villages. As Rao described it: "The leadership at all levels was involved not only in the inauguration of the campaign in their respective areas and also in repeated appeals, before and during the campaign, to the public through TV, radio, press for the success of the campaign."[39] He singled out the Director of Medical Services (Dr M. Kamatchi) and the District Leprosy Officer (Dr Andrews Deenabandhu), both of whom were tirelessly and successfully persuasive: "the volume of work involved in getting executive orders/letters issued from the ministers, the chief secretary, the health secretary ... was stupendous".[40]

Rao was also full of praise for those who worked at the district level: "The program leadership at the district level has also risen to the assigned tasks and successfully implemented the campaign, coordinating with all allied departments/NGOs for involvement of their staff, volunteers and mobilization of necessary logistics, including vehicles, for effective supervision."[41] The World Bank evaluation applauded the MLEC in Tamil Nadu, which involved the whole of government (both political and administrative). They also praised the use of both electronic and print media to create "unprecedentedly useful awareness about leprosy elimination and the role they had to play among the communities as well as the peripheral health workers, health guides, teachers, *panchayat* presidents, and members".[42]

These efforts set a precedent for other states – such as Bihar, Uttar Pradesh, West Bengal, Madhya Pradesh, and Orissa – where there had never been any comprehensive case detection, where communities were not well informed about leprosy, where there was stigma, and where the primary health centres were not yet involved.[43] In June 1997 in Geneva, representatives of the World Bank, WHO, and the government of India decided to prepare for MLECs in the states of India. Each of the states would hold two campaigns, one immediately and then a second one just before the year 2000. The second campaign was to find any hidden cases of leprosy. These campaigns would follow the pattern set in Tamil Nadu. They would involve all the health staff as well as volunteers from the community, who would receive an orientation session. They would also be accompanied by a drive to create community awareness amongst the whole population, which would be coordinated from a newly established centre at the National Headquarters.[44]

Community participation in these activities was quite extraordinary. In Madhya Pradesh, for example, people made pamphlets, cinema slides, wall paintings, and poster hoardings. Drawing upon popular religious festivals, they made a "Kustha Mukti Rath" or Leprosy Elimination Chariot displaying information about the disease with audiotapes of songs and information on a public address system that was moved from district to district. This was so popular that a prototype was created and sent out to all the districts.[45] There were over 45,500 teams made up of Anganwadi workers, teachers, students, and others. In total, 77,226 people took part in the MLEC.

The extent of the campaign became apparent when workers arriving at "an interior village of Dewas district" met a woman, "the lady of the household", who when a worker began to tell her about leprosy took over the instruction herself, automatically narrating all the symptoms. When asked how she knew about them already, she replied that she heard it on the radio.[46] People were getting the message. From the MLEC in Madhya Pradesh, out of the 20,248 new cases detected, 6,444 were diagnosed with MB leprosy and 744 with grade II deformities.[47]

The Bihar elimination campaign was delayed because some of the district teams had not yet been formed.[48] But by March, Dr N. S. Dharmshaktu, the Deputy Director from the Directorate General of Health Services in New Delhi, was able to report over the telephone to Denis Daumerie that, sensationally, the MLEC had started in Bihar four days previously, and 33,000 new cases of leprosy had been detected. Dharmshaktu expected that the MLECs for the year 2000 would find 140,000 new cases in total in the five states. This would bring the annual detection for 1999–2000 to about 400,000 new cases.[49] In the meantime, the WHO arranged with the government of India to appoint five leprosy consultants for the most endemic states. In order to enhance the IEC communication to communities, Daumerie and Dharmshaktu worked together on a new poster that was designed to make people aware that leprosy was treated without charge, and that treatment was available at the local health centre. All health centres that provided MDT services would display this poster in a prominent place.[50]

In 2001, about 760,000 new cases were detected in India, an increase on the 677,180 new cases for 2000.[51] This included 4%, or 24,649, with grade

II disability in 2000.[52] At this stage, in what the Leprosy Unit considered was the second phase of their elimination activities, the most difficult issue they were facing was the "highly vertical and centralized management structures composed of specialized staff" that still remained in the country.[53] They continued to envisage and encourage "a more simplified approach to diagnosis and treatment, using the general health worker at the village level".[54] Some of the staff in the already-existing vertical leprosy programme were not happy to involve outside staff, particularly those from primary healthcare centres, because to do so was seen "as a threat to their continuation in the existing position and place".[55] They were reassured that they would have a role to play, but would need to understand and receive more instruction about their respective roles.[56] These specialised staff presented a dilemma once World Bank funding came to an end, but efforts were made to retrain them so that they could be integrated into the primary healthcare and general medical services.

The numbers

For seven years, LECs had been carried out in more than twenty-five endemic countries, and over 1 million cases had been detected. But the numbers of new cases coming forward with leprosy were not declining, in India at least. As the leprosy elimination efforts in India were increasingly ramped up, making an accurate diagnosis became significant. M.T. Htoon, the WHO representative on the evaluation team, reported there was a great deal of overdiagnosis, especially in response to targets issued to the districts; the job was being done too well:

> Medak district has a registered prevalence of 673 cases (2.43/10,000 as of 31/12/99). During the period of April–Dec 1999, 803 new cases were detected through routine activities. … A sample of new cases and suspects that were identified during the campaigns were re-examined. Among the 17 new cases detected during the campaigns which were re-examined, 2 cases with single skin lesion were wrongly diagnosed as leprosy. Among the 25 suspects that were re-examined, none of them were found to have leprosy.[57]

Twelve months later, in Orissa, Htoon found that a significant number of the sample cases that were being treated were instances of overdiagnosis. He also found that some of the cases that had been referred to the primary healthcare centres for continued treatment, as well as the defaulter cases that were restarting treatment, had been reported as new cases.[58]

In May 2001, the government of India, WHO, ILEP, and the Sasakawa Memorial Health Foundation (SMHF) met to discuss their respective roles in elimination activities in India. Neira wrote to J. V. R. Prasada Rao, at the Ministry for Health and Family Welfare, to tell him that the new national leprosy elimination project supported by both the World Bank and SMHF included "improved and more accurate case finding". She was concerned that the number of new cases had remained relatively constant and pointed to questions about "the accuracy of diagnosis, the extent of re-registering of old cases as new, and whether the incentive structure (notably, annual targets), rather than the detection and treatment of the disease, have determined the annual case finding rate".[59]

The nagging issue of stable or even increasing new cases required elucidation. It was inevitable that new cases appeared, as the campaigns were covering previously inaccessible areas. Some of these newly diagnosed people may have contracted the disease earlier and remained undetected for some time. The Leprosy Unit continued to argue that only a small percentage of these new cases were actually "true incident cases": that is, those who had experienced the onset of the disease within the preceding year. In some countries, repeated MLECs showed a significant decline in detection trends, except for India, where 78% of the new cases were being detected. There were several possible explanations. The larger numbers of cases discovered in subsequent LECs may have meant that the campaigns had not been conducted properly in the first place. Or, with the increased awareness of leprosy, it was possible that more people were presenting themselves for treatment. Perhaps annual targets for detection may have encouraged overzealousness so that there was over-detection or re-registration of old cases. Or, the worst possibility of all: transmission continued to be high.[60]

A fourth and last MLEC was carried out in India during 2003 and 2004, in Delhi, Jharkhand, Maharashtra, Uttaranchal, and West Bengal. In Jharkhand, there were 9,939 new cases, and in West Bengal there were 6,139. This was 51% less than the previous MLEC. Immediately after the LEC, the quality of the diagnosis was verified in six random districts so that 47% of the suspected cases were identified and re-examined, and 21% were found not to have leprosy at all. Of the 267 who were newly diagnosed with PB leprosy, 12% did not have the disease and 5% were either recycled cases who had completed treatment or defaulters who had been re-registered as new cases.[61] Amongst the multibacillary cases, 8% were wrongly diagnosed and 9% were recycled.[62] This seemed to explain partly why the numbers were not diminishing, although not everyone was convinced of this as an explanation.

In his capacity as special consultant, Noordeen addressed the anomalies in the detection of leprosy in a letter to the Secretary of the Ministry of Health and Family Welfare, Prasada Rao. He identified the increasing tendency "to report cases which should not be reported". He cited a recent independent study in India that showed that over 45% of the currently reported cases were either over-diagnosed or re-registered cases that had already been fully treated. One reason for this problem was that a campaign was judged successful by the numbers of cases detected, irrespective of the quality of detection. With repeated MLECs in a district, the proportion of true new cases needing treatment diminished, while the proportion of unnecessarily detected "cases" greatly increased.

Even though successive MLECs did demonstrate a very steady fall in new cases, repeated campaigns were increasingly less cost effective. Noordeen therefore recommended cessation of mass screening through MLECs and other campaigns. Patients were best encouraged to self-report through appropriate IEC strategies. Health workers were better when not pressured through targets to detect "early leprosy" where the specificity of diagnosis was very low, and when they were carefully trained to be clear about making a diagnosis. Leprosy services that were truly integrated enabled leprosy patients to be properly diagnosed and treated within the PHC system. Noordeen concluded that "Attaining [the] elimination of leprosy in India hopefully by the end of 2005 would be a historic achievement hardly envisaged as a possibility by some of us who joined the fight against the disease nearly 50 years ago."[63]

A questionable victory

In 2003, the global leprosy programme moved from the WHO in Geneva to New Delhi, and a new goal for elimination was set for the year 2005. In April 2005, Pannikar reviewed the global strategy program with the national leprosy elimination programme authorities and ILEP. Together they decided to limit their activities to those directly relevant to attaining the elimination goal by the end of 2005. The LECs, SAPELs, validation, and monitoring exercises were postponed. Coordinators from the World Health Organization and ILEP were both congratulated for their excellent support of the efforts of various nations. The global leprosy programme was expressly judged to be on track.[64] Trevor Durston from the Leprosy Mission reflected with unmistakable satisfaction on the significance of this change for ILEP:

A change in leadership in the WHO and also in ILEP brought new opportunities and much hope. The top levels of the WHO had already ordered an evaluation of the Global Alliance which resulted in a very frank and open discussion allowing people to air their views and emotion. Dr Pannikar was appointed as the new leprosy team leader for the WHO and everyone made enormous efforts to try and rebuild the partnership that was so necessary in the global fight against leprosy. Therefore as the WHO developed its new global strategy it did so with significant interaction with ILEP, resulting in a strategy that the ILEP Technical Commission and ILEP members could fully endorse. Similarly the operational guidelines that give a framework for national programme managers to implement the strategy were also developed in the context of this close collaboration, and fully endorsed by the ILEP Technical Commission and the ILEP members. Full technical collaboration between ILEP and the WHO was re-established at this international level with much relief.[65]

ILEP members were particularly encouraged to see the new strategy and guidelines embrace the broader issues of leprosy like disability and stigma and recognise the need for a strong collaborative international partnership between all key players.

The new emphasis was on "sustainable leprosy control", an eloquent statement of something that could be relied on to continue. The differences in the politics of international health had robbed the elimination initiative of its final attempts at decisively pronouncing that the disease had been eliminated as a national public health problem in every country of the world. Whether or not that would have been possible is still a matter for debate. The Nippon Foundation continued to provide support to the tune of US$4 million a year, and Novartis continued to provide free drug supplies.

At the "Global Forum on the Elimination of Leprosy as a Public Health Problem" held in Geneva on 26 May 2006, the stakeholders were told that leprosy control had reached "a critical milestone".[66] The disease had declined dramatically, yet there were still pockets in some countries in Africa, Asia, and Latin America. Early diagnosis of people with the disease was more difficult, and as a result there was an increasing risk of deformities due to nerve damage. The Director–General at the WHO, Dr Margaret Chan, praised the public health approach to the disease that brought treatment to millions of people infected with leprosy. The Minister of Health from India pledged to continue the fight against the disease in his country. (India would announce that it had achieved elimination nationally at the end of December that same year, amidst much continuing controversy.) The Secretary of Health from Brazil confessed that "to be very honest, we wasted a lot of time in Brazil", but declared the country's commitment to elimination. At the beginning of 2009, Brazil announced that it had abandoned the goal of elimination, but in 2012 reaffirmed pursuit of elimination of the disease as a public health problem.

The new case-detection figures continued to decline, but some say that this decline reflects the decreased interest of national governments in pursuing the disease and recording new cases. In 2003, there were 514,718 new cases reported throughout the world; in 2004, there were 407,791; in 2005, there were 296,499; in 2006, there were 259,017; in 2007, there were 254,525; and in 2008, there were 249,007.[67] Today there are about 210,000 annually.[68]

Leprosy in the world in 2020

Leprosy has certainly not disappeared, and taking into account the fallibility of reporting, it may even be slowly creeping back. The old, much-maligned and misunderstood campaign to eliminate leprosy as a public health problem has shifted to specific efforts that are indicators of delayed diagnosis and infectivity. Endemic countries have embraced the WHO Global Leprosy Strategy 2016–20 of "Accelerating towards a leprosy-free world."[69] The new targets are to have no new cases of children with grade II disability by 2020; less than 1 per million of the population of any new leprosy cases with grade II disability; and no countries with laws or legislation that allow discrimination against people with leprosy.[70] Nonetheless, at the end of 2017, the WHO reported an increase in global prevalence across all the WHO regions since 2016:

> The registered global prevalence of leprosy was 192 713 cases (0.25/10 000 population) at the end of 2017, an increase by 20 765 cases over that in 2016. The increase was observed in all WHO regions: 42.8% (9189 cases) in AFR, 19.5% (5162 cases) in AMR, 42% (1303 cases) in EMR, 3.4% (3875 cases) in SEAR and 20.9% (1220 cases) in WPR.[71]

The disease persists in large numbers in India, Brazil, and Indonesia. Most concerning, the threat of drug resistance continues to trouble observers, and the WHO reports that tests for resistance raise concerns about the future of leprosy treatment.[72] The WHO guidelines for therapy remain, "The 3-drug regimen comprising rifampicin, dapsone and clofazimine is now recommended for all leprosy patients, with a duration of 6 months for PB and 12 months for MB leprosy."[73]

In 2020, the partnerships continue between national governments, the ILA and the Nippon Foundation, the WHO, ILEP, Novartis, and the newly created Global Partnership for Zero Leprosy (GPZL).[74] Efforts are focused on active case finding and contact tracing, analysis of transmission of the disease in clusters of the population, and post-exposure prophylaxis. Attention has also turned to stigma and discrimination, although no agreement about an end goal has been reached. Medical researchers also acknowledge the need to address the ongoing issue of the mental health of people either diagnosed with leprosy or living with the effects of the disease. In the laboratory, in the fields of molecular biology, immunology and vaccines, and microbiology, researchers are working on developing ways of diagnosing the disease in its early stages and monitoring the progress of treatment, especially the patient's response to MDT. Research into understanding the pathogenesis of *M. leprae*, which is ultimately about the immune response of the host to the bacillus, continues. Most importantly, researchers are concerned with drug resistance and exploring alternative drug regimens. At the 2019 International Leprosy Congress, Paul Saunderson reported that there was "not much eye-opening research", and no controversies or disagreements at the Congress, nor was there any public discussion about the WHO guidelines on the therapy of leprosy.[75]

Leprosy is a slow disease. It takes a long time to incubate, and it spreads selectively and opportunistically. It appears that transmission has not been interrupted, but one thing is certain: if provided early enough, there is a treatment that makes leprosy – this disease that has for so long caused so much grief, deformity, and suffering – nothing more than a short-lived infection. The most eloquent testimony towards this is that of the medical worker. In 2009, I asked a doctor in Cebu, in the Philippines, if she thought that the disease was declining. She replied strongly in the affirmative, adding that she was sure that never again would she see children cast out from their families with nowhere to go and no hope of escaping the inevitable disfigurement from the disease. She was also personally relieved that she was saved from the heartbreak of being unable to offer hope to anyone with leprosy because now she could treat the disease when she encountered it.

12

THE HUMAN RIGHTS OF LEPROSY-AFFECTED PEOPLE

One of the most common and persistent myths surrounding leprosy-affected people has been about their passivity. Religious ideas of leprosy as a divine punishment, the long history of the disease without either cure or comprehension, and the peculiar symptoms of slow wasting and destruction of the body all contributed to a picture of the sufferer as someone who was reduced to multiform debilitation. Social anathema and exclusion over the centuries only intensified this reduction of the individuals' agency and even identity. However, a closer look at people affected by the disease indicates that they have been and continue to be extraordinarily proactive in spite of their disempowerment on so many different fronts, constantly asserting their personhood and agitating for their rights and freedoms. So often they went unheard, and even though most of the world averted both their faces and their minds, leprosy-affected people never ceased expressing their demands for respect, dignity, and the opportunity to marry, to own property, to have children, and to earn a living: in short, to live as social beings and as citizens.

Bearing in mind the debate between those who prioritised public health measures against the disease and those who emphasised the importance of the whole person, this chapter will trace the outcome of the elimination campaign for those who were actually affected with leprosy. It will argue that the persistent and emerging voices of leprosy-affected people today, against all odds, have begun to be heard as they take on the power to represent themselves and reclaim their human rights. It will show that, as their human rights are increasingly foregrounded, a healing of the bifurcation between the two approaches to a cure (the public health approaches to the disease and the rehabilitation of the whole person) becomes evident – ironically but appropriately – in the politicised, proactive bodies of the people affected by the disease. They are themselves both appropriating approaches to their own experience of leprosy and fusing them in ways that fit themselves, their own local organisations, and their communities. This chapter describes how this fusion is taking place organically, from the ground up, ultimately changing the tenor of the international work against the disease.

Agency in the contest for ownership

This history has only so far alluded to the agency of leprosy-affected people because so much of the debates and politics around their treatment took place with little consideration for them as agents. This is not to say that those who were focused on treatment did not care about people. Their desire was to get multidrug therapy to as many people as needed it, as quickly as possible. It was a given that achieving this would be effective in eliminating stigma and making rehabilitation unnecessary, provided people could be diagnosed and treated before they contracted disabilities. As Noordeen expressed it: "In terms of the long-term future, the importance of the public health goal of elimination of leprosy far outstripped the human problems to be faced in the short and medium terms." If multidrug therapy was made available, the social and economic issues would become non-issues.

On the other hand, the anti-leprosy organisations that predated international efforts against the disease espoused the goal of restoring people to wholeness, if not physically, then socially, economically, and (most importantly) spiritually. As has already been demonstrated, the anti-leprosy organisations believed that they had a responsibility to the "whole person" affected by the disease, and they fiercely resisted attempts to see leprosy care circumscribed by clinical pathology. But the efforts of these organisations were also tinged with a degree of benevolence that fostered dependence and succeeded in ensuring their own sustainability, especially in the 1940s and 1950s, when efforts went into maintaining special places set aside for people with the disease.

These sites became and remained effectively "special" places where people would live through the generations, set aside because of the taint of leprosy. While the ILEP Medical Commission steered these organisations away from that model of leprosy care and into step with international health initiatives, many leprosy-affected people, when they were discharged, remained close to the old leprosy institutions in nearby settlements that retained the stigma of leprosy. Although this phenomenon bore eloquent testimony to the continuing stigma in the community, it also spoke of the dependence created by anti-leprosy work. It ensured that, in spite of a medical cure, leprosy continued to deal a fatal blow to one's social standing and economic capability.

As has already been shown in this history, as the meaning of a cure for leprosy changed and became increasingly politicised, the representation of the people affected by the disease also changed. These representations were not designed to hurt people, but they ultimately continued to disenfranchise individuals. Early on, amidst the eagerness and ambition of the medical people to secularise and professionalise the treatment of leprosy as a public health problem, the actual people afflicted with the disease were represented as victims who suffered a social toll on their lives that was perpetuated in their children. They were represented before the WHO as people without power, in need of rescue. These were people who had been cast out and neglected, not seen by the general medical profession as worthwhile recipients of medical attention or even of being included in an international health agenda, so such appeals were necessary; nonetheless, representation has its own interpellative power. If you are constantly represented as needing to be rescued, that is how you see yourself and that is what you become.

Under mass treatment, people became cases to be counted. With that came a loss of identity that was multifaceted. Leprosy had already robbed people of their physical and social identities. As has already been described, people would disguise themselves by taking on a new name when they entered a leprosarium in order to protect their family from stigma. Nonetheless, everyone in a leprosy colony was identified in the records and their symptoms and history described in detail. Records from these places speak eloquently of individuals with their own stories, unsilenced by the passing of time. But with mass leprosy campaigns, the names of people with leprosy were unimportant and personal identities disappeared altogether. If this meant that people could emerge from their everyday lives, take the medication, and re-enter their daily activities barely touched by the disease, this was a desirable outcome. But so often people remained as cases, forever on the register, drifting from one treatment centre to the next, restarting their drug regimens while the bacillus still lurked in their bodies, capable of resurging unpredictably.

In the contest between multidrug therapy for treatment and treatment of the whole person – including social and economic rehabilitation – for the most part, leprosy-affected people were represented as passive recipients, although they were expected, encouraged, educated, and trained to cooperate in their treatment, whatever it might include. They were co-opted to the plan and not expected to make any trouble. But while better outcomes for the lives of real people were implicit in this contest, it was also about the rivalry between the status of medicine and rehabilitation. This rivalry grew into a proxy for a struggle for ownership of anti-leprosy work, within which the people affected by the disease and all of its social and economic implications were somewhat incidental. Their views, opinions, and experiences were notably absent in this rivalry, and yet their representations were put to use in its service.

Yet as far back as 1978, following on from the aspirations of the Alma Ata declaration, the treatment of leprosy had been represented as the individual's personal responsibility at each stage, and this depended upon individual self-reliance or self-governance and upon community participation. People had to take ownership of their own health rather than passively relying on others to do it for them. Profoundly ironic, as is evident from the ILA Forum in 2001, was the lack of confidence in people to do this, especially those at the mercy of general medical services in third-world countries. Additionally, epidemiologists were concerned that people absorbed into the larger healthcare system would no longer be considered "cases" once they received their treatment. In short, the broad success of multidrug treatment in the community militated against monitoring the success or otherwise of individual cases. The Forum mourned the "loss" of the patient as "epidemiological evidence" for the way in which the anti-leprosy programme was developing. The "success" of the devolution and democratisation of treatment made it difficult to measure the treatment's success empirically and scientifically.

The Alma Ata declaration marks a moment of empowerment conferred upon the patient by the institution, and the state-wide elimination campaigns – in Tamil Nadu and other states of India especially – show its effects on the ground. But if you listen to the stories of individuals, you discover that even before this every single person diagnosed with leprosy was brought to a crisis point, to the edge of a cliff, where they would have to take control of their own well-being in the face of active discrimination and indifference, as well as medical stigma and societal disempowerment. If people were to survive in the face of ostracism, isolation, and discrimination, there was never a moment when they did not have to dig deep within themselves and find the courage to fight for respect and the means by which to live. Many were less successful at this than others because the opportunities were not there or their spirits failed in the face of overwhelming odds, but some – spectacularly and triumphantly, with superhuman strength – pulled themselves up from the edge of that cliff and remade their lives. The raw courage of people who salvaged their lives out of the damage that leprosy does – not only to their bodies, but to their relationships with their immediate family, their relatives, their villages, their social and economic status, their overall well-being, and most of all to their mental state – is exhilarating to witness.

Individual courage and dignity

Young women married into a family far away from their parents were more powerless than most. And yet, against the most overwhelming cruelty and discrimination, Afsana Begum found a way to live that grew out of her own agency and strength of spirit. She was married at fourteen years of age to a man twice her age, living in Bihar. After the birth of her son and six years into her marriage, she started to show patches on her face and hands. Without understanding why, she found that she was being treated like a pariah. When she gave birth to a sickly girl, she was locked up by her in-laws, starved, and refused contact with her parents. Fortunately, her brother visited and persuaded her in-laws to allow her to leave. They relented, but only on the condition that she abandon her 4-year-old son to the family.

Afsana returned to Calcutta with her baby girl to live with her parents, her siblings, and their partners, only to experience their silent rejection of her. This brought her to the courageous decision to leave her parents' home and live independently.

> I knew I had to, there was no other choice. But the big question that hounded me day in and day out, circling my mind like vultures atop a carcass was where would I seek shelter, considering my state and moreover, with my daughter in tow. I felt helpless, forlorn and resigned to fate.[1]

Her rescuer came in the form of Dilruba Begum, or Mamata Didi, a medical person at a GRECALTES dispensary, who explained to her that she was suffering from leprosy and treated her, even following her up if she missed her visits.[2] At first Afsana experienced reactions to the treatment that made her appearance worse, but within six months of taking the medication, her scars faded significantly. She felt as if she had been reborn: "I have no qualms in going out during the day time without covering my face and hands. I hold my head proudly and without being mortally afraid that somebody will point an accusing finger at my scars and ask with mock sympathy, 'What are those scars, Afsana?'" She learnt to sew and planned to work for a tailor. Her interviewer noted that she still longed for her son, but "From a girl in her teens fighting against all odds she has carved a place for herself as an ideal portrayal of a woman who fought for her self-respect and won it."[3]

So strong is the human spirit that someone like Anjan Dey, a Bengali from Orissa, the prized only son in his family who dreamed of becoming an engineer, who lost everything to leprosy, including his future, was able to regain a professional identity and claim his rightful place in society, refusing the dependency and helplessness that leprosy offered him. When he was diagnosed, like Stanley Stein, his imaginings of the taint of the disease descended on him. He pictured images of beggars with leprosy outside the temple: "the truth caught me in a stranglehold, a similar fate was awaiting me in the not-so-distant future".[4] He was deeply conscious of the impact of his condition on his immediate family, especially when his sister's wedding was called off, so he left his town without telling anyone.

In Bombay, he sought out treatment and was exiled to a cowshed by one doctor. He then went to Pune, to the Dr Bandorwalla Leprosy Hospital in Kondhwa, where for the first time a doctor actually touched him and treated him.[5] While he was there, he cleaned the floors to earn his living, but all the time he nurtured a burning desire to get his dignity back and lead the life he had dreamed of. He became interested in physiotherapy, and his doctor suggested he go to the Christian Medical College Vellore, where he was treated successfully and became a qualified physiotherapist.[6] He triumphantly returned home with a regained social status, owning his own house, a car, and the ability to educate his own children. He went on to head the department where he used to clean the floors. He stressed the importance of getting rid of the "special places" such as rehabilitation centres, leprosy colonies, homes, and vocational centres dedicated to people with leprosy. For him, real rehabilitation occurs when a person returns home and takes up their life from the point where they left it.[7]

So often people not only salvaged their own pride, dignity, and financial independence in the face of the most adverse circumstances, they also organised themselves into collectives in order to represent themselves politically. One of the common themes in the stories of these isolated and discriminated-against people is that they found strength in others who had had the same experience. Sanjiv Kakar argues that in India, in the 1930s and 1940s, there were visible and organised displays of protest from people with leprosy in a series of revolts in leprosy asylums across the country.[8] People agitated to have their living conditions improved, and they focused their demands on religious teaching, medical treatment, and segregation of the sexes.[9] As he points out, they did not agitate against confinement, for "Clearly living conditions outside were not favorable," but they resisted segregation of the sexes in whatever way they could.

Kakar argues that "by their actions" patients managed "to influence and modify asylum culture" so that in 1934, when the people in the Naini asylum protested, a whole new rights-based approach to their institutionalisation was forged between inmates and managers.[10] Kakar concluded that "This radically new stance on the part of the management allowed leprosy patients a freedom of mobility and of choice which had hitherto been denied."[11] And this legacy of activism persists: "Organized protest by handicapped persons (which includes leprosy patients with developed deformities) is not uncommon nowadays. Protest can take various forms, such as petitioning the state or initiating or implementing rehabilitation programmes. More assertive forms include conducting public demonstrations, at the risk of being arrested."[12]

M. Guruappa, from Haryana, is someone who was empowered as part of a collective. He was orphaned as a young boy and placed in the care of his stepbrother. In order to support his younger brother's education, he began to run a milk-supply business in his village, but when he began to experience loss of sensation in his hands and feet, he realised he had leprosy. He was "appalled, angry and apprehensive" and filled with self-disgust.[13] Becoming increasingly aware of discrimination from those closest to him and rejection from private doctors, he sought out and received medication from a German-supported hospital at Dichpali in Andhra Pradesh. He eventually exiled himself from his village and his brother's house so as not to be a burden and lived in a community of beggars on a train station platform in Bombay.

There he encountered a doctor, Dr Nelson, who was called Mataji (mother). "It was a place where we were treated like normal human beings, a place where we could freely talk about our pain and aspirations."[14] Inspired by her and with the support of other social activists, the community found strength in uniting and speaking with a single voice by forming a legally recognised collective (Samiti). This occurred in the same year that MDT began to be administered in India, and their settlement was chosen to pilot implementation. Their lobbying and protests succeeded in winning the monthly allowance, which made begging unnecessary. Guruappa concludes,

Two decades have passed since then and I am happy to say I am no longer a beggar. Granted, life is not a bed of roses, but I am happy because of the love and affection we get from people around. Today I live with my wife and our twelve-year-old adopted daughter. While working on my poultry farms, I often thank God for engaging me meaningfully in life to earn my livelihood.[15]

People afflicted with leprosy come from all walks of life, and the sense of indignation of those from more privileged families, when their social identity and sense of value is imperilled by a diagnosis of the disease – just as in our earlier example of T. N. Jagadisan who met Gandhi – informs their power to resist and overturn discrimination. Md Salaluddin came from a wealthy family in Hyderabad and cherished the dream of becoming a doctor.

A neighbourhood doctor noticed some red patches on his cheeks and alerted his father, who took him for further examinations. In spite of treatment, he started to lose sensation in his feet. He was denied entry to a medical college, and when he attempted to join the navy he was ostracised to the point that he withdrew.

Nonetheless, he was determined to make what he called a respectable livelihood, so he left home in search of a job. After several unsuccessful attempts, he decided to improve his educational qualifications while at the same time holding down several part-time jobs. His symptoms worsened, so he went to Victoria Hospital at Dichpally in Hyderabad. There he was met by one of the most famous leprosy specialists of the time, Dr Davey, who offered to take him into his own home.[16] As Salaluddin improved, he made plans to leave, but Davey asked him to take over the administrative work of the hospital. He also began to visit recovered, but disabled, patients in the colony outside the hospital. With Davey's support, he trained them to work as laboratory technicians, assistants, physiotherapists, non-medical assistants, and chemists.[17]

At the government's recommendation, Salaluddin further visited the rehabilitation centre of Moulali in Hyderabad, where people lived in appalling conditions. He set about to progressively change the predicament of these people by fighting for their right to register for employment, establishing a Council of Hansen's Social Welfare, and registering them as citizens with the right to vote. He succeeded in obtaining a grant of 56 acres of land for 300 families, and established childcare, healthcare, adult education programmes, *mahila mandalis* (women's organisations), and also succeeded in ensuring the education of the next generation. His dream was of "a world where there will be no more stigma and no fear of contempt and humiliation for those affected by leprosy".[18]

Each of these stories is about a courageous individual who against all odds salvages a life of which they are proud and forges a future which gives them hope. Moreover, each story also includes someone who reaches out to rescue the abandoned and despairing person. These rescuers come in many guises: a female medical worker who informs, watches over, and encourages, and who belongs to an international NGO (the then German Leprosy Relief Association [GLRA], which includes programmes for training people for employment and independence); a hospital specially dedicated to the care of people with leprosy, now a struggling government institution; a premier training college showcasing groundbreaking rehabilitation techniques (founded by British medical and rehabilitation specialists who were supported by the Leprosy Mission and BELRA); a local doctor and several social activists who found a place for displaced beggars and showed them a way forward to political representation and land ownership; an outstanding Wesleyan medical missionary who recognised the status and innate dignity of the person he was treating and who afforded him the respect he was used to and a direction for his talents, capability, drive, and an outlet for his social obligations and sense of entitlement.

Some of these rescuers were also the pioneers in the development of the drugs for successful treatment. Some were supported by the international anti-leprosy organisations. Some belonged to locally based humanitarian groups. By offering personal attention, a helping hand, appropriate and effective medical care, and vocational opportunities, they enabled leprosy-affected peopled to help themselves in order to regain their dignity and self-respect.

Human rights

The international discourse on human rights emerged after World War II, as a result of the work of the Commission on Human Rights and its Universal Declaration of Human Rights, which was proclaimed on 10 December 1948 (eight months after the beginning of the WHO). The principles of human rights for leprosy-affected people became a touchstone for their activism and advocacy towards the end of the twentieth century, bringing our history full circle, towards a reconciliation of the two impulses that have driven the efforts against leprosy: the public health approach and the holistic/humanistic approach. For while it is possible to produce a genealogy of human rights from the earliest examples of Buddhism, Judaism, Christianity, Confucianism, and Islam, the attachment of human rights to people with leprosy can also be traced back to such inspirational figures as Saint Damien de Veuster, Wellesley Bailey, Abbé Pierre, and Raoul Follereau, the respective founders of the anti-leprosy organisations. And yet the change from saving people to framing them within an international human rights perspective calls for a significant shift in understanding. Instead of "lifting up" the poor, benighted, abandoned leprosy sufferer, we are asked instead to see the "value and the dignity of each individual", and that they are armed with a right to self-determination, with basic social and economic rights as well as civil and political rights.

Enumerating these inalienable rights against the history of the lives of leprosy-affected people clarifies the magnitude of the sacrifice they were required to make for the sake of the greater good: a sacrifice of their humanity.[19] To be more precise, those rights include the right to work, the right to equal pay for equal work, the right to join trade unions, the right to social security, the right to protection of the family with special assistance to mothers and children, the right to an adequate standard of living and food, the right to the highest attainable standard of physical and mental health, the right to education, and the right to take part in cultural life.[20] The switch from victims to subjects was further secured in the Millennium Development Goals which, in Lauren's opinion, brought about "the transformation of individual victims from objects of international pity into subjects of international law".[21]

Several contemporary streams of collective representation emerged from the courageous and unrelenting activism of leprosy-affected people. These people's organisations changed the benevolent model of care into a demand for the restoration of basic human rights. In Brazil, the Movement of Reintegration of Persons Afflicted by Hansen's Disease (MORHAN), was established on 6 June 1981, by eight people in São Paulo.[22] This group consisted mainly of former patients and those still living in leprosy colony hospitals. Its founder and first National Coordinator, Francisco Augusto Vieira Nunes (Bacurau), had been diagnosed with leprosy when he was five years old, and like many children throughout the world grew up in a colony. MORHAN is notable for its activism and political strategy in public health policymaking, taking on and influencing the make-up of state technical commissions and municipal health councils.

Another influential organisation emerged with the work of Anwei Law. Her father had been a pioneering American medical missionary in China, and she began a lifelong mission of advocacy for leprosy-affected people by taking a small and rather motley group of leprosy-affected people to International Leprosy Congresses where all the medical and scientific experts on the disease gathered. These interventions proved to be rather embarrassing to the regular participants, but were nonetheless entirely appropriate. Her unrelenting advocacy, as a woman in a predominantly male-dominated group, earned her a grudging respect amongst those who worked in the field. Her presence and that of the people with her could not be ignored.

From her point of view, the medical conferences were mandarin affairs in which medical men exchanged scientific and medical knowledge in a disciplinary bubble of elite collegiality that was remote from the actual people who bore the burden of the disease. Her challenge to the attendees at the congresses occurred at a time not so far distant from when some medical professionals (not all) were careful to never actually touch a person with leprosy, relying on the nursing attendants (who were often the children born to leprosy-affected people, or people who had recovered from the disease) to do the hands-on nursing. There were still echoes of the old days when doctors walked through trays of water and disinfectant and wore special clothing when they examined people with the disease, thereby perpetuating the fear of leprosy and adding to its stigmatisation. As far as she was concerned, medical values left much to be desired when it came to respect for people affected by the disease.

In 1994, in Petropolis, Brazil, Anwei Law and forty-nine others from six countries, including representatives of MORHAN, gathered to form the International Association for Integration, Dignity and Economic Advancement (IDEA), a global forum to promote the human rights and dignity of individuals affected by leprosy. This group of people proclaimed that everyone, including people affected by leprosy, had the right to fully participate as social beings in their communities. They fostered an international network of support through which people could share their experiences. They exposed stigma, discrimination, segregation, isolation, and the derogatory terminology associated with the disease because of its profound effect on people's lives. They mounted an ongoing attack on the long history of damaging representations of leprosy-affected people by promoting the use of "positive images, inspiring words, artistic talents, and other ways of self-expression, to replace outdated images and stereotypes with a holistic understanding of individuals whose lives have been challenged by leprosy/Hansen's disease".

This organisation drew its strength from a human rights discourse that claimed the right to equal justice, equal opportunity, and equal dignity without discrimination.[23] People had the right to live where they chose, marry whom they wished, worship where they desired, provide for themselves and their families, and ensure that their children received an education. The organisation strove to restore to people the "identity, self-confidence and dignity" that leprosy had taken away from them, and they put this aspiration into action by giving people the opportunities to speak publicly, attend workshops with local and government officials, regain economic independence, and educate their children.[24]

IDEA's programmes included a global campaign to eliminate stigma and promote empowerment and self-sufficiency, as well as offer scholarship programmes, psychological support, professional and public education, and media awareness.[25] One of the interventions that IDEA created was the Quest for Dignity Exhibit, a travelling exhibition launched at the United Nations by the United Nations Secretary–General Kofi Annan.[26] Today, IDEA has members in more than thirty countries.[27] IDEA describes its priorities as follows:

> IDEA's approach is holistic – looking at the whole person through the lens of rights, rights related to health care, psychological well-being, education, marriage, voting, religious practices, housing and employment. It encompasses individuals' families and their communities, with a focus on those facing challenges to regain their rightful place in society.[28]

Legal challenge from residents of Japanese Sanatoria

One of the first events that brought the human rights of leprosy-affected people to wider national and international attention occurred when surviving residents of the leprosy sanatoria in Japan successfully launched a class action against the Japanese government, challenging the policies that restricted and limited their human rights and caused them pain and suffering. On 11 May 2001, Kumamoto District Court ruled on the Hansen's Disease Government Liability Lawsuit, instructing the government not to launch an appeal against the ruling but to "effect a swift and comprehensive resolution to the issue" in order to provide compensation to all the patients and former patients throughout the country regardless of whether they had been involved in the class action.[29] Following on from the successful ruling, the Ministry of Health, Labor and Welfare commissioned the Japan Law Foundation to form a verification committee charged with investigating why people had been segregated for so long and what human rights violations they had experienced.[30]

The Verification Committee visited all of the thirteen national sanatoria in Japan as well as the two private sanatoria and two sanatoria overseas (Korea and Taiwan) in order to carry out their task.[31] They interviewed 841 people in total. "758 of these people were those living in the 13 national sanatoria for Hansen's disease across the country; 9 of them were those living in two private sanatoria for Hansen's disease; 69 were those who had left sanatoria for Hansen's disease; and 5 were family members."[32] The investigation encouraged people to tell the story of their lives.[33] They were aware that "this study has only scratched the surface and [can be] seen [to offer] a glimpse of the deep and dark cave of the damage".[34] Out of the 3,500 residents of the fifteen sanatoria, only those who volunteered were interviewed. Many of those who had experienced the worst of the segregation policies were too elderly and too difficult to interview. Furthermore, many people did not want to be identified as belonging to this group because "a large number of victims remain unknown within families of Hansen's disease patients".

So great was the continuing stigma in Japanese society that many people refused to admit any connection to the sanatoria. The committee members conceded that "many families suffered just as much damage as the patients themselves".[35] People feared the repercussions and had no hesitation in resorting to the extreme of suicide if exposed. As the report indicated, "One former resident responded: 'If they ever find out, I plan even now to sit on a JR railroad track with my hands put together (praying), even though I know this will cause trouble to JR.' (male, placed in sanatoria in 1944)."[36]

The final report of the "Verification Committee Concerning Hansen's Disease Problem" which followed on the lawsuit and concluded in March 2005 contained harrowing reading. The unique tone of this report gives an insight into the discoveries of the investigators and their collective remorse. Overall, the investigators noted the extreme social disruption produced by the confinement in sanatoria: "basic acts of normal life in a normal community, such as going to school, getting a job, falling in love, getting married, and even clothing and food were suspended by placement in sanatoria, and they were restarted or 'created' in a new form inside the sanatorium".[37] They concluded that people had endured disadvantage in every aspect of lives, suffering financial, physical, and psychological damage amounting to the "violation of the right to live peacefully in society".[38]

The most harrowing discoveries made by the Verification Committee evidenced damage done to residents' right to marry and reproduce. If a man in the sanatoria sought permission to marry, he had to "choose" to be sterilised. (The Commission adds that the number of women in the sanatoria was much smaller than the men, so there were actually many men who never had "the luxury" [my words] of such a choice.)[39]

They also discovered the tragic remains of foetuses. The Committee commented that "Among the items of this verification task, nothing has damaged and continued to damage the human dignity of residents more than the problem of these fetus samples."[40] Bearing eloquent testimony to the eugenic policies against the reproduction of people with leprosy and to the scientific research initiatives that were a by-product of the sanatoria, these remains were preserved indefinitely, with no respect to the truncated lives they represented. They found "a large number of samples, in formalin, of fetuses and newborn babies". These resulted from artificial abortions, natural miscarriages, and artificially induced births.[41] The date of discovery, the locations, and the numbers of these remains were as follows:[42]

25 June 2003:	National Sanatorium Oku Komyo En	49
12 November 2003:	National Sanatorium Hoshizuka Keia i En	17
8 December 2003:	Research Center for Hansen's Disease of the National Infectious Disease Research Center	2
1 March 2004:	National Suruga Sanatorium	10
1 June 2004:	National Sanatorium Matsuoka Hoyo En	1
31 July 2004:	National Sanatorium Tama Zensho En	35

Even more shocking, at least 25% of the foetuses were not the result of abortions but were the result of induced early births or natural, mature births: that is, amongst the remains, a quarter were of children born alive who had been killed at birth. Additionally, the evidence indicates that the remains were "left without any purpose or application". Sixty per cent were abortions performed before the enactment of the 1948 Eugenic Protection Law, but because abortions were mandatory in the sanatoria, and performed without consent, they were illegal regardless of whether they were performed before or after that law. Finally, for those children born alive, the committee concludes,

> If a fetus was born alive, the question is how the life was stopped after the birth. It is extremely difficult now to speculate how it was done, but there are some cases where the only imaginable thing is, at least for some newborn babies, that workers at sanatoria were committing murders in the sense of the Penal Law.[43]

In addition to the remains of foetuses, many body parts were discovered stored in various leprosaria: "many other surgery-extracted body parts were randomly placed in large polyethylene buckets in a careless manner".[44] This was as a result of a policy of automatic autopsy. The Committee concluded this section of their report with the following:

> At any rate, the 114 fetus samples, many surgery-extracted materials, and over 2000 pathological samples, all resting in silence at national sanatoria for Hansen's disease, etc. – what are they saying to us quietly? Are they not powerfully asking us the question "What have they done?" – to all those who have been involved in the medical treatment of Hansen's disease in this country until now? Even if these corpses are carefully commemorated and respectfully buried, these facts must never be trivialized or forgotten by any means.[45]

The court action and the report of the Verification Committee further provoked attention on the human rights of leprosy-affected people throughout the world.

Yohei Sasakawa and Human Rights

In the midst of the Nippon Foundation and Sasakawa Memorial Health Foundation's donations to the WHO, Yohei Sasakawa, the son of Ryoichi Sasakawa, became increasingly aware of the continuing social conditions of leprosy-affected people throughout the world. People were receiving MDT, but they were still not accepted back into society. This failure to reintegrate people was for Sasakawa a violation of human rights, so in concert with IDEA and other advocacy organisations, in his capacity as the WHO's Goodwill Ambassador for Leprosy Elimination, he began to draw international attention to the human rights of people with leprosy.

In speaking about leprosy, Sasakawa argued that both the disease and discrimination against the disease had to be tackled concurrently. His favourite analogy was the motorcycle (an accessible image for India in particular, and third-world countries in general). He explained, "If the front wheel represents medical activities, and the back wheel [the] efforts to address the social issues, the wheels must be the same size and rotate at the same speed if the motorcycle is to move forward."[46] To achieve this balance in effort, his strategy to address discrimination was threefold: first, to focus attention on leprosy as a human rights issue by making political appeals to international organisations and national governments to take action; second, to build awareness by launching a Global Appeal to End Stigma and Discrimination Against People Affected by Leprosy; and, finally, to support the empowerment of people affected by leprosy.

Early responses by the other organisations to Yohei Sasakawa's stated intentions were respectful but underwhelming. In the political maelstrom of the elimination campaign, his focus on human rights seemed irrelevant and attracted the criticism that had always been levelled at Japanese contributions to anti-leprosy work. The donations to the WHO had always been appreciated, but with that financial support came the power to influence the direction of the work in ways that critics charged benefitted the reputation of the Nippon Foundation and of Japan. Yohei Sasakawa's efforts in the arena of human rights seemed guaranteed to work towards that end as well. But with the benefit of hindsight, this approach has proved prescient and efficacious. Not only did it accomplish a resolution of the competing ideological and methodological impulses in the work against leprosy, but it did so by passing ownership of the treatment, and thereby empowerment, to the very people whose bodies were affected by the disease.

In July 2003, Yohei Sasakawa approached the Office of the High Commission on Human Rights (OHCHR), asking that the Commission take up the issue of leprosy-affected people's human rights.[47] He was invited to make a presentation to the Sub-Commission on the Promotion and Protection of Human Rights the following month. He prepared to address a large group of people, but only ten people were in the audience.[48] Suppressing his disappointment, he argued that unless the discrimination against leprosy was eliminated, the elimination of the disease could not be achieved. From his perspective of thirty years' work, he described the long and continuing history of discrimination and prejudice experienced by people with leprosy, especially their loss of social identity, to the extent that even when they died they could not be buried with family. In the words of one woman, "We will only be able to go home when we leave the crematory chimney as smoke."

Sasakawa told the listeners of his efforts as the WHO's Special Ambassador for the Elimination of Leprosy, in concert with the elimination campaign. He spoke of how he was acting with IDEA to give people the opportunity to empower themselves and to support each other.[49] In closing, he cited the words of one of the victorious plaintiffs in the court case in Japan: "Human rights are like air. I feel that today is the first time that I can breathe freely." He closed with the poetry of Akashi Kaijin, a poet from the 1920s who knew what it was to have leprosy: "Unless I illuminate myself like a deep sea fish, nowhere will I find even a glimmer of light." Sasakawa concluded with the request, "I strongly wish that the Human Rights Commission will take this issue up as a vital human rights issue and bring this to the attention of other relevant human rights agencies and to the wider public."[50] This was the first time that leprosy had been raised as a human rights issue at the United Nations.

The following year, the issue was introduced before the Sub-Commission on the Promotion and Protection of Human Rights at its fifty-sixth session.[51] The Commission then began a fact-finding survey. Yozo Yokota's resulting report found that "If one tries to list human rights that are denied to leprosy-affected persons, almost all categories would apply."[52] It expresses the injustices suffered in the following terms:

> The way leprosy patients and their families have been treated by Governments, communities, schools, companies, hospitals and other organizations, including religious institutions, involves serious human rights violations.

Forced lifelong hospitalization in isolated leprosy facilities, abandonment and rejection of close contact, neglect, lack of adequate health care and social welfare, discrimination in family, social and public life and discrimination in employment are some features of human rights violations against leprosy patients commonly found in almost any country or any community. In some cases, leprosy-affected persons have been the targets of abuse or even physical attack. For a long time, leprosy patients and their families have been discriminated against in marriage and social life. This kind of discrimination still exists today in many parts of the world.[53]

In August 2005, the United Nations Sub-Commission on Human Rights adopted a resolution based on the recommendations of the survey requesting that all governments act to end discrimination against leprosy-affected people.[54] As the Special Rapporteur, Yozo Yokota began a comprehensive study on discrimination against leprosy victims and their families.[55]

In the meantime, from 2006 until the present day, Yohei Sasakawa held annual "Global Appeals to End Stigma and Discrimination Against People Affected by Leprosy" in order to raise public awareness through the media, and win support from world leaders and organisations generally concerned with human rights.[56] Different groups of people in positions of authority and influence were asked to become signatories to these appeals. He began with world leaders and Nobel Peace Prize laureates, working his way through levels and layers of society in order to awaken people to the rights of leprosy-affected people.[57]

Guidelines to address discrimination

The open-ended consultation to exchange views on the impact of discrimination on the human rights of persons affected by leprosy and their family members, held on 15 January 2009 by the Office of the High Commissioner on Human Rights, provides a concerning snapshot of the continuing conditions for leprosy-affected people.[58] While all countries purported to be following the WHO guidelines with respect to treatment, and in most cases with respect to rehabilitation and reintegration, it was obvious that the idea that leprosy-affected people had a right to a normal life had not entered their purview. Admittedly in some of the countries represented, there were very few people, if any, with leprosy, and some only had a few very old people left. Many countries stated that because of measures already in place, there were no grounds for discrimination, and therefore there was no discrimination. The invisibility of people's experiences enabled such a response.

In contrast, when leprosy-affected people were given the floor at the meeting, the perspective was very different. IDEA had by that point attained consultative status with the Economic and Social Council, and they told another story of institutionalised stigma and discrimination. People from Angola continued to isolate themselves out of fear of rejection. People in Brazil experienced subtle and silent discrimination, such as social rejection as well as "dismissal from work, verbal abuse and eviction from rented flats".[59] In China, people affected by leprosy and their families still experienced social discrimination, especially in areas surrounding villages historically related to the disease. This led to delayed medical treatment. Medical staff were reluctant to treat people affected by leprosy, even if their disease was a thing of the past. People in leprosy villages also suffered from separation from their families for decades, and children of people with the disease experienced "restrictions in education, employment and other areas of life".[60]

In Ethiopia, people had been resettled en masse in 1960 and then relocated again in 1991 at the administrative fiat of the newly established regional governments. People in Ethiopia also had to carry the burden of guilt, believing that they had merited the disease as a curse resulting from their sins. This prejudice impacted on their social status and especially their marriage prospects. In Ghana, social rejection was an everyday part of the life of a leprosy-affected person because they were seen as bearers of bad luck. In Orissa in India, people were not entitled to contest elections or hold the post of councillor of a municipality. There were also discriminatory provisions relating to marriage and divorce, juvenile justice, transportation, life insurance and industrial disputes.[61]

In Kenya, people were "expected to stay in their homes and avoid attending public and social functions such as meetings, markets, churches and schools". They were generally debarred from taking part in commercial activity, and because many people lived in remote rural areas, they did not have access to treatment. Within tribal groups in Kenya,

> the disease was equated with witchcraft, and people affected by it were thought to be paying for their sins. In some clans, isolation in life followed them to their grave. Furthermore, they were not buried within the homestead like other members of the family, but in shallow graves in the bushes. Other tribes did not mourn the death of a person affected by leprosy.[62]

Land was administrated through communal and tribal inheritance systems, which in most cases discriminated against these individuals, and when "people affected by leprosy were excommunicated, their land was taken over by their relatives. This forced people affected by leprosy to live in poverty".[63] People in Mali and Mozambique faced discrimination in the health system and were unable to work or sell their products.[64] People in Nepal were denied the right to food, clothing, and shelter. They were denied access to religious services, social and community functions, and family property. They still came under legislation that could require their separation from family and enable divorce upon diagnosis. Because "leprosy had been categorized as a highly contagious disease, interaction with people affected by leprosy in public places was forbidden".[65]

In Niger, because of rejection at general health centres, people had to go to one of three medical centres that treated leprosy "and had formed communities in different regions of the country".[66] People were reduced to poverty, begging being their only option, with few of their children given the chance of secondary schooling.[67] In Nigeria, "in some parts of the country, if someone had leprosy, family members would hide or kill and burn them in order to avoid shame for the family. People affected by leprosy were denied participation, socially, politically and economically, and some committed suicide". In Indonesia, a hotel refused to accommodate people affected by leprosy, "even after having received objective information from authorities and experts participating in a workshop about the disease, its treatable and curable characteristics and the lack of risk for the hotel staff and other guests".[68]

At its third session, the Advisory Committee endorsed the draft set of principles and guidelines.[69] The guidelines begin with the most fundamental statement, but one that represents a hard-won victory for leprosy-affected people: "Persons affected by leprosy and their family members should be treated as people with dignity and are entitled, on an equal basis with others, to all the human rights and fundamental freedoms proclaimed in the Universal Declaration of Human Rights." A follow-up resolution, together with principles and guidelines, was adopted by the United Nations Human Rights Council in September 2010, and this paved the way for the resolution to be adopted by the United Nations General Assembly in December that year.[70]

Yohei Sasakawa's hope continues to be that leprosy-affected people use the resolution to ask what is being done to help them become independent and gain the employment to which they are entitled. He envisages a world in which organisations of leprosy-affected people will have the same status as other interest groups so that they can negotiate for their rights and for their social and economic rehabilitation: that they be "negotiating partners with the provincial and state governments of each nation". In doing this, they would also be able to ensure the dissemination of accurate information about leprosy in order to eliminate stigma. In his mind, this then balances out the medical efforts with the social efforts.

To further this work, Sasakawa continued to visit countries where leprosy was a problem or even where it was being pushed aside as a priority because of larger health issues, in order to bring the rights of leprosy-affected people to governmental attention. When Brazil decided to shelve the goal of elimination, he persisted in visiting and succeeded in having it made a health priority. Similarly with Mozambique, he kept going back for years, even in the face of much procrastination, until they achieved elimination at the national level. In his position as Goodwill Ambassador, Sasakawa was able to meet heads of state, especially in Africa. He said, "I speak with heads of state as an individual. And I can really talk with them in a very close way, and I can build a close relationship because I am not representing the government."[71] While he continued to be aware of the long time it would take to convince governments to take the United Nations resolution seriously, he was content that there was a way forward:

> I will continue as long as I live with this work. And after I am no longer able to continue this work, of course, there will be people that will follow in my footsteps as the work of the Nippon Foundation. ... Now I can clearly say that we have a clear direction of the path that we will follow to eliminate discrimination and stigma of the leprosy-affected people. Of course we don't know how fast it will be resolved or if it will be resolved after many many years. We don't know the time it will take, but we at least know the direction to follow.[72]

His guiding rationale has been to put people first; because leprosy-affected people were the main players, "They must be in the forefront."

Community self-help, Microeconomics

Without doubt, as people became freed of leprosy infection – if not freed of the disabilities associated with the disease – due to treatment with MDT, they were in a better condition to claim back their rights and take control of their lives. As they found strength within organised and officially recognised collectives, they also drew support from IDEA, Sasakawa Health Foundation, members of the ILEP federation, and local support groups. There are many people's organisations of varying sizes and different composition scattered throughout the world. Some are very small, others comprise an extensive network organised through a central committee.

In all, irrespective of their local character, we can see how both impulses towards a cure (the public health, chemotherapeutic impulse, and the holistic impulse) are embodied as leprosy-affected people appropriate and publicly articulate their fundamental human rights. They appropriate these rights in grounded instances by participating in society, living and laughing and helping each other, picking up whatever traces of life that they can salvage. As they progressively become, or are already, independent, these groups, in ways that are unique to them and their culture, exemplify the self-empowerment of leprosy-affected people.[73]

As an example of a large network, in China, where there are still about 200,000 people affected by leprosy, HANDA (standing for HANsen and DAmien) has over 5,000 members, twenty-two full-time staff – including three persons affected by leprosy – and thousands of volunteers.[74] Originally the members on their board of directors were entirely leprosy-affected people, but now they include up to one-third non-leprosy-affected members.[75] They work in the southern provinces of Guangdong, Yunnan, and Guangxi, and also with some mobile services in eleven other provinces.

HANDA involves itself in leprosy services such as finding people with possible signs of leprosy, supporting people who have let their treatment lapse, helping people avoid developing disabilities, providing counselling for people affected by leprosy and their families, fostering socioeconomic development, making people aware of the truth of leprosy in order to dispel prejudice and stigma, and acting as advocates. HANDA teaches villagers to supervise and take responsibility for the recurrent injuries to hands and feet that can occur as a result of the nerve damage in the aftermath of the disease by forming self-care groups. They have a mobile prosthetic workshop that can reach people in remote areas and provide protective shoes and tailor-made prostheses.[76] These initiatives amongst the local leprosy-affected people have begun to spill over into the general community.[77]

HANDA has helped villagers develop their own community enterprises that have grown into sustainable community development projects. They began in 1995 in three villages with chicken breeding, fish farming, and growing herbs for Chinese medicine. This was a staged process that involved oversight and ongoing encouragement:

> Initially, we conducted field surveys and met with local governments to get their approval for using their land. We had to ensure the active participation

of the villagers and enable them to take part in the decision-making process and elect their own leaders for the enterprises. We conducted skill training and study tours, and provided people with knowledge and skills in product packaging, marketing, and sales. Every week we travelled to the villages to monitor and support their economic activities. When people dropped out in the middle of the process, we tried to spend more time with them and build up their confidence.[78]

Today eighty people affected by leprosy and 150 family members are involved.[79]

HANDA also runs empowerment workshops along the lines pioneered by IDEA. These connect people and develop leaders. People share a newsletter and can also attend other recreational groups so that they share their experiences and build psychological support. Mr Feng Keteng, President of HANDA, says: "Participating in HANDA opened my eyes to the wider world. My work is now respected by my peers; my voice is heard and responded to carefully. I realized that I have rights and I have the confidence to ask for them and to voice my needs." Mr Yuan Yahua, a leprosy-affected prosthetic technician, similarly finds meaning in his work: "My participation in leprosy rehabilitation activities gives me positive energy. When seeing that people affected by leprosy are able to walk freely and comfortably with suitable prostheses, I consider my job a meaningful one. I feel surrounded by positive energy and even my family and friends feel this energy."[80]

As an example of a smaller group, in Indonesia, the Enterprise and Self-Care Group (KUK) is located in a former leprosy settlement named Jongaya in Makassar, South Sulawesi. This was once one of the largest leprosy settlements in Indonesia. There are now 32 members who are active in KUK. Most of them are middle-aged or elderly, and the majority are women. They live together in one settlement and know each other well. Such a small group creates "group coherence as well as group pressure". The KUK members emphasise how important it is "to support each other".

They started out as a self-care group in 2005. Typically, many suffer nerve damage and the resulting changes to their hands and feet, as well as recurrent wounds. As a result of self-care sessions, instead of ignoring their wounds, they manage to keep them under control, "We became aware and more confident that we can deal with our wounds. We would not hide our feet and hands anymore but accept them as they are and care for them as much as possible." Those who have been successful in managing their nerve-damaged hands and feet and healing their wounds have become role models for others. The group describe how their self-care group developed and how it conducts its activities:

In the beginning, we met in an empty community room and brought our soaking basins with us from home every time. Later we decided that to attract more people, we should have our own permanent meeting place. The city health services allowed us to use the veranda of their unused health station, located centrally in the settlement. The provincial leprosy control program built concrete soaking basins and later added a roof to shield against the sun and rain. Today we have three permanent soaking places with roofs. We take the water to fill the basins from a neighboring house and all of us contribute some money to pay for the water. When we started, three of us volunteered as "self-care assistants" to keep the meeting place in order, remind members of the meeting schedule, help them with self-care, footwear and other problems, and keep record books for all our members. As self-care assistants we had special t-shirts and our position was acknowledged in the settlement. The provincial leprosy control program paid us small fees in the early years. We also had external help from an NGO, which visited regularly to provide guidance. For self-care we use materials that everybody can afford, like strips of cloth to cover wounds. If people need new special footwear or help with their prosthesis, we rent a car using our own group money and make an appointment with the local leprosy hospital. At times, the hospital team has even come to the settlement, and announced their visits through KUK. Over the years we have received many visitors from all over Indonesia and even from abroad, who came to see and learn from our group.[81]

In 2008, the women began a savings and loan scheme. This enables them to borrow money with very little interest. Many members have taken out one or several loans and started successful enterprises. Their success serves as an example for others, and also makes it possible for them to use the income to help others in need.[82] While they are not officially registered as a collective and do experience the internal politics of any small group, they have their own regulations, goals, and work plans, and this makes it possible for them to run their activities successfully and sustainably, without having to look for continuous external support. They find their strength in their communality: "We are friends and we help each other."[83]

2020: The special rapporteur's report to the United Nations

Alice Cruz, the United Nations Human Rights Council Special Rapporteur, insists that people must be the "leading protagonists" in eliminating stigma and discrimination.[84] In April 2020, she presented a policy framework for the future to the Human Rights Council for the General Assembly of the United Nations. In signalling her disregard for a "well-intentioned discourse", she threw down the gauntlet to the member nations, calling for their progressive, but expeditious and effective, realisation of equality for persons affected by leprosy and their family members, and for the assurance of adequate standards of living and economic autonomy for the sake of their personal development. She called for social protection, including social security (that incorporates access to healthcare, shelter, housing, water, and sanitation), so that those affected by leprosy could live in and be included in the community without discrimination, as participating citizens. The report also challenged States to be proactive in eliminating stereotypes, affording the right to truth and memory, and empowering people, especially those in vulnerable groups.[85]

In conclusion, it is worth reflecting back on the long journey since the first representation made in 1949 to the WHO. Then the medical advocates were asking for the most basic considerations: inclusion in an international health agenda. Today, before the United Nations, the Rapporteur presents a strategy that also asks for the most basic considerations. While the Rapporteur distinguishes the journey to human rights as distinct, preliminary, and fundamental for a cure for leprosy, something that cannot be provided by medical means alone, history also shows that a cure for leprosy cannot be provided without medical means either. Both the medical body and the social body are one, embodied in the person with the disease who lives and participates in society, surrounded by like-minded others, and who uniquely synthesises the competing interests that bring themselves to bear on their own bodies to fit their own purposes.

CONCLUSION

The events recounted in this history of international efforts against leprosy are open to several interpretations. In one version, the extra-budgetary funding for anti-leprosy work was accompanied by unwarranted interference in the WHO programme, resulting in an over-hasty, acrimonious, and ultimately unsuccessful elimination campaign. In another version, a great work of disease control in the twentieth century was accomplished by a combination of extraordinary philanthropy, visionary courageousness, and wily and pragmatic diplomacy. In yet another version, experienced, self-sacrificing anti-leprosy experts refused to abdicate their professional responsibilities to populist campaigns that cared more for statistics than people, risked patients with under-trialled drug therapies, and irresponsibly entrusted patients with medication without supervision. Each version of the story invokes a specific perspective and perhaps a corresponding label: bureaucratic, triumphalist, elitist. But just as these labels are not fully separable, neither are the versions themselves. If not for the intervention of donors, a great work of disease control could not have been accomplished, even if it was at the expense of a closer degree of expert medical oversight. None of the versions exists independently of the other. None of the versions is without credit, and none is to the complete credit of all involved. Yes, they can exist side by side.

Decisions about when and how the work against leprosy should proceed have always been at the mercy of political and economic contingencies. Although this is something that is true of any disease to some degree, with leprosy those decisions were also freighted with emotional intensity which was upon occasion harnessed to potent figurations of institutional and national identity and value. At the same time, as the work against leprosy became an international initiative, the notion of a "cure" for the disease developed in such a way that it too became politicised. The politics of different and eventually competing notions of a "cure" for leprosy have been central to this narrative.

223

Implications for the historiography

An overview of the history of the WHO shows that efforts to control leprosy were influenced by the overall trajectory of the organisation just as much as any other disease control effort, something not always appreciated by those immersed in working against leprosy. Yet while the overall trajectory of the WHO determined what happened to international work against leprosy, the uniqueness of leprosy's social and representational aetiology calls for a degree of nuance in charting its recent history.

Much of the critical literature on the history of international health measures since World War II is, not without reason, underpinned by a critique of international paternalism and a narrow technological view of medicine.[1] These scholarly works see the biomedical (magic bullet) models of disease control of the 1950s and 1960s being orchestrated at the expense of a more rounded and contextualised approach to international health that would take into account the social, cultural, economic, political, and national conditions in which people live.[2] Packard argues that "International Health interventions during most of the 20th century have focused on preventing the transmission of infectious agents and on treating those who are infected with specific curative agents."[3] He emphasises the focus of tropical medicine on the health of populations in underdeveloped but richly resourced colonised nations, citing the efforts of the Rockefeller Foundation in the 1920s and 1930s against yellow fever and malaria in Latin America and demonstrating how these connections became even more pronounced after World War II.[4]

Leprosy is a little different. While the case for international efforts against leprosy made to the WHA did indeed include arguments about the cost to nations and societies of permanently disabled people, leprosy also presents another perspective on third-world poverty. To be afflicted with leprosy could cause disability and make it difficult for people to earn a living, but the stigma associated with the disease inevitably brought about a loss of both social and economic status. So addressing the early onset of the disease with medication (the magic bullet of DDS) could prevent people from slipping out of their place in society. If all went well, they could even continue to make a contribution to their and their family's livelihood. Equally, the biomedical model or magic bullet of medication made a difference to stigma.

When people were confident that there were medications to deal with the disease, the disease was de-demonised. Improving a leprosy-affected person's social and economic conditions robbed the disease of its power over the imaginary. Later, after 1991, community-based rehabilitation efforts also provided micro credit for cured patients to establish their own small businesses.[5] In this instance of disease control, the biomedical model had a direct impact on individual well-being, for even if the disease itself was not eliminated, the misery produced by the disease in individual lives was reduced. Admittedly, a productive third-world country with fewer disabled people would only perpetuate the exploitation of the third world for the sake of the first world's needs for resources and for markets. But clearly different diseases require different approaches, and the experience with leprosy shows that it is simplistic to oppose the biomedical model to the socially and economically contextualising models. In leprosy control, at least, they are interconnected.

The scholarly critique of international health efforts also focuses on oppositions between vertical and horizontal approaches to disease control. Birn argues that this was encapsulated in the contradictions between the success of smallpox eradication and the aspirations of Alma Ata/primary healthcare.[6] Two models of healing are opposed to each other: on the one hand, vertical, technical, centrally driven, disease-based, doctor-centred healing and on the other hand, horizontal, social, locally defined, health-based, individual community-based healing.

In international anti-leprosy efforts, both models of healing were deployed selectively throughout the long history of encounters with the disease. Public health administrators were pragmatic about whether to mobilise the resources of primary healthcare. If multidrug therapy could be furthered by community involvement, then so be it. If a specialised vertical programme would make a difference, then they did not hesitate. If a large and populous country with poor infrastructure at the periphery had a vertical programme for leprosy, then the transition to primary healthcare was deliberate and measured. At the same time, administrators mobilised volunteers and the whole community, from the most influential businessperson to the humblest villager. To implement the drug regimes, they drew on primary healthcare workers to entrust the medication to people for self-administration. Similarly, they simplified chemotherapeutic regimens in keeping with the values of primary healthcare. They also simplified administrative procedures, much to the chagrin of the epidemiologists. Yet special targeting and very local vertical campaigns were deployed as well, in spite of the criticism that this might undermine primary healthcare. In all, there was a pragmatic blend of whatever approach was feasible, and, at the same time, a progressive assimilation/integration of medical services into the periphery.

Rosenberg et al. claim that "participants in global health have been left with an exquisite horizontal–vertical balancing act, and the outcome is still being played out".[7] I would argue that this balancing act was important to the success of the leprosy elimination efforts in countries such as India. The combined vertical campaigns that were mobilised using volunteers from all sections of society were spectacular successes and managed to orient both health professionals and the community to the disease and its treatment. In addition, speaking leprosy's name in public, owning it as a health problem that could be addressed, robbed the stigmatising disease of its power.

Debates about the shortcomings of single-disease eradication efforts constantly dogged the leprosy elimination campaign. In an extended analysis of polio eradication, Muraskin argues strongly that disease eradication yields benefits to the Western world and puts the burden of costs of eradication on underdeveloped countries. He maintains that this incurs the likely risk of a loss of interest once the threat is reduced and offers a short-term investment, low risk, and big returns, in alignment with a Wall Street investment credo.[8] Such campaigns are by their nature top-down, undemocratic blame-and-shame affairs which twist and distort national priorities in the interest of a public good defined by those outside the nation.[9]

Although no one wants to stir up past acrimonies gratuitously, it should be now possible to debate dispassionately the value of what has taken place and the policies that underpinned that. And people are now prepared to weigh up the advantages and disadvantages of the policies. As Diana Lockwood writes: "It is important that we should discuss the elimination strategy and its strengths and weaknesses because we can then use the parts that worked and develop alternatives for the aspects that did not work." She argues that there is still a lack of evidence to justify the policy itself, for modelling shows that leprosy cases will continue to present for decades yet, and studies in Bangladesh and India reveal that there are still many undetected cases of leprosy in the community.[10] Cairns Smith recognises the political advantages that the campaign won for a relatively unimportant disease. He contends that "The elimination strategy was highly successful in providing a focus for leprosy and in securing political and financial commitment leading to a dramatic reduction in registered prevalence by the end of 2000."[11]

Has the elimination initiative done more harm than good? Admittedly, spending for further research diminished; national programmes shifted their focus to other pressing concerns; and people still continue to be infected. But in the face of these significant issues, the millions of people who have been cured of leprosy and the many saved from disability remain a vivid testimony to a public health initiative that was arguably a compelling moral imperative. The voices of the people who experienced the regimes of the past throw into sharp contrast the very different scenario that the present holds for anyone now diagnosed with the disease.

From a medical point of view, should there have been a more measured approach to treatment so that multidrug therapy was not introduced until it had been subjected to extensive clinical trials? Should integration of leprosy into general medical services and into primary healthcare have taken place step by step so that the full measure of procedures such as laboratory tests were preserved? If normal cautions had prevailed, dapsone monotherapy may have been extended another decade, with all of the disastrous consequences of drug resistance.

Leprosy elimination in the era of COVID-19

In the midst of the COVID-19 global pandemic, the efforts to control leprosy infection throughout the world offer uncanny resonances and a microcosm of issues that have since only intensified in magnitude and seriousness. So far, the only measures available for public health disease control, whether viral or mycobacterial, still involve isolating populations. As always, the most vulnerable, the poorest, the most disadvantaged, are those who fall victim to the disease. Meanwhile the race for a vaccine being conducted at "warp speed" is sweeping aside the usual protocols for trials in a way that makes the "deft strategy" used to win approval for MDT a relatively minor irregularity by comparison. The sacrifice of human rights expected of leprosy-affected people echoes some of the measures employed to contain COVID-19. On the other hand, in liberal democracies where people insist on their individual freedoms, infection rates have soared with fatal results. The criticism of the WHO's response to the pandemic dwarfs the resentment towards the WHO in the leprosy elimination campaign.

What lessons have we learned from the leprosy elimination campaign? Not very many, from what I can see. While we are warned that no pandemic is ever the same — and, furthermore, I stress that leprosy is an endemic disease, not a pandemic — it is impossible not to compare the public health measures against the mycobacteria and the virus.[12] Both have infected millions, although COVID-19's impact seems more dramatic, unless you take a long view of the history of leprosy. COVID-19 continues to spread swiftly through the world's population, killing a relatively small percentage of those infected, and although leprosy does not kill its host, COVID-19 may not yet have infected as many people as leprosy has in its long coexistence with mankind.[13] Additionally, while COVID-19 has disrupted the world's economy dramatically, leprosy was also perceived as a similar threat in the late nineteenth century.

In this reading, the isolation measures against leprosy, before efficacious drugs were introduced and especially before MDT, seem today to be antiquated and unscientific, and inhumane. Yet the current control measures available against COVID-19 are not all that different. People with leprosy were isolated from society. People with COVID-19 are required to self-isolate, or they are quarantined; people with leprosy were isolated for a lifetime until efficacious drugs became available; self-isolation with COVID-19 is short, by comparison, yet today whole cities have shut down, streets have been emptied, and places of commerce have been abandoned.[14] The side effects of leprosy isolation continue. Stigma persists in the subsequent generations. The effects of repeated bouts of isolation because of COVID-19 are yet to be determined, although the impact of isolation on mental health is spreading throughout the community.

At the same time, and in spite of the long-term damage that COVID-19 may do to individual health, the infection does not produce visual effects comparable with leprosy. And although some people who are infected have been subject to discrimination and marginalisation to some extent in different countries, that stigma will be different and possibly less than anything like the life-altering stigma experienced by people affected by leprosy. And while self-isolation and quarantine for those with COVID-19 have lasted for shorter periods, earlier releases from region-wide lockdowns seem guaranteed to produce further flare-ups of the virus and ensure ongoing requirements for isolation. Leprosy infection worldwide is not over, and we have no idea when, or even if, there will be an end to the current COVID-19 pandemic.

Testing, tracing, and isolating remain the mainstays in the attempts to control COVID-19, just as they were originally against leprosy. It seems certain that the efforts to produce a vaccine against leprosy will be overtaken by a successful vaccine against COVID-19. This raises a question: is differential time lag in vaccine development due to the differences in behaviour in the laboratory between the bacillus and the virus, or is this also about the financial energy and political will for countering COVID-19, as opposed to the complacency still swirling around leprosy?

As has already been observed, the story of disease in society is mostly about the politics. As this narrative demonstrates, leprosy has been heavily politicised. Equally, as contemporary history demonstrates, the COVID-19 pandemic is also infused with politics to the extent that whether an individual wears a mask has become a badge of their political allegiance. What lessons can we take from comparing the politics of disease control measures against leprosy and COVID-19? First, COVID-19 vividly demonstrates what we already knew about leprosy: disease discriminates on the basis of socio-economic status and ethnicity. We have seen socio-economic and racial discrimination experienced with leprosy reveal their full-blown effects in the differential spread and containment of COVID-19 in different nation–states, especially those that were most vigilant in guarding against leprosy. In "Flailing States," Pankaj Mishra writes, "Covid-19 has exposed the world's greatest democracies as victims of prolonged self-harm; it has also demonstrated that countries with strong state capacity have been far more successful at stemming the virus's spread and look better equipped to cope with the social and economic fallout."[15]

But our global interconnectedness brings us back to the raison d'être for the WHO in the first place, that the right to health of the individual is a fundamental right that cannot be achieved without ensuring the health of all. In addition, as pointed out by the United Nations and the WHO, "human wealth depends upon nature's health".[16] We still know so little about diseases like leprosy and the recent coronaviruses, not just as human-infecting pathogens but as elements in a global ecosystem. While we show little regard for our natural environment, we seem helpless in the face of disease. Leprosy and COVID-19 make us reconsider our relationship to our natural environment, as well as to each other, and the use we make of others and of the natural world as a resource. How much has changed in the thousands of years between *M. Leprae*'s and COVID-19's respective emergences from our ecosystem, and how have we responded to their promptings to rethink our coexistence with pathogens?

NOTES

PROLOGUE

1. Queensland State Archives 15 May 1891 (Col Sec 264: No. 05874).
2. In the face of this reluctance to leave, administrators complained that people had become used to the luxuries of the asylum.

INTRODUCTION

1. Hansen and Looft, *Leprosy*, 86.
2. Hastings, *Leprosy*, 32.
3. See Dharmendra in Hastings, "The various clinical manifestations in leprosy are the results of the variations in the tissue response of the host to the presence of leprosy bacilli in the body. In other words, they are determined by the host–parasite relationship," 88.
4. Birn, "The Stages of International Health," 62.
5. This is the story for malaria, although recently McMillen's *Discovering Tuberculosis* has nuanced the story of anti-tuberculosis efforts.
6. Skinsnes, "Leprosy in Society I," 23.
7. Skinsnes, "Leprosy in Society I." The descriptions that he identifies refer to leprosy amongst other diseases, but he qualifies the specifics of the disease in each of these instances.
8. Skinsnes, "Leprosy in Society II," 121.
9. This occurred at the Fifth International Congress of Leprosy, held in Havana. *IJL* 16, no. 2 (1948): 184 and 243–44.
10. Sontag, *Illness as Metaphor*, 3–4.
11. Sontag, *Illness as Metaphor*, 58.
12. Di Giacomo, "Metaphor as Illness," 109.
13. Scheper-Hughes and Lock, "Speaking 'Truth' to Illness," 137–40.
14. Martin, *Miracle at Carville*, and Berthelsen, *The Lost Years*.
15. Mark, "Alexander the Great," 286. This idea began with Johs Andersen's "Studies in the Medical Diagnosis of Leprosy in Denmark," *Danish Medical Bulletin* 16, supplement 9 (1968): 10–45 and 123. In contrast, Mark, "Alexander the Great," argues that leprosy came with children and slaves.
16. Douglas, "Witchcraft and Leprosy," 723–36.
17. Douglas, "Witchcraft and Leprosy," 734.

18. Douglas, "Witchcraft and Leprosy," 731–3.

19. Vaughan, *Curing Their Ills.*

20. Vaughan, *Curing Their Ills,* 88 and 83.

21. BELRA Annual Report 1935. Unpublished. LEPRA Archives, Colchester, UK.

22. Vaughan, *Curing Their Ills,* 79.

23. Smith Kipp, "The Evangelical Uses of Leprosy," 166.

24. Smith Kipp, "The Evangelical Uses of Leprosy," 175.

25. Anderson, "Leprosy and Citizenship," 720, and *Colonial Pathologies: American Tropical Medicine, Race, and Hygiene in the Philippines.*

26. Obregón, "The State Physicians and Leprosy in Modern Colombia," 130–57.

27. Adams, *The Seven Books of Paulus Ægineta.*

28. Hebra and Kaposi, *On the Diseases of the Skin*, 118–19. They list a bewildering variety of names from different countries: "Lepra Arabum, Elephantiasis Graecorum, Leprosy of the English, Spedalskhed of the Norwegians; Aussatz, Maltzey (of the Middle Ages), Limafalsk (Iceland), Malum mortuum, Malmorte (Salernitan school), Mal rouge (de Cayenne), Mal rosso, juzam (Arab) Krimskaia, Lepra taurica, Rosa asturiensis, Kushta (India), Fa-fung (China), Koban (Africa), Kokobay (West Indies), Ngerengere and Tuwhenna (New Zealand) Morbus Phoenicius, Morbus herculeus, Satyriasis, Leontiasis (of the old Greeks), Zaraath (Hebrew), Morphoea, Spiloplaxia, Tyria &c., &c."

29. "Elephantiasis, Vitiligo, Alphos, Leuke, Melas," in Hebra and Kaposi, 121 and 125.

30. Hebra and Kaposi, *On the Diseases of the Skin*, 125–7.

31. Danielssen and Boëck, *Traite de la Spedalskhed ou Elephantiasis de Grecs*, 138.

32. Their most notable publication was *Om Spedalskhed*, Christiania 1847, which was translated into French as *Traité de la Spedalskhed ou Elephanthiasis des Grecs*, Paris, 1848. This was accompanied by an *Atlas Colorié de Spedalskhed (Elephantiases des Grecs)* which contained twenty-four lithographs by J. L. Losting (1810–76). Their studies of the pathological anatomy of the disease classified two principal types: the tubercle and the anaesthetic.

33. Hansen observed and dated his discovery, in English, as follows: "If one examines, microscopically, sections or teased preparations of fresh nodules, one sees little else but cells, with distinct nuclei, usually of the size of a white blood corpuscle, or rather larger … With a higher power, one sees in the fluid of the preparation small straight rods, which are not destroyed by addition of potash. These are the lepra bacilli, and thus they were discovered in the year 1871." Hansen, *Leprosy: in its Clinical and Pathological Aspects*, 31. See Worboys, "The Colonial World as Mission and Mandate," 207–18; "Was There a Bacteriological Revolution in Late Nineteenth-Century Medicine?" 20–42; and Edmond, *Leprosy and Empire.*

34. Hebra and Kaposi, *On the Diseases of the Skin*, 131.

35. Gussow, *Leprosy, Racism and Public Health,* 6–7.

36. Categories for the clinical signs of the disease were debated up until the 7th International Leprosy Congress (Tokyo, 1958), and until a classification system

was arrived at that was based on the body's immune response to the disease, in 1962.

37. Dyer, "The Berlin Leprosy Conference," 357–68.

38. World Health Organization, *Leprosy: A Survey of Recent Legislation*, 6.

39. World Health Organization, *Leprosy: A Survey of Recent Legislation,* 4–5.

40. In 1941, Robert Cochrane stated that "leprosy is a child's disease". Cochrane, *The Epidemiology, Pathology and Diagnosis of Child Leprosy*; Robertson, "The Leprosy-Affected Body as a Commodity," 131–64.

41. Rogers and Muir, *Leprosy*, 11.

42. Rogers and Muir state that "in three of these the symptoms appeared respectively ten months, one year and two years after such exposure to infection" (80).

43. Studies demonstrated the vulnerability of young children living in houses with people suffering from lepromatous leprosy: the most infective form of the disease (72–3).

44. This practice is well documented in the secondary literature; for example, the legend that tells of the cure of Rama, the king of Benares, in Parascandola, "Chaulmoogra Oil and the Treatment of Leprosy," 47–57; Buckingham traces the use of chaulmoogra oil in the Ayurvedic tradition in *Leprosy in Colonial South India*; also Greenwood, *Antimicrobial Drugs,* 190–4.

45. Mouat, "Notes on Native Remedies," 646–52.

46. Rogers and Muir, *Leprosy*, 242.

47. The usual dose was between 0.5 cc to 6 cc once or twice weekly. Rogers and Muir, *Leprosy*, 251. At the turn of the twentieth century, a chemical analysis of the seeds of *Taraktogenos kurzii* from Assam and Burma was carried out by Frederick B. Power at the Wellcome Chemical Research Laboratories in London, in 1904. He isolated an unsaturated fatty acid named chaulmoogric acid. Further analysis of *Hydnocarpus wightiana*, from south-west India, and *Hydnocarpus anthelmintica*, from Siam (Thailand) and Indochina (Vietnam), produced oils that were similar in physical characteristics and chemical analysis. From these, the chemical analysts at Wellcome also obtained a new acid, which they named hydnocarpus acid. Parascandola, "Chaulmoogra Oil," 7.

48. "Recoveries from Leprosy," 667–88. The authors were Oswald E. Denny, the medical officer in charge of the National Leprosy Home at Carville; Ralph Hopkins, the Professor of Dermatology at Tulane University, Louisiana, and attending Dermatologist; and Frederick A. Johansen, the Acting-Assistant Surgeon at Carville.

49. Information about these cases was presented to the American Association of Tropical Medicine, in Miami, Florida, in November 1930. The accounts of recoveries rely on the premise that "a cure, once mutilation had occurred" was impossible. A cure, in this instance, is defined as the restoration of physiological function.

50. Twenty-eight of those released were female. All were designated as white. Their ages ranged from sixty-six years to three. Eight were 50 years and over, seven were 40 years and over, and six were 30 years and over. In addition to the

3-year-old, the youngest were thirteen, seventeen, and nineteen. There were three women in their twenties (twenty, twenty-three, and twenty-four years). There were thirty-seven men who were designated as belonging to a variety of racial categories. Twenty-three were described as white, six as Negro, four were Filipino, and there were also individuals designated as Chinese, Brown, Mexican, and Hawaiian. Their ages ranged from sixteen to sixty-seven. The majority, nine, were in their thirties. Three were under twenty, twelve were between twenty and thirty, nine were between thirty and forty, eight between forty and fifty, three between fifty and sixty, and only two who were older than sixty. The youngest were sixteen, seventeen, and nineteen.

51. Denny et al.
52. Case 14-12, Denny et al., "Recoveries From Leprosy," 671.
53. Case 32-87, Denny et al., "Recoveries From Leprosy," 675.
54. Case 64-40, Denny et al., "Recoveries From Leprosy," 685.
55. Case 33-118, Denny et al., "Recoveries From Leprosy," 676.
56. Case 34-84, Denny et al., "Recoveries From Leprosy," 676. Case notes indicate that she was unable to tolerate chaulmoogra for any length of time.
57. Case 5-76, Denny et al., "Recoveries From Leprosy," 668.
58. Burnet, *Report of the Study Tour*.
59. The use of the term "bleach" here is unusual in medical terms associated with leprosy. It may be a very literal translation of the French term, *blanchir*, to whiten.
60. Burnet, *Report of the Study Tour*, 39.
61. About this time, medical people recognised that the disease was sometimes "self-arresting", particularly in what was known as neural forms of leprosy (and are now known as paucibacillary leprosy or PB). This was most common in children.
62. Burnet, *Report of the Study Tour*, 39.
63. Muir, *Manual of Leprosy*, 169–78. The layout can be seen on p. 171.
64. This is evident in the earliest editions of *Leprosy Notes* which were published by the *British Empire Leprosy Relief Association*.
65. Pandya, "Ridding the Empire of Leprosy."
66. Rogers and Muir, *Leprosy*, 248.
67. Rogers and Muir, *Leprosy*, 254.
68. Stein, *Alone No Longer*, 40.
69. Stein, *Alone No Longer*, 39.
70. Stein, *Alone No Longer*, 56–7.
71. Burnet, *Report of the Study Tour*, 41.
72. Stein, *Alone No Longer*, 217.
73. Stein, *Alone No Longer*, 218.
74. Greenwood, *Antimicrobial Drugs*, 53 and 66–70.
75. Greenwood, *Antimicrobial Drugs*, 74; and Doull, "Sulfone Therapy of Leprosy," 143. Domagk was eventually awarded a Nobel Prize after the war for his discovery, despite the best efforts of the Nazi regime to deny him the honour.

76. Buttle, "Viewpoint," 443; Greenwood, *Antimicrobial Drugs*, 70–1; the patent was filled out by Mietzsch and Klarer (the chemists who had actually synthesised and tested the chrysoidine analogues, substance Kl 730).

77. Buttle, "Viewpoint," 464.

78. Greenwood, *Antimicrobial Drugs*, 195; Doull, "Sulfone Therapy of Leprosy," 143–4.

79. Buttle, "Viewpoint," 464; Doull writes that Rist, who was at the Institut Pasteur, found the stronger bacteriostatic effect of DDS and also the results against experimental avian tubercle bacillus infection in the rabbit, both in 1939. Clinical results against infections were reported by Heitz Boyer and Palazzoli and Bovet in 1937. Trials of Promin had shown that it was successful against experimental pneumonia in guinea pigs.

80. Cited in Doull, "Sulfone Therapy of Leprosy," 145–6.

81. Doull, "Sulfone Therapy of Leprosy," 145.

82. Faget, Johansen, and Ross, "Sulfanilamide in the Treatment of Leprosy," 1892–9.

83. WHO describes lepra reactions as follows: "During the course of leprosy, immunologically mediated episodes of acute or subacute inflammation known as reactions may occur in up to 25% of patients with paucibacillary leprosy and as much as 40% in multibacillary leprosy. Clinical indications of a reaction are nerve pain, loss of sensation and loss of function. The reactions may rapidly cause severe and irreversible nerve damage and must always be treated promptly. If a patient does not respond to lepra reaction treatment within 4 weeks or his/her condition deteriorates at any time during lepra reaction treatment, send that patient immediately to the nearest specialist centre. During a lepra reaction, do not interrupt leprosy multidrug therapy. Treatment with multidrug therapy reduces the frequency and severity of lepra reactions." http://apps.who.int/medicinedocs/en/d/Jh2988e/4.html#Jh2988e.4

84. Faget et al., "Sulfanilamide in the Treatment of Leprosy," 489.

85. Martin, *Miracle at Carville*, 181.

86. Doull, "Sulfone Therapy of Leprosy," 149.

87. Faget et al., "The Promin Treatment of Leprosy"; Faget, "The Story of the National Leprosarium," 649.

88. Faget et al., "The Promin Treatment of Leprosy," 298. In 1945, Faget again reported on the Promin trials. The improvements had continued, although he did not claim that it was a specific for leprosy. He continued to hope for a faster-acting drug. Faget also tried diasone, pencillin, and promizole. In 1946, in "The Story of the National Leprosarium", he stated that the public should know that "recent improvement in the treatment of leprosy renders it no longer a hopeless disease". Faget and Pogge, "The Therapeutic Effect of Promin in Leprosy" and "Penicillin Treatment of Leprosy"; Faget et al., "Promizole Treatment of Leprosy"; Faget, "The Story of the National Leprosarium, 1871–1883."

89. Faget began with oral dosages even though Sharpe had recommended against it. Stein, *Alone No Longer*, 221.

90. Faget et al., "The Promin Treatment of Leprosy," 303. Case 1206.
91. Faget et al., "The Promin Treatment of Leprosy," Case 1032.
92. Faget et al., "The Promin Treatment of Leprosy," Case 869.
93. Faget et al., "The Promin Treatment of Leprosy," Case 864.
94. There were sixteen for whom treatment had to be discontinued. Five had refused to participate and two had absconded. In addition, four had suffered from ENL reactions and four others had suffered from complications such as exfoliative dermatitis, leucopenia, and previously advanced nephritis, and one was still suffering from hepatitis induced by the sulphanilamide trial. Faget et al., "The Promin Treatment of Leprosy," 308.
95. Faget et al., "The Promin Treatment of Leprosy," 309–10.
96. Stein, *Alone No Longer*, 222.
97. Stein, *Alone No Longer*.
98. Martin, *Miracle at Carville*, 197–8.
99. Martin, *Miracle at Carville*, 202.
100. Stein, 223.
101. John Lowe, "Treatment of Diamino-Diphenyl Sulphone by Mouth," 145–50. Lowe's paper would not be published in *Lancet* until 1950.
102. Cochrane, "Correspondence," 195; Lowe, "Treatment of Leprosy," 145.
103. Cochrane, "The Use of Diaminodiphenyl Sulfone," 98.
104. The only other report about the toxicity of the drug came from Long and Bliss in 1939, cited in Feldman et al., 1944.
105. Lowe, "Treatment of Leprosy," 145.
106. Lowe, "Treatment of Leprosy," 146.
107. Lowe, "Treatment of Leprosy," 147.
108. Lowe, "Treatment of Leprosy," 149.
109. Lowe, "Treatment of Leprosy," 27.
110. The derivative was sulphetrone.
111. "The Use of Diaminodiphenyl Sulfone," 91–3.

1. WINNING PRIORITY FOR LEPROSY AT THE WORLD HEALTH ORGANIZATION

1. The WHO Constitution states that "Unequal development in different countries in the promotion of health and control of disease, especially communicable disease, is a common danger". Constitution of the World Health Organization. Basic Documents, 45th edition. Supplement October 2006. http://www. who.int/governance/eb/who_constitution_en.pdf

The United Nations Conference equated political stability with health and well-being at their 1945 meeting in San Francisco. At that same conference, approval was given to form an international health organisation. The International Health Conference opened in New York on 19 June 1946, the WHO Constitution was drafted and an Interim Commission was established to prepare for the WHO. The Interim Commission, which lasted two years, convened the first World Health Assembly on 24 June 1948, in Geneva. Previous international health organisations were as follows: the fourteen International Sanitary Conferences, held in Europe between 1851 and 1938; the Office International d'Hygiène Publique, which was convened in 1907 and based in Paris to oversee international rules regarding quarantine and to administer other public health conventions, being eventually absorbed into the Interim Commission; and the Health Committee of the League of Nations, which lasted from 28 June 1919 until 20 April 1946, and was formed to oversee the health work of the League of Nations, conduct inquiries, and prepare work to be presented to the Health Council. "Work of the Interim Commission," 75, 77, and 91.

2.   "Constitution of the WHO," 1.

3.   WHO, First World Health Assembly, Geneva, 24 June to 24 July 1948, Verbatim Records of the Plenary Meetings: First Plenary Meeting, 24 June 1948, 25.

4.   WHO, "First World Health Assembly," 24.

5.   These ideals were formulated in the shadow of "biological warfare, like that of the atomic bomb", for there was an all-pervasive sense that humanity was at risk of "total annihilation". WHO, *Chronicle* 1, no. 1 (1947): 5.

6.   WHO, *Chronicle* 2, no. 8–9 (1948): 179; Minutes and Documents of the Fifth Session of the Interim Commission, held in Geneva from 22 January to 7 February 1948.

7.   The Interim Commission stated that the diseases that took the greatest toll on health and life were malaria, venereal diseases, tuberculosis, ankylostomiasis, filariasis, leishmaniasis, leprosy, schistosomiasis, trypanosomiasis, influenza, trachoma, and cancer, just as leprosy was showing a response to Promin and associated sulphones. WHO, *Chronicle* 2, no. 8–9 (1948): 171.

8.   Raj Kumari Amrit Kaur had been elected as one of three vice presidents of the inaugural assembly in Geneva on 24 June 1948. WHO, *Chronicle* 2, no. 8–9 (1948): 164.

9.   He writes: "The question of further simplifying my life and of doing some concrete act of service to my fellowmen had been constantly agitating me, when a leper came to my door. I had not the heart to dismiss him with a meal. So I offered him shelter, dressed his wounds, and began to look after him. But I could not go on like that indefinitely. I could not afford, I lacked the will to keep him always with me. So I sent him to the Government Hospital for indentured labourers." Gandhi, *Autobiography*, 202.

10. "Sanskrit scholar Dattatray Parchure Shastri, a leprosy patient, asked to be admitted to Sevagram ashram. Some members objected as they feared infection. Gandhi not only admitted him; he attended to his needs. In his letter to Shashtri he writes, 'Shastriji, You have fallen ill! It is not good if it is from worry. But if it is death calling, there is no harm. You must go with a smile on your lips. And that too from a Lepers' House. Whatever it may be, remain calm and sing Tukaram's abhangs. Blessings from BAPU.'" http://www.tukaram. com/gujarati/gujarat.asp

11. Diwan, "The Three All India Leprosy Workers Conferences," 128. Gandhi spoke of the neglect of people with leprosy in India, saying: "It is largely the missionary who, be it said to his credit, bestows care on him. The only institution run by an Indian, as a pure labour of love, is by Shri Manohar Diwan near Wardha. It is working under the inspiration and guidance of Shri Vinoba Bhave."

12. Raj Kumari Amrit Kaur to T. N. Jagadisan, 28 October, 1949, in Jagadisan, *Fulfilment Through Leprosy*, 159.

13. Erikson, "On the Nature of Psycho-Historical Evidence"; Trivedi, "Visually Mapping the 'Nation'"; *Khadi* is any cloth that is hand-spun or woven. The Khadi movement refers to the boycotting of British cotton and the spinning and wearing of the homegrown product. Followers of Gandhi and the movement to independence took to spinning their own clothing as a form of resistance. Many of the leprosy workers wore *khadi*.

14. Gandhi composed *Constructive Programme: Its Meaning and Place* on the train from Sevagram to Bardoli, in which he listed thirteen items as national priorities: "(1) Communal Unity; (2) Removal of Untouchability; (3) Prohibition; (4) *Khadi*; (5) Village Industries; (6) Village Sanitation; (7) *Nai Talim* or Basic Education; (8) Adult Education; (9) Uplift of Women; (10) Education in Health and Hygiene; (11) Provincial Languages; (12) National Language; (13) Promotion of Economic Equality. Later he added five more: (1) *Kisans*; (2) Labour (3) Adivasis (4) Lepers (5) Students." Narayanaswamy, "Constructive Programme Towards Twenty First Century."

15. Gandhi, *Constructive Programme: Its Meaning and Place*.

16. Raj Kumari Amrit Kaur to T. N. Jagadisan, 28 October 1949, in Jagadisan, 159.

17. There is a debate around the concrete application of the symbolism. Arnold, *Gandhi*, 127.

18. Editorial, "Constructive Programme and Leprosy," 41. This editorial adds a correction to the statement that there was only one leprosy institution in India, run by an Indian. In addition to that run by Manohar Dewan near Wardha, there were several others: the colony of Zahirabad, near Hyderabad (Deccan) (1936); the Naba Kushta Nibas, run by Jimut Bahan Sen, Purulia, Bengal (1937); and the Kala Kala Health Home, founded by Lakshmi Narayan Sahu, a member of the Servants of India (1944).

19. Jagadisan, *Fulfilment Through Leprosy*, 61–3.

20. Jagadisan, *Fulfilment Through Leprosy*, 81. The Board to which he referred was the Kasturba Gandhi National Memorial Trust.

21. Cochrane, "Opportunity in India," 286.

22. Some of the attendees were M. B. Diwan, R. V. Wardekar, W. Bailey, E. Andersen, Dr Sushila Nayyar, R. G. Cochrane, Shrikrishnadas Jaju, Jivraj N. Mehta, A. V. Thakkar, A. D. Miller, Dharmendra, I. Santra, M. S. Kaka Kalekar, V. N. Das, Laury Baker, T. N. Jagadisan, and David Molesworth.

23. Jagadisan, 124–5. Although the conference had been organised at short notice, those who could attend felt a keen sense of the momentous and extraordinary significance of the gathering. This feeling was bolstered by supportive messages

from Mahatma Gandhi and the governors and health ministers of various provinces, as well as a broadcast message from Rajkumari Amrit Kaur. Diwan, 128–9.

24. India Council of the British Empire Leprosy Relief Association, "All-India Leprosy Conference, Wardha," 1.

25. India Council of the British Empire Leprosy Relief Association, "All-India Leprosy Conference, Wardha," 3–4. He was another close associate of Gandhi. He had left his lucrative practice as an advocate in 1921 and worked with Gandhi to spread the khadi movement. http://www.gandhi-manibhavan.org/gandhicomesalive/comesalive_associates_india.htm#Jaju, Shrikrishnadas

26. India Council of the British Empire Leprosy Relief Association, "All-India Leprosy Conference, Wardha," 5–6. Even at this enlightened moment, the people affected by the disease, apart from the highly educated Jagidisan, were not afforded agency.

27. "Leprosy Relief on Humane Understanding Lines," *Madras Information Fortnightly* 3, no. 14 (1949): 62–4. This article does not have an author, but it would not be surprising to discover that the author was T. N. Jagadisan.

28. The Leonard Wood Memorial was established as a philanthropic and non-profit appeal for support for the scientific and medical work conducted against leprosy in the large leprosy colony situated on the island of Culion, in the Palawan group of islands in the Philippines, in memory of Major–General Leonard Wood who had been the Governor–General of the Philippines between 1921 and 1927. Perry Burgess had been the national campaign manager for a New York fundraising firm. He left this position to dedicate his time exclusively to assisting Dorothy Paul, the wife of Dr Herbert Windsor Wade. They assembled an American Committee for the Eradication of Leprosy and succeeded in enlisting the support of New York capitalist Eversley Childs. Long, "Forty Years of Leprosy Research," 241–2; League of Nations, Health Organization, Leprosy Commission, "Report on the Programme of Work of the Leprosy Commission," 2–3; Appeal Pamphlet, "The Leonard Wood Memorial for the Eradication of Leprosy." RG 3.2, Series: Medical Interest 160, Sub-Series: Philippines. Rockefeller Archive Center, New York.

29. The leprosy-affected people on Culion did not see much of him, as he spent much of his time in his laboratory.

30. Robert Cochrane, "The Campaign Against Leprosy," *BMJ* (18 April 1931): 681.

31. Chagas's address to the Health Committee of the League of Nations emphasises this.

32. "Obituary: James Angus Doull," *Leprosy Review* 34.3 (1963): 115. His international influence and the role that he played in getting leprosy onto the WHO agenda will be dealt with later; Long, 251; Brand, "The United States Public Health Service," 590.

33. Browne, "Ernest Muir: Obituary," 1–3.

34. Jagadisan, "Ernest Muir: Obituary," 3.

35. He wrote *La Lèpre* when he was head of the Leprosy Service at the Institut Pasteur. It was favourably reviewed in "Three French Monographs" in the *British Medical Bulletin* 7.3 (1951): 221. His primary focus in leprosy research concerned BCG as a vaccine. He became secretary for a Panel of Experts on Leprosy for the WHO. *International Journal of Leprosy*, Centennial Festskrift edition, 41, no. 2 (1973): 181.

36. After the First International Leprosy Congress was organised by the International Leprosy Association in Cairo in 1938, Etienne Burnet wrote of the "happy circumstance that an International Society was spontaneously formed, which aims at drawing together and coordinating the work of the various institutions concerned in leprosy". In his view, the "moving spirits" were "a group of well-known leprologists ... notable for their experience, knowledge and geniality, and their zeal ... in the case of anti-leprosy work generally". Burnet, "Report Upon the Position of the International Leprosy Association," 4. League of Nations Archives, Geneva.

37. "Société des Nations: Organisation D'Hygiène, "Rapport au Conseil sur Les Travaux de la Vingt-Huitème Session du Comité d'Hygiène," Genève, 30 juin/2 juillet 1938. League of Nations Archives, Geneva.

38. "The World Health Organization and the ILA," 129–30. "A draft resolution will be submitted to the Assembly calling for approval of the principles laid down by the Executive Board for the collaboration of WHO with the Council for the Coordination of International Congresses of Medical Sciences (Medical Congress Council)," 105.

39. "Leprosy News and Notes: The International Leprosy Association: Minutes of the Association Meeting at Havana," 249ff.

40. "Leprosy News and Notes: The International Leprosy Association: Minutes of the Association Meeting at Havana," 249ff. The International Leprosy Association also entered into a relationship with the permanent Council for the Coordination of International Congresses of Medical Sciences. *IJL* 17, no.1–2 (1949):104.

41. "Editorial: The Centenary Year," 75.

42. The varied characters and complexities of the non-governmental organisations such as the Mission to Lepers, BELRA, the Leonard Wood Memorial, the American Leprosy Missions (ALM), and other philanthropic organisations that emerged at a later date will be examined further in Chapter 3.

43. "News and Notes: The International Leprosy Association and the United Nations," 480. WHO, First World Health Assembly, Programme Committee: Preliminary Report 12.1.7 Other Activities. A/Prog/66, 13 July 1948, 12.1.7.4.4 Leprosy: "It is recommended that the World Health Organization should continue the international work on leprosy, including investigations on epidemiology, treatment and prophylaxis," p. 5; Working Party and "Other Activities," 12.1.7. A/Prog/71, 16 July 1948, Note 2: 12.1.7.44 Leprosy: Referral to Epidemiological section recommended p.3; Committee on Programme: Twentieth Meeting, Monday, 19 July 1948, at 10 am. A/

Prog/72, 17 July 1948, 12.1.7.4.4 Leprosy: "It is recommended that this item be entrusted to the Epidemiological division." A/Prog/73, p. 11; Interim Commission, *Official Records of the World Health Organization No 10: Report of the Interim Commission to the First World Health Assembly: Part II Provisional Agenda Documents and Recommendations.* 13–14. WHO Archives, Geneva.

44. "Report from Chaussinand, Paris (ILA) to WHO re leprosy situation." 471/1/1. WHO Archives, Geneva.

45. WHO, Technical Questions: "Leprosy: Correspondence with Dr R. Chaussinand, Paris," 471/2/2. WHO Archives, Geneva.

46. "News and Notes: The International Leprosy Association and the United Nations," 479.

47. Doull, "World Health Organization: First Meeting of the Assembly," 468–72: "On November 2, 1948, at its Second Session, the Executive Board of the WHO adopted a report of the standing committee on nongovernmental organizations recommending that the WHO establish a relationship with *inter alia*, the ILA," 472.

48. "News and Notes: The International Leprosy Association and the United Nations," 480.

49. WHO, Second World Health Assembly, June 1949, "Leprosy: Item 8.15.3.15 of the Agenda," 2. A2/Prog/min/17. WHO Archives, Geneva.

50. WHO, Second World Health Assembly: 1 June 1949, "Leprosy: Memorandum Submitted by the Delegation of the Government of India" (A2/40 1 June 1949, Supplementary Agenda Item 8.15.3.15. (471/1/1), 1. WHO Archives, Geneva.

51. WHO, Official Records of the World Health Organization, No 21, *Second World Health Assembly*, Rome, 13 June–2 July 1949: Decisions and Resolutions; Plenary meetings (Verbatim Records); Committees (Minutes and Reports) (WHO, Geneva, December 1949) Fourth Plenary Meeting, 76. WHO Archives, Geneva.

52. WHO, "Leprosy: Memorandum Submitted by the Delegation of the Government of India," 2–3. WHO Archives, Geneva.

53. WHO, "Leprosy: Memorandum," 4.

54. WHO, Tenth Report of the Committee on Program A2/102, (5); A World Research Centre was considered premature, and the request for drugs was modified so that new leprosy drugs would be available for control trials under conditions laid down by the Expert Committee. WHO Archives, Geneva.

55. WHO, *Chronicle of the World Health Organization* 3, no. 8–10 (1949): 173.

56. "News and Notes: Leprosy at the Second World Health Assembly," 321–6.

57. "Coordination of Medical Congresses," 130–1.

58. "WHO Program and Budget Estimates for 1950," 129–33.

59. "The Third World Health Assembly," 273.

60. "News and Notes: Leprosy at the Third World Assembly," 411 and "Organization of WHO and Its Budget," 418.

61. WHO, Executive Board, "Proposed Programme and Budget Estimates for the Financial Year 1 January–31 December 1950," EB 3/37, February 17, 1949, 288–9. WHO Archives, Geneva.

62. "The Third World Health Assembly," 274. Dr Roland Chaussinand of the Institut Pasteur in Paris represented the ILA at the Third Assembly.

63. "Leprosy at the Third World Health Assembly," 413–14.

64. "Leprosy at the Third World Health Assembly," 418.

65. WHO, Executive Board, Seventh Session, "An Overall Discussion or Symposium on the Different Phases of the Leprosy Problem throughout the World: Memorandum Submitted by the Government of the Republic of the Philippines," EB7/17, 15 December 1950.

66. This memorandum was quite specific about the information that many governments needed in order to clarify the new treatment for people with leprosy. The delegation estimated the numbers of leprosy-affected people in the world as 8 million (the Indian delegation had stated 5 million, although they had said that this was an underestimation). Clearly, no one really knew how many people were in fact affected by the disease.

67. They needed to know the differing effects of the various sulphone preparations as well as the necessary dosages; side effects of the treatment; and how the various sulphones compared with DDS, the "mother sulphone", the cost of which made it possible to reach poor patients and for poor governments to treat their own people. The classification scheme for leprosy had been a subject of fierce debate since 1938. It was imperative to establish fundamental principles as a guide for leprosy control in endemic countries so that medical and public health people knew the basics for treating people.

68. WHO, Executive Board, Seventh Session, "Resolution on Leprosy," EB7/R/1 23, January 1951.

69. WHO, Official Records of the World Health Organization, "Proposed Programme and Budget Estimates for the Financial Year 1 January–31 December 1952 With the Proposed Programme and Budget Estimates for Technical Assistance for Economic Development of Under-developed Countries," March 1951, 546. US$12,728 was allocated.

70. "Leprosy at the Third World Health Assembly," 413.

71. "News and Notes: WHO and Leprosy," 229–30.

72. "Editorials: Establishment of a Consultative Group of Leprosy Experts by the WHO," 75–8. The experts were E. Agricola (Brazil), R. Boenjamin (Indonesia), R. Chaussinand (France), R. Cochrane (UK), M. A. K. El Dalgamouni (Egypt), Dharmendra (India), J. A. Doull (United States), A. Dubois (Belgium), F. A. Johansen (United States), John Lowe (Nigeria), E. Muir (UK), J. N. Rodriguez (Philippines), H. W. Wade (Philippines).

73. "News and Notes: WHO and Leprosy," 230.

74. "WHO and Leprosy," 115–16.

75. "The World Health Organization and Leprosy," 78–81.

76. "Review of Relationship with ILA, 2 April 1952," CC44. WHO Archives, Geneva.

77. H. W. Wade, President of the ILA, to Dr P. Dorolle, ADG WHO, 6 April 1952. CC 4.4 Int. Leprosy Assn Liaison and Relations with Non-Governmental Organizations. WHO Archives, Geneva.

78. Dr A. M. W. Rae was the Deputy Chief Officer, Colonial Office, London.

79. "ILA Relationship With WHO," 549. Affiliated organisations: The British Empire Leprosy Relief Association; The Mission To Lepers; HKNS; American Leprosy Missions; Federação das Sociedades de Assistencia aos Lazaros e Defesa Contra a Lepra, Rio de Janiero; Patronato de Leprosos de la Republica Argentina, Buenos Aires; Société contre Lèpre de Meshed, Teheran; Associação Brasileira de Leprologia, Rio de Janeiro; Japanese Leprosy Association, Tokyo; Sociedad Cubana de Leprologia, Havana; and the Indian Association of Leprologists, Calcutta.

80. Packard, "Malaria Dreams," 282; Litsios, "Malaria Control," 255–78; Brown, "Malaria, Miseria," 239–54; Packard and Brown, "Rethinking Health, Development, and Malaria," 181–94; Packard, *The Making of a Tropical Disease*; Birn, "The Stages of International (Global) Health."

81. Szlezák, *Globalizing Public Policy*, 13.

82. Packard and Brown, "Rethinking Health, Development, and Malaria," 184.

83. Packard, "Malaria Dreams," 282.

2. THE MOBILE LEPROSY CAMPAIGN

1. WHO, Eleventh World Health Assembly, "Committee on Programme and Budget Provisional Minutes of the Third Meeting," 24.

2. These two decades stretched from 1952, when the first WHO-appointed Expert Committee on Leprosy was set up, to 1973, when the International Leprosy Association's Tenth International Leprosy Congress was held in Bergen, 100 years after Hansen's discovery of the leprosy bacillus.

3. This proscription was accomplished at the International Leprosy Association's Congress in Havana in 1948.

4. Black, *The Children and the Nations*; Black, *Children First: The Story of UNICEF.*

5. UNICEF–WHO Joint Committee on Health Policy, "Fifth Session Provisional Summary Record of the Second Meeting," 4; "Fifth Session Provisional Summary Record of the Third Meeting," 11.

6. UNICEF–WHO Joint Committee on Health Policy, "Leprosy: Note by the World Health Organization; Agenda Item 4.4," 3.

7. UNICEF–WHO Joint Committee on Health Policy, "Leprosy: Note by the World Health Organization; Agenda Item 4.4," 3.

8. UNICEF–WHO Joint Committee on Health Policy, "Leprosy: Note by the World Health Organization; Agenda Item 4.4," 4.

9. UNICEF–WHO Joint Committee on Health Policy, "Leprosy: Note by the World Health Organization; Agenda Item 4.4," 7.

10. *Expert Committee on Leprosy: First Report*, 14 and 11 respectively.

11. UNICEF–WHO Joint Committee on Health Policy Sixth Session, "Provisional Summary Record of the Third Meeting," 7.

12. UNICEF–WHO Joint Committee on Health Policy Sixth Session, "Provisional Summary Record of the Third Meeting," 2.

13. WHO, Eleventh World Health Assembly, "Committee on Programme and Budget Provisional Minutes of the Third Meeting," 24.

14. WHO, *Expert Committee on Leprosy: First Report*, 13.

15. WHO, *Expert Committee on Leprosy: First Report*, 14.

16. WHO, *Expert Committee on Leprosy: Second Report*, 18.

17. WHO, *Expert Committee on Leprosy: First Report*, 19.

18. UNICEF–WHO Joint Committee on Health Policy, "Leprosy: Note by the World Health Organization; Agenda Item 4.4," 7.

19. "Leprosy and the WHO Board," 219.

20. "Leprosy and the WHO Board," 219.

21. WHO. Resolutions of the Executive Board. "Leprosy Control Programmes," EB17.R29. 30 January 1956. WHO Archives, Geneva.

22. WHO, Tenth World Health Assembly, "Committee on Programme and Budget Provisional Minutes of the Second Meeting," 10 and 17–18; "Committee on Programme and Budget Provisional Minutes of the Fourth Meeting"; "Review of work during 1956: Annual Report of the DG" and "Committee on Programme and Budget Provisional Minutes of the Third Meeting," 28; "Committee on Programme and Budget Provisional Minutes of the Eighth Meeting," 8; and UNICEF/WHO Joint Committee on Health Policy, Eleventh Session Geneva, 20–21 October 1958, "Review of Leprosy Control Activities," 17 December 1958, 2.

23. In Angola 13,000 people out of a possible 20,000 were receiving treatment, and in Mozambique 90% of the known 59,000 were being treated. In the Federation of Mali, 990,000 inhabitants had been examined and 55,000 were being treated. India had examined 12 million people and detected 80,000 with leprosy. In Ghana and Niger, leprosy treatment was being vigorously pursued. In the Republic of the Congo, the number of arrested cases or those under observation without treatment was greater than the new cases being reported. Similarly, reports were proffered by other African countries such as what was then the Central African Republic, Cameroon, Northern Nigeria, and Upper Volta. The Americas reported preliminary surveys in Central America, Mexico, Colombia, and Ecuador in preparation for control programmes in 1960. WHO, Thirteenth World Health Assembly, "Committee on Programme and Budget Provisional Minutes of the Seventh Meeting," 16 May 1960, 27.

24. WHO, Eleventh World Health Assembly, "Committee on Programme and Budget Provisional Minutes of the Third Meeting," A11/P&B/Min/4, 7 and UNICEF–WHO Joint Committee on Health Policy Eleventh Session, "Review of Leprosy Control Activities," 1 September 1958, 3. The projects were in French Equatorial Africa, French West Africa, Ghana, Nigeria, Uganda,

Ethiopia, Iran, Burma, Indonesia, Thailand, the Philippines, the Solomon Islands, and Paraguay.

25. News and Notes, "Seventh International Congress of Leprology," *IJL* 406.

26. "News and Notes: Reports of the Technical Committee on Education and Social Aspects," 510.

27. WHO, *Third Expert Committee on Leprosy*, 18.

28. WHO, *Fourth Expert Committee on Leprosy*, 26.

29. WHO, Eleventh World Health Assembly, "Committee on Programme and Budget Provisional Minutes of the Fourth Meeting," 9.

30. WHO, Eleventh World Health Assembly, "Committee on Programme and Budget Provisional Minutes of the Fourth Meeting," 9.

31. WHO, *A Guide to Leprosy Control*, 4.

32. UNICEF–WHO Joint Committee on Health Policy Tenth Session, "Minutes of the Fourth Meeting," 23 September 1957.

33. WHO, "WHO Inter-Regional Leprosy Conference Report," WHO/Lep. Conf/21, 24 November 1958, 9–10.

34. By 1958, surveys were required to determine the prevalence rate within a specific area, to classify patients by race, sex, age, and the proportions of different clinical forms of the disease, as well as degree of disability and the number of new cases in a year. The survey would also track the contacts of people who were infectious. The results of treatment were also broken down to register tolerance for the treatment, reactions to the treatment, frequency of attendance, changes to bacteriology and histopathology, the numbers of those who were free from active symptoms, those classed as "under observation without treatment" (UOWT), as well as the numbers in a year whose disease had undergone a relapse in either or both clinical and bacteriological senses. UNICEF–WHO Joint Committee on Health Policy Eleventh Session, "Review of Leprosy Control Activities," 18.

35. "Editorial: Information and Comments on Development of International Leprosy Activities (November 1958–May 1960)," 20.

36. WHO, Executive Board 29, 15–26 January 1962, 2.

37. "News and Notes: Research Activities," 232 and 236.

38. "Leprosy Advisory Team: Reports and Related Correspondence," L4/451/2 (a) J1. Leprosy Archives, Geneva.

39. Bechelli and Martínez Domínguez, "The Leprosy Problem in the World."

40. Bechelli and Martínez Domínguez, "The Leprosy Problem in the World," 821.

41. Bechelli and Martínez Domínguez, "The Leprosy Problem in the World," 822.

42. Bechelli and Martínez Domínguez, "The Leprosy Problem in the World," 823.

43. "Reports of Speciality Panels: Committee 5: Advances in Epidemiology," 461.

44. "Reports of Speciality Panels: Committee 5: Advances in Epidemiology," 462.

45. Wade, "Editorial," 349.

46. WHO, Second World Health Assembly: 1 June 1949, "Leprosy: Memorandum Submitted by the Delegation of the Government of India"; "News and Notes: Leprosy at the Second World Health Assembly," 322.

47. "News and Notes: Sixth International Congress of Leprosy," *IJL*, 517–18.

48. "Leprosy News and Notes: Sixth International Congress of Leprosy," 517.

49. Camus, *The Plague*.

50. They add, "Such findings have led to the suggestion that after long treatment, sulphone resistance may develop in the bacilli. There is no strong evidence for or against this idea.""Leprosy News and Notes: Sixth International Congress of Leprosy," 517.

51. "Leprosy News and Notes: Sixth International Congress of Leprosy," 517–18.

52. UNICEF–WHO Joint Committee on Health Policy Tenth Session, "Minutes of the Fourth Meeting," 10.

53. Dr P. Laviron, "Organization of Leprosy Control," WHO Inter-Regional Conference Tokyo, 20–24 November 1958, WHO/Lep. Conf./3, 23 September 1958 (1). WHO Archives, Geneva.

54. WHO, Fourteenth World Health Assembly, "Committee on Programme and Budget Provisional Minutes of the Ninth Meeting," A 14/P&B/Min 9, 22. WHO Archives, Geneva.

55. Dr P. Laviron, "Treatment," WHO Inter-Regional Conference Tokyo, 20–24 November 1958, WHO/Lep. Conf./2 23 September 1958, 6. WHO Archives, Geneva.

56. Dr P. Laviron, "Treatment," WHO Inter-Regional Conference Tokyo, 20–24 November 1958, WHO/Lep. Conf./2 23 September 1958, 9. WHO Archives, Geneva.

57. "News and Notes: Second WHO Expert Committee on Leprosy," *IJL* 27, no. 4 (1959): 389.

58. WHO, Executive Board, 35/31, 11 December 1964; Provisional agenda item 2.4 "Report of the Study Group on the Introduction of Mass Campaigns against Specific Diseases into General Health Services." WHO Archives, Geneva.

59. WHO, Eighteenth World Health Assembly, "Committee on Programme and Budget Provisional Minutes of the Ninth Meeting," A18/P&B/Min/9, 11. WHO Archives, Geneva.

60. WHO, "Suggestions from the Director–General for the Consideration of the Executive Board," *Fifth General Programme of Work Covering a Specific Period (1973–77 inclusive)*, 10 December 1970, EB 47/23, 2. WHO Archives, Geneva.

61. Jacobson and Trautman, "The Treatment of Leprosy with the Sulfones," 726–37.

62. Jacobson and Trautman, "The Treatment of Leprosy with the Sulfones," 736.

63. Bechelli, "Advances in Leprosy Control," 294; "Reports of Congress Committees: Committee 5: Advances in Epidemiology," 461.

64. "As I am writing these lines, on an historical Sunday, two men will actually land on the moon within the next twelve hours." Lechat, "Editorial," 191–3.

65. Webb, "Malaria Control and Eradication Projects in Tropical Africa," 35–56; Webb, *The Long Struggle Against Malaria*.

66. Birn, "The Stages of International (Global) Health," 56.

67. Birn, "The Stages of International (Global) Health," 70.

68. Birn, "The Stages of International (Global) Health, 125.

69. "News and Notes: Sixth International Congress of Leprosy," *IJL*, 517–18.

3. OWNERSHIP OF LEPROSY TREATMENT (1966–73)

1. Gussow, *Leprosy, Racism, and Public Health*, 23–4.

2. I use the word "leper" here to capture the mentality of those donating, but refrain from using that word due to its damaging impact on people who suffer from the disease and who continue to be branded, defined, and constrained by their illness.

3. van den Wijngaert, "Comment j'ai fondé 'Les Amis du Père Damien'," 33. Initially, Les Amis du Père Damien (APD) amalgamated with Damiaanaktie, and then Fondation Belge pour la Lutte contre la Lèpre joined them. The Damien Foundation International for Leprosy Control became international, entering into cooperative relations with third-world countries. It also became a completely lay organisation.

4. van den Wijngaert, "Comment j'ai fondé 'Les Amis du Père Damien'," 43. Damien Foundation, Brussels.

5. van den Wijngaert, "Comment j'ai fondé 'Les Amis du Père Damien'," 45.

6. Robertson, "The Leprosy Asylum in India."

7. Askew clearly indicated that the Mission "does not use its medical services as a tool for pressurized or indiscriminate evangelism, but believes that the effectiveness of modern treatment is increased when it is allied with a concern for the total personality of each patient: true happiness demands physical, mental, and spiritual fulfilment". Askew, "The Leprosy Mission – A Crucial Dimension of Service," 171.

8. At Karigiri in India, Addis Ababa in Ethiopia, Bauru in Brazil, Caracas in Venezuela, and Carville in Louisiana, United States. The William Jay Schieffelin Leprosy Research and Training Centre at Karigiri in south India became an outstanding model of an institution dedicated to complete physical, social, and economic rehabilitation. This is where Paul Brand carried out his work in surgical rehabilitation.

9. In 1968, Follereau legally made the children of two people who had sheltered him in Saint-Étienne during the war his heirs, and their son-in-law, André Récipon, took responsibility for the running of the foundation. *Association Internationale des Fondations Raoul Follereau: Son histoire; Ses buts* (Paris), 21. Follereau Foundation, Paris.

10. ILEP, "From Leprosaria to Vaccine Trials."

11. This was actually the seventh World Leprosy Day ever held. Follereau introduced Jacques Vellut at this time. Vellut and his wife Francine would leave in 1962 for Polambakkam, where his aunt Claire Vellut was working. This would head off potential conflict with Wijngaert, p. 25. The recipients were Ben-San (Vietnam); Polambakkam (India); Tshombe (Zaire); Bunia-Ituri (Zaire); Ouidah (Benin); Orofara (Tahiti). From 1960, Franz Hemerijckx was

the President of the Comité d'Honneur and Raoul Follereau was one of its members. van den Wijngaert, "Comment j'ai fondé 'Les Amis du Père Damien," 21. Damien Foundation Archives, Brussels.

12. Abbé Pierre, born Henri Marie Joseph Grouès, in Lyon in 1912, was a "father figure" par excellence and without exaggeration "a legend in his own lifetime".

13. "Marcel Farine – Des Paroles et des actes," http://www.marcelfarine.ch/index_fr_02.htm.

14. It expressed its mandate in the following terms: to "initiate and support measures to combat leprosy, to foster medical and social rehabilitation, to support leprosy research and training, and also to promote health education and information and a heightening of public awareness." ILEP, "From Leprosaria to Vaccine Trials".

15. ILEP, "From Leprosaria to Vaccine Trials," 166.

16. Robertson and McDougall, "Leprosy Work and Research in Oxford."

17. ILEP, "From Leprosaria to Vaccine Trials."

18. At this point a distinction needs to be made between the international members of the anti-leprosy organisations (those based in the donor countries, mostly Europe) and those who were based in the recipient countries (usually third-world countries).

19. Thévenin, *Raoul Follereau*, 363.

20. van den Wijngaert, "General Secretary's Report," 7–9 April 1972. The first meeting was held in Brussels on 2 October 1965. The second meeting was held in Berne. ILEP Archives, London.

21. ELEP, "Minutes of the Meeting Held in Bern, 24–25 September 1966," 2. ILEP Archives, London.

22. ELEP, "Minutes of the Meeting Held in Bern, 24–25 September 1966," 3. ILEP Archives, London.

23. In 2007, membership was as follows: Association Française Raoul Follereau (AFRF) now Fondation Raoul Follereau, France (1966); Associazione Italiana Amici di Raoul Follereau (AIFO), Italy (1966); Aide aux Lépreux Emmaüs-Suisse (ALES), now FAIRMED Health for the Poorest, Switzerland (1966); American Leprosy Missions (ALM), United States (1975); British Leprosy Relief Association (LEPRA), UK (1976); Comité Exécutif International de l'Ordre de Malte pour l'Assistance aux Lépreux (CIOMAL), Switzerland, now the Order of Malta, France (1966); Deutsches Aussätzigen-Hilfswerk (DAHW) (1966), now Deutsche Lepra- und Tuberkulosehilfe; Damien Foundation Belgium (DFB), Belgium (1966); Fondation Luxembourgeoise Raoul Follereau (FL), Luxembourg (1966); Fondation Père Damien pour la lutte contre la Lèpre (FO), Belgium, (1966); Fontilles Lucha contra la Lepra (SF), Spain (1969); Leonard Wood Memorial (LWM), United States (1982); Netherlands Leprosy Relief (NLR), Netherlands (1966); Sasakawa Memorial Health Foundation, Japan (1975); Le Secours aux Lépreux – Leprosy Relief (SLC), Canada (1980); The Leprosy Mission International (TLMI), UK (1966);

Taiwan Leprosy Relief Association (TLRA), Taiwan (1988). See also http://www.who.int/lep/partners/ilep/en/

24. Askew, *Edge of Daylight*, 108.

25. Askew, *Edge of Daylight*, 109.

26. Askew, *Edge of Daylight*, 108.

27. Askew, *Edge of Daylight*, 109.

28. Askew, *Edge of Daylight*, 109.

29. Paul Sommerfeld, Secretary–General of ILEP (1988–98) in discussion with the author. May 2010.

30. Interview with Paul Sommerfeld.

31. ILEP, "From Leprosaria to Vaccine Trials."

32. In the instance of Polambakkam, India, Emmaüs-Suisse contributed US$48,000; Deutsche Aussätzigen Hilfwerk US$ 22,000; Les Amis du Père Damien US$ 15,000; Le Secours aux Lépreux US$ 10,000; and Association Française Raoul Follereau [AFRF] US$ 5,000). Minutes from the Third ELEP General Assembly London, 21 April 1968, Work Session (Sunday, 21 April), ILEP Archives, London.

33. Minutes from the Third ELEP General Assembly London, 21 April 1968, ILEP Archives.

34. Minutes from the Third ELEP General Assembly London, 21 April 1968, ILEP Archives.

35. ELEP, "Minutes of the Meeting Held in Bern, 24–5 September 1966." ILEP Archives, London.

36. Medical Commission of the European Leprosy Relief Associations, General Report of the Medical Commission for 1971, 2. ILEP Archives, London.

37. Minutes of the Seventh Medical Commission of ELEP, 6 November 1968; S. G. Browne, "The Integration of Leprosy into the General Health Services," An annex to the Minutes of the Medical Commission of ELEP; Minutes of the Fourteenth Medical Commission of ELEP, 16 April 1971, 2. ILEP Archives, London.

38. Minutes of the Sixteenth Medical Commission of ELEP, 18 December 1971. ILEP Archives, London.

39. General Report of the Medical Commission, 1971, 21. ILEP Archives, London.

40. Minutes of the Twentieth Medical Commission of ELEP, 7–8 April 1973, 7. ILEP Archives, London.

41. During a journey to India in 1960, Dr Ruth Katherina Martha Pfau visited the Marie Adelaide Leprosy Clinic in Karachi, run by the Order of the Daughters of the Heart of Mary in the "Beggar Colony" off McLeod Road. On seeing the plight of the people there she decided to stay on. From its early days of a "Hut" made from fruit crates, Marie Adelaide Leprosy Centre now has a main hospital with eighty beds and a large OPD with all necessary service facilities. The training centre is recognised by the government as the National Training Institute. http://leprosyhistory.org/database/person184

42. Minutes of the Eleventh or Twelfth Medical Commission, 20 March 1970 or 23–4 October 1970, Item 5. ILEP Archives, London.

43. Minutes of the Eleventh or Twelfth Medical Commission, 20 March 1970 or 23–4 October 1970, Item 5. ILEP Archives, London.

44. Minutes of the Fifth Medical Commission 13 October 1967, 3. ILEP Archives, London.

45. General Report of the Medical Commission for 1971, 6. ILEP Archives, London.

46. I owe this observation to Paul Sommerfeld.

47. "The World Health Organization and Leprosy," *IJL*, 78–81.

48. "The World Health Organization and Leprosy," *IJL*, 78–81.

49. Dr L. M. Bechelli, Chief Medical Officer, Leprosy, Division of Communicable Diseases to Dr M. Gilbert, Secretary General, Ordre Souverain de Malta, Comité Exécutif International pour l'Assistance aux Lépreux, 9 December 1963. L4/372/7, Leprosy, WHO Archives, Geneva.

50. Bechelli to Dr Gilbert, Ordre Souverain de Malta, Comité Exécutif International pour l'Assistance aux Lépreux, 27 January 1964. F4/180/13 (E) Special Account for Leprosy Programme – Order of Malta J1 1965–1979; R. Vernet, President, Ordre Souverain de Malta, Comité Exécutif International pour l'Assistance aux Lépreux, to the Director General, WHO, 30 September 1964; M. Farine to Bechelli, 17 October 1964. WHO Archives, Geneva.

51. Memorandum from Chief, LEP/HQ to RD, SEARO "Burma 0017 – Leprosy Control Voluntary Contribution, Emmaüs-Switzerland." F4/180/13 (1). WHO Archives, Geneva.

52. Dr L. M. Bechelli to Dr Gilbert, 13 June 1967; "Leprosy – Coordination with the Order of Malta"; Memorandum Dr Martínez Domínguez, LEP to the Director, CD, 22 March 1968. "Contribution by the Order of Malta," L4/372/7; "Utilization of Funds Contributed by the Deutsches Aussätzigen Hilfswerk Wursburg (DAHW) and the Order of Malta to the Leprosy Control Project, Republic of Korea," Annex III (to the Master Plan of Operation for General Health Services Development in the Republic of Korea). F4/180/13 (2) Voluntary Funds for Health Programmes Special Account for Leprosy Programmes – Korea 4. WHO Archives, Geneva.

53. Minutes of the First Medical Commission of ELEP, 27 September 1966. ILEP Archives, London.

54. Minutes of the Second Medical Commission of ELEP, 6 January 1967. ILEP Archives, London.

55. Minutes of the Second Medical Commission of ELEP, 6 January 1967. ILEP Archives, London, 2.

56. Handwritten report "Visit of ELEP's Medical Commission to the World Health. Organization (18 December 1972), ILEP Archives, London.

57. Minutes of the Eighth General Assembly of ELEP, 6–8 April 1973, 6. ILEP Archives, London.

58. Minutes of the Twentieth Medical Commission of ELEP, 7–8 April 1973, 2. ILEP Archives, London.

4. OF MICE, *M. LEPRAE*, AND THE LABORATORY

1. Cochrane, *Leprosy in Theory and Practice*, 7; Ryan and McDougall, *Essays on Leprosy*.
2. Cochrane, *Leprosy in Theory and Practice*, 13.
3. World Health Organization, "International Work in Leprosy 1948–1959," 3–39.
4. Cochrane, *Leprosy in Theory and Practice*, 14.
5. Cochrane, *Leprosy in Theory and Practice*, 14.
6. Cochrane, *Leprosy in Theory and Practice*, 7.
7. Cochrane, *Leprosy in Theory and Practice*, 22.
8. Cochrane, *Leprosy in Theory and Practice*, 11.
9. Cochrane, *Leprosy in Theory and Practice*, 13.
10. Cochrane, *Leprosy in Theory and Practice*, 15.
11. Cochrane, *Leprosy in Theory and Practice*, 111.
12. Cochrane, *Leprosy in Theory and Practice*, 19 and 52.
13. Cochrane, *Leprosy in Theory and Practice*, 52.
14. "International Work in Leprosy 1948–1959", 3–39.
15. Cochrane, *Leprosy in Theory and Practice*, 53–4.
16. Cochrane, *Leprosy in Theory and Practice*, 56.
17. Cochrane, *Leprosy in Theory and Practice*, 75–6.
18. Cochrane, *Leprosy in Theory and Practice*, 69.
19. Cochrane, *Leprosy in Theory and Practice*, 115.
20. Cochrane, *Leprosy in Theory and Practice*, 19.
21. Cochrane, *Leprosy in Theory and Practice*, 118.
22. World Health Organization, "International Work in Leprosy 1948–1959."
23. Cochrane, *Leprosy in Theory and Practice*, 55.
24. Cochrane, *Leprosy in Theory and Practice*, 57.
25. The Mitsuda preparation contained bacilli and various tissue substances; the Dharmendra preparation contained separated bacilli. When used, they gave later and early responses respectively. Cochrane, *Leprosy in Theory and Practice*, 32, 117, and 18.
26. Long, *Forty Years of Leprosy Research*, 245–6.
27. Cochrane, *Leprosy in Theory and Practice*, 12.
28. "Leprosy Activities of WHO, 1960–1961," 231.
29. Long, *Forty Years of Leprosy Research*, 242. H. W. Wade was its first medical director in 1931.
30. Long, *Forty Years of Leprosy Research*, 242–3.
31. Long, *Forty Years of Leprosy Research*.
32. Long, *Forty Years of Leprosy Research*, 253. He had left Western Reserve University and had taken a commission in the USPHS in the office of the Surgeon General, Thomas Parran, where he held the rank of Medical Director and where he had been part of the team responsible for setting up of the post-war international agencies such as the WHO, as described in an

earlier chapter. He was granted leave from the service to become the Medical Director of the LWM.

33. Initial recipients were James Doull, who received funding for clinical evaluation studies and also for research and teaching in leprosy; Hanks, who received funding to study the metabolism of non-cultivable mycobacteria, and to further the epidemiological studies of leprosy; and Mason and Bergel, at the University of Rochester, to study the survival of the Hansen's bacillus in laboratory animals. "News and Notes: Government-Aided Leprosy Research Projects," 471.

34. "News and Notes: Government-Aided Leprosy Research Projects," 281.

35. Shepard, "Acid-Fast Bacilli in Nasal Excretions," and "The Experimental Disease."

36. Shepard, "Multiplication of *Mycobacterium Leprae* in the Footpad of the Mouse."

37. Shepard, "The Experimental Disease," 450; F. Fenner, "The Pathogenic Behaviour of *Mycobacterium ulcerans* and *Mycobacterium balnei*."

38. Charles C. Shepard, "Acid-Fast Bacilli in Nasal Excretions," 148.

39. I am indebted to Professor Lou Levy for this description of Shepard's laboratory procedure.

40. An aliquot is a sample or a portion of the total amount of a solution. The supernatant is the liquid lying above a layer of precipitated insoluble material.

41. Shepard, "Acid-Fast Bacilli in Nasal Excretions," 149.

42. Draper, "Editorial: The Mouse Footpad Model," 3.

43. WHO, *Multidrug Therapy against Leprosy*, 4. The minimal inhibitory concentration (MIC) is the lowest concentration of an antimicrobial that will inhibit the visible growth of a microorganism.

44. Draper, "Editorial," 4.

45. WHO Expert Committee on Leprosy Geneva, 27 July–2 August 1965: R. J. W. Rees, "Transmission of Human Leprosy to Experimental Animals," 1. LEP/WP/4.65. WHO Archives, Geneva.

46. "Proceedings of a Conference on Research Problems in Leprosy," 780–1.

47. Shepard concentrated on the bacteriology of the infection, Dick Hilson and Lou Levy on its use in developing and comparing anti-leprosy drugs, and Dick Rees and Graham Weddell on the immunology and pathology of the infection. (Many others were involved; those named may be regarded as "team leaders"). Draper, "Editorial," 3–4.

48. Cochrane, "Summary of the Activities of the Leprosy Research Unit."

49. Details supplied to the author by Hilary Morgan.

50. "Editorial," *Leprosy Review*, 110. "Experimental Leprosy," 1040. Confirmed by Pattyn, "Current Literature, 522." The Eighth International Leprosy Congress accepted that the infection produced was the human leprosy bacillus.

51. Rees, "New Prospects for the Study of Leprosy in the Laboratory," 136–54.

52. From Hilary Morgan to the author, 2003.

53. *Transactions of the Leonard Wood Memorial: Symposium*, 108.

54. *Transactions of the Leonard Wood Memorial: Symposium*, 88. Several research directions were pursued from Sungei Buloh; for example, the following drugs

were trialled: DDS, DDS and Etisul, CIBA 1906, B663, Rifampicin, and B 671 (Thalidomide); in addition to studies in the cultivation of *M. leprae;* and immunological studies to do with lepromin and BCG.

55. Rees and Valentine, "The Appearance of Dead Leprosy Bacilli by Light Electron Microscopy"; "News and Notes: CIBA Symposium on Pathogenesis," 248–9.

56. Rees and Valentine, "The Appearance of Dead Leprosy Bacilli by Light Electron Microscopy," 8; Rees and Waters, "Applicability of Experimental Murine Leprosy," 43.

57. Rees and Waters, "Applicability of Experimental Murine Leprosy," 48.

58. "Resume of Papers: Dr R. J. W. Rees, 'Recent Applications of Experimental Human Leprosy in the Mouse Foot-Pad'": "Seventh Scientific Session: Experimental Studies in Leprosy," 163.

59. "Seventh Scientific Session: Experimental Studies in Leprosy," 166–7.

60. I am indebted to Professor Lou Levy for this clarification.

61. Rees, "Recent Applications of Experimental Human Leprosy," 163.

62. Waters et al., "Ten Years of Dapsone in Lepromatous Leprosy," 288–98.

63. Rees, "Experimental Studies in Leprosy," 339.

64. "CTS Agreement with the Medical Research Council, London, UK–WHO Collaboration Centre with Reference and Research on *M. Leprae,*" L4/181/37; "Designation and Activities of the WHO Collaborating Centre for Reference and Research on *Mycobacterium Leprae*–Laboratory for Leprosy and Mycobacterial Research National Institute for Medical Research, London, UK," 3 L4/286/4 (A) 9. WHO Archives, Geneva.

65. "Designation and Activities of the WHO Collaborating Centre," (A) 9.

66. Joshua-Raghavar, *Leprosy in Malaysia*, 97.

67. Joshua-Raghavar, *Leprosy in Malaysia*, 97.

68. Joshua-Raghavar, *Leprosy in Malaysia*, 98.

69. Shepard, "The Development of DADDS and Its Application," 20. QIMR/0360. Douglas Russell Collection. Queensland Institute of Medical Research, Brisbane.

70. "Karimui BCG and DADDS Treatment Project–Miscellaneous Lists, Registers and Papers–Douglas Russell." QIMR/0360. Douglas Russell Collection. Queensland Institute of Medical Research, Brisbane.

71. D. H. McRae, D. A. Russell, D. R. Vincin, G. C. Scott, and C. C. Shepard, "Bacteriologic Results at 5 years in Lepromatous Patients in the Acedapsone (DADDS) Trial in the Karimui, New Guinea," Karimui BCG and DADDS Treatment Project–Articles and Drafts with Correspondence–Douglas Russell," QIMR/0361. Douglas Russell Collection, QIMR, Brisbane.

72. Levy, "Relationships Among Laboratory Research, Chemotherapy and the Control of Leprosy."

73 Shepard, "The Development of DADDS and Its Application," 21. QIMR/0361. Douglas Russell Collection. Queensland Institute of Medical Research, Brisbane.

74. "Experimental Chemotherapy in Leprosy," *Bulletin WHO* 53 (1976): 425–33.

75. Sansarricq, "My Interventions in Leprosy Work: 1972–1984."
76. Sansarricq, "My Interventions in Leprosy Work: 1972–1984."

5. THE JAPANESE DELEGATION TO THE WORLD HEALTH
   ORGANIZATION

1. The International Affairs Division of the Ministry of Health and Welfare of the
   Japanese Government formally introduced the new organisation; Dr Morizo
   Isidate, Chairman of the Sasakawa Memorial Health Foundation to Dr Masuo
   Takabe of the Division of Communicable Diseases, 30 May 1974. L4/348/1.
   WHO Archives, Geneva.

2. Dr Morizo Isidate, Chairman of the Sasakawa Memorial Health Foundation to
   Dr Masuo Takabe of the Division of Communicable Diseases, 30 May 1974.
   L4/348/1. WHO Archives, Geneva.

3. Dr Morizo Isidate, Chairman of the Sasakawa Memorial Health Foundation to
   Dr Masuo Takabe of the Division of Communicable Diseases, 30 May 1974.
   L4/348/1. WHO Archives, Geneva.

4. Memorandum from Director, CDS, to Dr L. Bernard, ADG, 18 June 1974, Re:
   Sasakawa Memorial Health Foundation of Japan. L4/348/1 WHO Archives,
   Geneva.

5. Memorandum from Director, CDS, to Dr L. Bernard, ADG, 18 June 1974, Re:
   Sasakawa Memorial Health Foundation of Japan. L4/348/1 WHO Archives,
   Geneva.

6. Frank Gibney, "Preface," in Sato Seizaburo, *Sasakawa Ryoichi*.

7. Seizaburo, *Sasakawa Ryoichi*, 51–2.

8. Yuma Totani, *The Tokyo War Crimes Trial: The Pursuit of Justice in the Wake of World War
   II*, Cambridge (Massachusetts) and London: Harvard University Asia Center
   (2008), 74.

9. Sasakawa, *Sugamo Diary*, 79.

10. Sasakawa, *Sugamo Diary*, 84.

11. Sasakawa, *Sugamo Diary*, 100.

12. Sasakawa, *Sugamo Diary*, 116.

13. Sasakawa, *Sugamo Diary*, 136.

14. Sasakawa, *Sugamo Diary*, 79.

15. Swenson-Wright, "Sasakawa Ryoichi: Unraveling an Enigma," 136.

16. Seizaburo, *Sasakawa Ryoichi*, 51–2.

17. Memorandum, 18 June 1974. The other two members were Professor Kiikuni
    (a disarmingly charming man who would figure as one of the main points of
    contact with WHO), who was tasked with ensuring that Ryoichi Sasakawa's
    wishes and agenda came to fruition, and Dr Saikawa, who was enthusiastic
    about establishing outpatient clinics in Japan, although most Japanese patients
    continued to be admitted to leprosaria. Saikawa left Mitsuda and went to
    Taiwan to work for WHO. He furthered the idea and practice of outpatient
    clinics in Taiwan. (Author Interview; Dr Yo Yuasa; Geneva, 2009.)

18. Author Interview; Dr Yo Yuasa; Geneva, 2009.

19. SMHF had a president who was an honorary non-voting member of the Board (this was a post held by Ryoichi Sasakawa); Professor Ishidate was the Chairman of the Board of Directors and bore the primary responsibility for running the Foundation; the Board of Directors itself consisted of leprosy or medical experts and several businessmen associated with the Nippon Foundation (Dr Hinohara, Yohei Sasakawa, and Professor Kiikuni were original members); the General Secretary was Mr S. Tsurusaki. As described in Yuasa, *Towards a World Without Leprosy*, 5–6.

20. Yuasa, "Synthesis of Promin."

21. Yuasa, "Synthesis of Promin."

22. Yuasa, *Towards a World Without Leprosy*, 7.

23. "Message" from Ryoichi Sasakawa. A handwritten note on the same page as the message indicated that the "shrine [was] presented, together with attached brochures on the Sasakawa Memorial Health Foundation, to Dr Mahler by Dr Ishidate and Dr Kiikuni of the Sasakawa Memorial Health Foundation, when they came to see DG on 28 June 1974," Warner, DG's Office. L4/348/1 WHO Archives, Geneva.

24. Dr Takabe to Dr M. Ishidate, 11 July 1974. L4/348/1. WHO Archives, Geneva.

25. The urgent need for "target-orientated research work" was emphasised. This would be work that could be coordinated by the Leprosy Unit at WHO, "to find practical breakthroughs in the leprosy control measures available at present". Dr Takabe to Dr M. Ishidate 11 July 1974. WHO Archives, Geneva.

26. He noted that this included US$45,000 for IMMLEP and that WHO would also like some of the money for THELEP. Both of these programmes will be discussed in the next chapter. The future programme for 1977 included a symposium with representatives of the benevolent organisations, WHO, and governments. Lechat, *Commission Médicale de l'ILEP to Pierre van den Wijngaert, Secrétaire Général*, ILEP, 1 March 1976. ILEP Archives, London.

27. "Informal Consultation on the Development and Implementation of MDT over the last 25 Years," 2. Unpublished.

28. Morizo Ishidate, Chairman, SMHF to Dr Takabe, Director, Division of Communicable Diseases, 25 July 1974. L4/348/1 WHO Archives, Geneva.

29. "Informal Consultation on the Development and Implementation of MDT," 2. Unpublished.

30. Olof Stroh, Secretary–General, Central Committee of the Swedish Red Cross, to the Director–General of WHO, Dr M. G. Candau, 15 April 1961. L4/348/1. WHO Archives, Geneva.

31. Olof Stroh, Secretary–General, Central Committee of the Swedish Red Cross, to the Director–General of WHO, Dr M. G. Candau, 15 April 1961. L4/348/1. WHO Archives, Geneva.

32. Olof Stroh, Secretary–General, Central Committee of the Swedish Red Cross. "Plan for a Swedish Red Cross Project within the Frame of the Overall Leprosy Program in India," 1 October 1961, 4. L4/348/1 WHO Archives, Geneva.

33. SEARO Memorandum from the Regional Director to the Director–General HQ, Re: "Sasakawa Memorial Health Foundation," 8 August 1974. L4/348/1. WHO Archives, Geneva.

34. WPRO – Memorandum from Regional Director WPRO to Director–General, HQ 8 July 1974, Re: "Sasakawa Memorial Health Foundation, Japan." L4/348/1. WHO Archives, Geneva.

35. WPRO – Memorandum from Regional Director WPRO to Director–General, HQ 8 July 1974, Re: "Sasakawa Memorial Health Foundation, Japan." L4/348/1. WHO Archives, Geneva.

36. Yo Yuasa, "TNF(JSIF)/SMHF's Contributions 1974–2005." Unpublished.

37. Yuasa states that this allocation has not even doubled over the last thirty years.

38. Yo Yuasa, "TNF(JSIF)/SMHF's Contributions."

39. "Informal Consultation on the Development and Implementation of MDT," 2; Yuasa, "TNF(JSIF)/SMHF's Contributions," 2–3.

40. Yo Yuasa, *Towards a World Without Leprosy*, 9.

41. Morizo Ishidate, Chairman of the Board of Directors, Sasakawa Memorial Health Foundation, to Dr H. Sansarricq, Chief Medical Officer, Leprosy Division of Communicable Diseases, WHO, 17 July 1975; "International Seminars on Leprosy Control Co-Operation in Asia, Organized by the SMHF." L4/440/11. WHO Archives, Geneva

42. Correspondence from Suminori Tsurusaki, General Secretary, Sasakawa Memorial Health Foundation, to Dr H. Sansarricq, Chief Medical Officer, Leprosy Division of Communicable Diseases, WHO, 17 July 1975. WHO Archives, Geneva.

43. WHO, "Report on the Attendance of the First Seminar on Leprosy Control Cooperation in Asia: Sasakawa Memorial Health Foundation, Japan, 28 November–3 December 1974," 23 January 1975 (WP). L4/61/2; Dr H. Sansarricq, Chief Medical Officer, Leprosy Division of Communicable Diseases, WHO, to Morizo Ishidate, 27 August 1975; Dr H. Sansarricq to Professor K. Kiikuni, 27 August 1975. L4/440/11. WHO Archives, Geneva. Needless to say, WHO were anxious to see the money as the letter to Ishidate indicates: "In particular, when the reply from Mr Sasakawa to Dr Mahler's letter of 19 August has been received, I am sure we shall be able to develop and implement, in cooperation with you, various fruitful projects." And to Kiikuni: "Regarding the use of the one million dollar donation … I have reported on our discussion with Mr Sasakawa to Dr Mahler, Director–General. He is now awaiting Mr Sasakawa's reply to his letter of 19 August 1975." WHO Archives, Geneva.

44. Warren W. Furth, Assistant Director–General, to Mr Ryoichi Sasakawa, President JSIF, 9 September 1975. L4/440/11. WHO Archives, Geneva.

45. Ryoichi Sasakawa, President, The Japan Shipbuilding Industry Foundation, to Dr H. Mahler, Director–General, WHO, 28 August 1975. F4/180/3 C Special Account for Leprosy Programme – Japan Shipbuilding Foundation (Sasakawa Health Fund). WHO Archives, Geneva.

46. Tropical Disease Research (TDR) received US$500,000 and the Western Pacific received US$330,000. Leprosy received US$670,000, and smallpox US$500,000.

47. H. Mahler, Director–General WHO to Mr R. Sasakawa, Chairman, JSIF, 23 September 1976. F4/180/3 C Special Account for Leprosy Programme – Japan Shipbuilding Foundation (Sasakawa Health Fund). WHO Archives, Geneva.

48. It was allocated in the following way: Leprosy Programme US$900,000; smallpox eradication: US$500,000; extended programme on immunisation: US$80,000; TDR US$400,000; miscellaneous designated contributions to support projects in the WPR: US$450,000. The total was US$2,330,000. Warren W. Furth, Assistant Director–General to Mr R. Sasakawa, President, JSIF, 17 August 1977. L4/348/1 Leprosy – Relations with NGOs – General (J2). WHO Archives, Geneva.

49. H. Mahler, Director–General, WHO to Mr R. Sasakawa, President, Japan Shipbuilding Industry Foundation, 5 November 1979. F4/180/3 C Special Account for Leprosy Programme – Japan Shipbuilding Foundation (Sasakawa Health Fund). WHO Archives, Geneva.

50. Memorandum from Chief LEP to Dr L. Bernard, ADG, Re: "Contribution by the Japan Shipbuilding Industry Foundation (JSIF) to the VL (Leprosy) Account," 17 September 1976. F4/180/3 C Special Account for Leprosy Programme – Japan Shipbuilding Foundation (Sasakawa Health Fund). WHO Archives, Geneva.

51. "Proposed Leprosy Contribution by the Sasakawa Foundation: Preliminary Proposals." L4/348/1. Leprosy – Relations with NGOs – General (J2). WHO Archives, Geneva.

52. "Informal Consultation on the Development and Implementation of MDT," 1; Leprosy – Relations with NGOs – General (J2). L4/348/1. WHO Archives, Geneva.

53. SMHF, "International Seminars on Leprosy Control Co-Operation in Asia, Organized by the SMHF." L4/440/11. WHO Archives, Geneva. The first seminar went from 28 November to 3 December 1974. The Second Seminar on Leprosy Control Cooperation in Asia (Training) went from 20–22 August 1975. Nine workshops would follow. Yuasa, *Towards a World Without Leprosy*, 34; SMHF, *The 1st International Workshop on Chemotherapy*.

54. SMHF, *The 1st Seminar on Leprosy Control*.

55. SMHF, *The 1st Seminar on Leprosy Control*, foreword.

56. SMHF, *The 1st Seminar on Leprosy Control*, foreword; SMHF, *The Second Seminar on Leprosy Control*.

57. Yo Yuasa, *Towards a World Without Leprosy*, 26.

58. Before very long, Taiwan, South Korea, and Singapore were working partners rather than recipients of support from SMHF. He recalls "close and effective working relationships" with South Korea, Taiwan, China, Philippines, Indonesia, Thailand, Vietnam, Myanmar, Nepal, Papua New Guinea, Micronesia, and Mexico "at some time in the past". Later work was also conducted with

Zambia, Nigeria, Mexico, and Brazil ... and even more recently, with DR Congo, Mozambique, Angola, Madagascar, and East Timor. Yo Yuasa, *Towards a World Without Leprosy*, 27.

59. Yo Yuasa, *Towards a World Without Leprosy*, 28.
60. Yo Yuasa, *Towards a World Without Leprosy*, 3.
61. Yo Yuasa, *Towards a World Without Leprosy*, 7.
62. Yuasa comments that the French influence in ILEP was quite strong at this time. The ILEP office was in Amiens, and every December the meeting was held in Paris.
63. In Upper Volta, a combined leprosy and TB survey was being conducted between mid-1975 and early 1976, so that people in twenty-nine villages were examined for both tuberculosis and leprosy. Only seven new cases of leprosy were found, but 202 people manifested tuberculosis. The small numbers of people with leprosy were the first indication of a successful reduction of over 70% in leprosy control in Africa. The report confessed that "There has been some delay in the SEARO request for the issuing of these allotments, due to the more extensive development in SEARO country health programming including leprosy." The programme in SEARO countries was still being planned, but leprosy was now "a high priority programme". WHO had held a meeting in December 1975 with countries in the region, and it seemed that WHO would release the allocations once the countries adopted the "relevant recommendations". Nonetheless, promoting the programmes through seminars, workshops, and consultants in the region was certainly enhanced by the available funds. "The Leprosy Program" in "Statement of Allocations and Obligations ..." L4/440/11. WHO Archives, Geneva; Memorandum from Chief, Budget to Chief FIN, Re: "1975 Contribution by the Japan Shipbuilding Industry Foundation," 18 February 1977. F4/180/3 C Special Account for Leprosy Programme – Japan Shipbuilding Foundation (Sasakawa Health Fund). WHO Archives, Geneva.
64. This included formulating programmes and managing them, developing an information system, and developing manpower and research in the TDR/ IMMLEP and THELEP programmes (which will be described in the next chapter). Some of the money allocated to HQ was to go towards drug trials being developed by Dr Iyer at Chingleput and for the supply of drugs and equipment.
65. "Leprosy Programme (VL): Contributions from Japanese Shipbuilding Industry Foundation," Special Account for Leprosy Programme – Japan Shipbuilding Foundation (Sasakawa Health Fund). F4/180/3 C. WHO Archives, Geneva.
66. "Progress Report for the Year 1978 on JSIF Contributions to the WHO Leprosy Programme," in "Japan Shipbuilding Industry Foundation (JSIF) Contribution to Special Account for Leprosy Programme," 5. Special Account for Leprosy Programme – Japan Shipbuilding Foundation (Sasakawa Health Fund) F4/180/3 C. WHO Archives, Geneva.

258

67. Surveys were planned for Liberia and Swaziland in December 1978 and February 1979.

68. Annual courses were planned for Dakar, Senegal, and ALERT in Ethiopia for 1977 and 1978. Thirteen training centers had been identified and were being strengthened as a matter of priority. "Progress Report for the Year 1978 on JSIF Contributions to the WHO Leprosy Programme," 6. Special Account for Leprosy Programme – Japan Shipbuilding Foundation (Sasakawa Health Fund) F4/180/3 C. WHO Archives, Geneva.

69. Sierra Leone, Ethiopia, Cameroon, Zambia, Botswana, Mauritania, Mali, Zaire, Mozambique, and the Central African Republic.

70. "Progress Report for the Year 1978 on JSIF Contributions to the WHO Leprosy Programme," 6. Special Account for Leprosy Programme – Japan Shipbuilding Foundation (Sasakawa Health Fund) F4/180/3 C. WHO Archives, Geneva.

71. "Progress Report for the Year 1978 on JSIF Contributions to the WHO Leprosy Programme," 16. Special Account for Leprosy Programme – Japan Shipbuilding Foundation (Sasakawa Health Fund) F4/180/3 C. WHO Archives, Geneva.

72. "Progress Report for the Year 1978 on JSIF Contributions to the WHO Leprosy Programme." Special Account for Leprosy Programme – Japan Shipbuilding Foundation (Sasakawa Health Fund) F4/180/3 C. WHO Archives, Geneva.

73. "Progress Report for the Year 1978 on JSIF Contributions to the WHO Leprosy Programme," 6. Special Account for Leprosy Programme – Japan Shipbuilding Foundation (Sasakawa Health Fund) F4/180/3 C. WHO Archives, Geneva. The proposal for 1978 was for US$1,470,000 which would be broken up into US$250,000 for AFRO; US$200,000 for AMRO; US$300,000 for SEARO; US$500,000 for WPRO; and US$220,000 for HQ.

74. "Informal Consultation on the Development and Implementation of MDT," 3.

6. MULTIDRUG THERAPY

1. His project was supported by the Order of Malta, the German Leprosy Relief Association (DAHW), the Public Health Service in Malta, and the Maltese Government. The "therapy" involved a combination of anti-leprosy drugs: "rifampicin, isoniazid, ethionamide/prothionamid, sulfones, and long-term sulphonamides, and trimethoprim-sulphonamide combinations". These were to be administered "as second and third combination partners if possible" and would be tailored to the "individual requirements of each single patient". Professor Freerksen, Institut für Experimentelle Biologie und Medizin, Borstel, to Hubert Sansarricq, 29 March 1973; and "The Malta Leprosy Eradication Program: Interim Report March 1973," in "Analyse Test and Experiments – Clinical Trials of Anti-Leprosy Drugs." L4/446/2 (J2). WHO Archives, Geneva.

2. This was a combination of Prothionamid, Isoniazid, and Diamino-diphenyl-sulphone PTH+INH+DDS.

3. Sansarricq wanted to know the average BIs and MIs of the negative cases compared to those cases that were still BI-positive. Hubert Sansarricq to

Professor Freerksen, Institut für Experimentelle Biologie und Medizin, Borstel, 25 April 1973, 28 November 1973, and 25 February 1974; "Interim Report on the Leprosy Eradication Programme in Malta," 10 February 1975; Professor Freerksen, Institut für Experimentelle Biologie und Medizin, Borstel, to Hubert Sansarricq, 4 December 1973 and 6 August 1974. "Analyse Test and Experiments – Clinical Trials of Anti-Leprosy Drugs." L4/446/2 (J2). WHO Archives, Geneva.

4.   Jacques Grosset would go on to test these combinations.

5.   WHO, Special Programme for Research and Training in Tropical Diseases: TDR/THELEP/76.1–78.2, 4.

6.   "Informal Consultation on the Development and Implementation of MDT over the last 25 Years," 4. Unpublished.

7.   G. Torrigiani, WHO/UNDP Meeting of Heads of Agencies in Connexion with the Special Programme for Research and Training in Tropical Diseases, "Strategy for A Special Programme for Research and Training in Tropical Diseases," 3. TDR/WP/75.4. WHO Archives, Geneva.

8.   The research on the immunology of leprosy was possible when Eleanor Storrs demonstrated that the armadillo was extraordinarily susceptible to *M. leprae*. This ensured "unprecedented amounts of *M. leprae* for laboratory tests", and in the words of the IMMLEP committee, ensured a "concerted attack on this ancient disease". "News and Notes,"159; "Reprinted Article: Immunological Problems in Leprosy Research," 244–72 and 257-72.

9.   "Informal Consultation on the Development and Implementation of MDT," 2–4; THELEP Scientific Working Group (chemotherapy), M. Rosenfeld, "Report of the First Meeting of the THELEP Scientific Working Group," Geneva 25–9 April 1977. TDR/SWG-THELEP (1)/77.3; Special Programme for Research and Training in Tropical Diseases, *Book 3: STRC Report on the Leprosy Component of the Special Programme*, p. 3, STRC Reports UNDP/World Bank/WHO. WHO Archives, Geneva.

10. "Report of the Fifth Meeting of the Steering Committee of the SWG on the Chemotherapy of Leprosy," Geneva, 30–31 March 1979. TDR/THELEP-SC(5)/79.3; "Informal Consultation on the Development and Implementation of MDT," 4; "Report of the Fifth Meeting of the Steering Committee of the SWG on the Chemotherapy of Leprosy," Geneva, 30–31 March 1979. TDR/THELEP-SC(5)/79.3. WHO Archives, Geneva.

11. "TDRs Contribution to the Development of MDT for Leprosy," 24.

12. "Report of the Fifth Meeting of the Steering Committee of the SWG on the Chemotherapy of Leprosy," Geneva, 30–31 March 1979. TDR/THELEP-SC(5)/79.3. WHO Archives, Geneva.

13. "Report of the Sixth Meeting of the Steering Committee of the SWG on the Chemotherapy of Leprosy," Geneva, 16–17 October 1979. TDR/THELEP-SC(6)/80.1. WHO Archives, Geneva.

14. "Report of the Sixth Meeting of the Steering Committee of the SWG on the Chemotherapy of Leprosy," Geneva, 16–17 October 1979. TDR/THELEP-SC(6)/80.1. WHO Archives, Geneva.

15. K. L. Hitze to H. Sansarricq, Re: "Fifth Expert Committee on Leprosy, October 1976: Opinions expressed in respect of integration of leprosy control programmes into the general health services and the combination of tuberculosis and leprosy control programmes," 25 November 1975. Expert Committee 1976. L4/81/5 J2; also L4/81/5, J1, 4/7/1975–31/10/1975; J2, 1/11/1975–29/2/1976; J3, 1/3/1976–6/6/1977. WHO Archives, Geneva.

16. "Informal Consultation on the Development and Implementation of MDT," 3.

17. "Informal Consultation on the Development and Implementation of MDT over the last 25 Years," 5. The objectives were as follows: to review the information on problems related to chemotherapy and on chemotherapeutic regimes for leprosy, which has accumulated since the fifth meeting of the WHO Expert Committee; to recommend alternative multidrug regimens for dapsone-treated and new multibacillary cases in control programmes; to recommend regimens for clinically suspected dapsone-resistant multi-bacillary cases in control programmes; to recommend regimens for paucibacillary cases in control programmes; and to identify further research needs in clinical and operational aspects of chemotherapy of leprosy; "WHO Study Group on Chemotherapy of Leprosy for Control Programmes – Geneva, 12–16/10/1981." L4/522/6. WHO Archives, Geneva.

18. "Informal Consultation on the Development and Implementation of MDT over the last 25 Years."

19. "Informal Consultation on the Development and Implementation of MDT over the last 25 Years."

20. Memorandum from Chief, LEP to Dr I. D. Ladnyi, ADG, Re: "Proposed Study Group on Chemotherapy," 13 May 1981. WHO Archives, Geneva.

21. LEPRA, "Extracts from Minutes of Ex Co Meetings. Held on 22 March and 13 July 1978"; "Joint MAB_ILEP Medical Commission Meeting File" 197A#5F74; Dr Yo Yuasa, Medical Director, Sasakawa Memorial Health Foundation to G. F. Harris, Director, LEPRA, 11 November 1977. Box 18, LEPRA Collection, Wellcome Archives, London; Sasakawa Memorial Health Foundation, *Proceedings of the 1st International Workshop on Chemotherapy in Asia.*

22. At the SEARO Intercountry Consultative Meeting on Leprosy (2–7 June 1980) and the WPRO Working Group on Drug Policy and Operational Research in the Leprosy Programme, Manila (16–18 February 1981).

23. Memorandum from Chief, LEP to Dr I. D. Ladnyi, ADG, Re: "Proposed Study Group on Chemotherapy," 13 May 1981. WHO Archives, Geneva.

24. L. Levy, "Design of Chemotherapeutic Regimens for the Control of Leprosy." "WHO Study Group on Chemotherapy of Leprosy for Control Programmes – Geneva, 12–16/10/1981." L4/522/6. WHO Archives, Geneva.

25. L. Levy, "Design of Chemotherapeutic Regimens for the Control of Leprosy." "WHO Study Group on Chemotherapy of Leprosy for Control Programmes – Geneva, 12–16/10/1981." L4/522/6. WHO Archives, Geneva.

261

26. L. Levy, "Design of Chemotherapeutic Regimens for the Control of Leprosy." "WHO Study Group on Chemotherapy of Leprosy for Control Programmes – Geneva, 12–16/10/1981." L4/522/6. WHO Archives, Geneva, 7.

27. L. Levy, "Design of Chemotherapeutic Regimens for the Control of Leprosy." "WHO Study Group on Chemotherapy of Leprosy for Control Programmes – Geneva, 12–16/10/1981." L4/522/6. WHO Archives, Geneva, 10.

28. G. A. Ellard, "Available Drugs for the Treatment of Leprosy," 2. "WHO Study Group on Chemotherapy of Leprosy for Control Programmes – Geneva, 12–16/10/1981." L4/522/6. WHO Archives, Geneva.

29. Louis Levy, Department of Comparative Medicine, the Hebrew University–Hadassah Medical School – Jerusalem to H. Sansarricq, Chief LEP, 12 July 1981. "WHO Study Group on Chemotherapy of Leprosy for Control Programmes – Geneva, 12–16/10/1981." L4/522/6. WHO Archives, Geneva.

30. WHO, *Chemotherapy of Leprosy for Control* Programmes, 24.

31. Sansarricq, "The Study Group," in WHO, *Multidrug Therapy Against Leprosy: Development and Implementation over the Past 25 Years*, 35.

32. Sansarricq, "The Study Group," in WHO, *Multidrug Therapy Against Leprosy: Development and Implementation over the Past 25 Years*, 35.

33. Lechat, "Some Important Factors Contributing to the Implementation of WHO MDT," in WHO, *Multidrug Therapy Against Leprosy*, 58.

34. "The Role of WHO Including TDR," in *Multidrug Therapy against Leprosy*, 149.

35. "The Role of WHO Including TDR," in *Multidrug Therapy against Leprosy*, 150.

36. "Informal Consultation on the Development and Implementation of MDT," 5.

7. WHO, MDT, AND PRIMARY HEALTHCARE

1. Cueto, "The Origins of Primary Health Care and Selective Primary Health Care," 11.

2. The polarisation between comprehensive and selective primary healthcare that would develop soon after Alma Ata is a case in point.

3. WHO, "Primary Health Care," 49–50.

4. This was outlined in the constitution and was reiterated in the Alma Ata declaration.

5. WHO, "Primary Health Care," 3.

6. WHO, "Primary Health Care," 3–4.

7. WHO, "Primary Health Care," 40.

8. WHO SEARO, "Control and Prevention of Leprosy in the Context of Primary Health Care: Working Paper for the Technical Discussions," 35th session, 21 July 1982: Provisional Agenda item 9," 8. SEA/RC35/14. SEARO Archives, New Delhi.

9. Birn, "The Stages of International (Global) Health," 58.

10. Webb, *The Long Struggle Against Malaria*, 107.

11. Webb, "Malaria Control and Eradication Projects," 54.

12. McMillen, *Discovering Tuberculosis*, 160.

13. McMillen, 165, *Discovering Tuberculosis*, 183.

14. Dr S. K. Noordeen in conversation with the author.

15. Secondary dapsone resistance was first officially recognised in 1964 amongst patients in Malaysia who had been treated for more than ten years, although Robert Cochrane noted the possibility as early as 1959. Primary resistance was documented for the first time in 1977. Lechat, "The Saga of Dapsone," *Multidrug Therapy Against Leprosy: Development and Implementation Over the Past 25 Years*, 4.

16. Sansarricq, "The Study Group," in *Multidrug Therapy Against Leprosy*, 32.

17. WHO, "Global Medium-Term Programme Leprosy," 2–3. LEP/MTP/80.1.

18. The other long-standing problem of inadequate data would be addressed though a newly developed standard recording and reporting system, OMSLEP, which had been devised at the University of Louvain as a collaborative research project. The OMSLEP forms would collect data that could be assessed by the relevant country and also be used for international assessment.

19. "Global Medium-Term Programme Leprosy," 6.

20. WHO, *Chemotherapy of Leprosy for Control Programmes*, 18.

21. WHO, *Chemotherapy of Leprosy for Control Programmes*, 30.

22. That is rifampicin given at set intervals.

23. WHO, "Global Medium-Term Programme: Programme 13.9: Leprosy," 22 August 1983, 2. LEP/MTP/83.1.

24. Antia, "Leprosy and Primary Health Care," 208.

25. Antia, "Leprosy and Primary Health Care," 209.

26. McDougall, "Editorial,"163.

27. Bijleveld, "In Reality: A Medical Anthropologist's Reservations," 184.

28. Bijleveld, "In Reality: A Medical Anthropologist's Reservations," 187.

29. Ross, "Leprosy and Primary Health Care," 201–4.

30. National Leprosy Control Program, Department of Health, Philippines, "Final Report: The Pilot Study for MDT Implementation in Ilocos Norte and Cebu: 1984–88," 3.

31. National Leprosy Control Program, Department of Health, Philippines, "Final Report: The Pilot Study for MDT Implementation in Ilocos Norte and Cebu: 1984–88," 5.

32. National Leprosy Control Program, Department of Health, Philippines, "Final Report: The Pilot Study for MDT Implementation in Ilocos Norte and Cebu: 1984–88," 4.

33. National Leprosy Control Program, Department of Health, Philippines, "The Pilot Study for MDT Implementation in Ilocos Norte and Cebu," 1. The Philippines Leprosy Mission had played a significant role in supporting work against leprosy from as early as the 1960s. Initially, they raised funds to help people in sanitaria, particularly the Central Luzon Sanitarium in Ilocos Norte. They also liaised with the ALM and served as an advocate for the leprosy-affected Protestant minority in the Philippines. Mrs Soledad S. Griño and her husband, Enrico E. Griño, carried much of the responsibility for the initiatives

and activities of the PLM. They occupied an office in the Department of Health so that they could promote contact throughout all levels of government and link up with Dr Yo Yuasa and Dr Lee Jong-wook when he was at WPRO. When SMHF was established, as a preliminary to their first SMHF workshop in Manila some members of the foundation, most notably Professor Ishidate, travelled around Manila and Luzon as guests of the Philippine Leprosy Mission. Members of the working group were Dr Aurora Villarosa (Director, Bureau of Public Health Services), Dr Jose N. Rivera (Head, Leprosy Control Service), Dr Marcial P. Carrillo (Medical Specialist, Leprosy Control Service), Dr Pedro Vilela (Medical Specialist, Leprosy Control Service), Dr Cesar J. Viardo (Chief, Eversley Child Sanitarium, Cebu), Mrs Teresita R. Posis (Health Education Adviser, DRTS), Mrs Soledad S. Griño (Executive Director, Philippines Leprosy Mission). The WPRO provided technical and financial support. "The History of the Philippine Leprosy Mission, Inc: Compiled and Annotated by Soledad S Griño."

34. "The History of the Philippine Leprosy Mission, Inc: Compiled and Annotated by Soledad S Griño." 12.

35. "The History of the Philippine Leprosy Mission, Inc: Compiled and Annotated by Soledad S Griño." 18.

36. "The History of the Philippine Leprosy Mission, Inc: Compiled and Annotated by Soledad S Griño." 32.

37. "The History of the Philippine Leprosy Mission, Inc: Compiled and Annotated by Soledad S Griño." 12.

38. C. J. Viardo, "Philippines National Leprosy Control Program (NLCP)," in "JCT Steering Committee Meeting, 26, 27 and 28 May 1987, LWM Centre, Cebu," 1. Leonard Wood Memorial Archives, Cebu, the Philippines; "The Pilot Study for MDT Implementation in Ilocos Norte and Cebu," 12.

39. Leung, *Leprosy in China: A History*, 177.

40. J. Abella, R. Frankel, R. Farrugia, and R. Jacobson, "Evaluation of MDT Implementation in Leprosy Control Programme, China," 14 September to 8 October 1991, 1. L4/370/6 CHN Programme of Leprosy Control – China J 7, April 84–April 93. A 2654. WHO Archives, Geneva; Haide and Ye Ganyun, "Editorial: Leprosy Work in China," 82.

41. One of the key people in this work against leprosy in China was a Lebanese-American doctor, George Hatem. Sun Yunshan, et al., *Dr Ma Haide (George Hatem)*, 32.

42. This Institute was originally established as the India Centre of JALMA in 1966. This was renamed as Central JALMA Institute for Leprosy in 1976. It was renamed National Jalma Institute of Leprosy and Other Mycobacterial Diseases in 2005. http://www.jalma-icmr.org.in/

43. Leung, *Leprosy in China*, 193; and Sun Yunshan et al., *Dr Ma Haide*, 32.

44. Drs Wang Jian, the Director of the Bureau of Preventative Medicine, and Li Huan-Ying from the Beijing Tropical Medicine Research Institute to Dr Andrea A. Galvez, WPRO Regional Adviser in Chronic Diseases, 24 December 1984,

"Programme of Leprosy Control – China," CHN L4/370/6, J 7, April 84–April 93. A 2654. WHO Archives, Geneva.

45. Drs Wang Jian, the Director of the Bureau of Preventative Medicine, and Li Huan-Ying from the Beijing Tropical Medicine Research Institute to Dr Andrea A. Galvez, WPRO Regional Adviser in Chronic Diseases, 24 December 1984, "Programme of Leprosy Control – China," CHN L4/370/6, J 7, April 84–April 93. A 2654. WHO Archives, Geneva, 2.

46. "Draft Plan for Action of a Leprosy Control Programme with Multidrug Therapy in Yunnan, Guizhou and Sichuan Provinces, China, 1985–1989," 1; WPRO Memorandum: WRC/Beijing to CHD/WPRO, Subject: "Leprosy Control Programme with Multidrug Therapy," 7 January 1985. "Programme of Leprosy Control – China," CHN L4/370/6, J 7, April 84–April 93, A 2654. WHO Archives, Geneva.

47. "Draft Plan for Action of a Leprosy Control Programme with Multidrug Therapy in Yunnan, Guizhou and Sichuan Provinces, China, 1985–1989," 13. Programme of Leprosy Control – China.

48. "Draft Plan for Action of a Leprosy Control Programme with Multidrug Therapy in Yunnan, Guizhou and Sichuan Provinces, China, 1985–1989," 15.

49. "Draft Plan for Action of a Leprosy Control Programme with Multidrug Therapy in Yunnan, Guizhou and Sichuan Provinces, China, 1985–1989," 3, 4.

50. "Draft Plan for Action of a Leprosy Control Programme with Multidrug Therapy in Yunnan, Guizhou and Sichuan Provinces, China, 1985–1989," 5.

51. This would be accompanied by in-service training, health education, active case finding of contacts, and a survey of those between the age of four and fourteen with the aim of covering more than 70% of the population.

52. "Draft Plan for Action of a Leprosy Control Programme with Multidrug Therapy in Yunnan, Guizhou and Sichuan Provinces, China," 5.

53. Dr Andre Galvez, "Notes on a Field Visit to the People's Republic of China," 1–10 September 1985, 4. "Programme of Leprosy Control – China," CHN L4/370/6, J 7, April 84–April 93. A 2654. WHO Archives, Geneva.

54. "Draft Plan for Action of a Leprosy Control Programme with Multidrug Therapy in Yunnan, Guizhou and Sichuan Provinces, China," 7.

55. Robert R. Jacobson, "MDT Implementation and the Eradication of Leprosy in the People's Republic of China by the year 2000," 6–29 November 1990. "Programme of Leprosy Control – China," CHN L4/370/6, J 7, April 84–April 93. A 2654. WHO Archives, Geneva.

56. J. Abella, R. Frankel, R. Farrugia, and R. Jacobson, "Evaluation of MDT Implementation in Leprosy Control Programme, China," 14 September to 8 October 1991, 1. L4/370/6 CHN Programme of Leprosy Control – China J 7, April 84–April 93. A 2654. WHO Archives, Geneva.

57. "Travel Report Summary Submitted by Dr S. K. Noordeen, Visit to SEARO, New Delhi, MDT Projects in the Districts of Varanasi (UP) etc.," 14 July to 31 July 1986; "Report of Visit to MDT Leprosy Projects in India, 14–31 July 1986." "Dr S. K. Noordeen's Various Duty Travels," December 1984–October

1991. L4 44 11, J1; B. N. Mittal (Dy Director–General (Leprosy) to Dr S. K. Noordeen, 17 May 1990 in "Programme of Leprosy Control – India." L4/370/6 IND. WHO Archives, Geneva.

58. "Travel Report, 24 June–21 July 1990: Dr S. K. Noordeen's Various Duty Travels," L4 441 11, J1. WHO Archives, Geneva.

59. "Travel Report, 24 June–21 July 1990: Dr S. K. Noordeen's Various Duty Travels," L4 441 11, J1. WHO Archives, Geneva.

60. "Review of Activities of the NLEP Consultants for the Month of September '88 …" SEARO L4/27/1–IND vol. 1, no. 6. SEARO Archives, New Delhi.

61. Dr T. Verghese Dy Dr Gen (Lep) Directorate General of Health Services (Leprosy Division) to Dr N. K. Shah, WHO SEARO, 25 December 1988. SEARO Archives, New Delhi.

62. "Issue wise comments on DDG (LEP)'s letter of 21 June 1989 regarding NLEP meeting on 28 July at Nirman Bhawan, New Delhi." "Leprosy: Group Consultations & Training Activities – General L4/48/1 vol. 1, no. 12 Jan 1989–Feb 1991." SEARO Archives, New Delhi.

63. Rao, "Implementation of WHO MDT in India 1982–2001," in *Multidrug Therapy Against Leprosy*, 95.

64. C. K. Rao, "Integration of Leprosy Eradication Activities in Leprosy Endemic Districts Under MDT for Over 7 Years into the Primary Health Care System in India," 16 July–29 August 1990. "Programme of Leprosy Control – India." L4/370/6 IND. SEA/Lep/114 pub. 4 December.

65. Rao, "Implementation of WHO MDT in India," 93. These districts were mainly in the States of Bihar, Uttar Pradesh, Madhya Pradesh and West Bengal.

66. Rao, "Implementation of WHO MDT in India," 97.

67. WHO, "Report of a Coordinating Meeting on Implementation of Multidrug Therapy in Leprosy Control," 8.

68. WHO, "Report of a Meeting on Action Plans for Leprosy Control," New Delhi, 23–5 August 1982; Action Plans for Leprosy Control (WHO/LEP/83.1). WHO Archives, Geneva.

69. Lopez Bravo noted: "Surprisingly enough, Dr Opromolla was a member of the WHO Study Group on Chemotherapy of Leprosy for Control Programmes."

70. L. Lopez Bravo, "Travel Report Summary," 24 November 1983, 3. L4/441/10. WHO Archives, Geneva, 3.

71. L. Lopez Bravo, "Travel Report Summary," 24 November 1983, 3. L4/441/10. WHO Archives, Geneva, 3.

72. These were Manaus in Amazonas and Bauru, in Sao Paulo.

73. L. Lopez Bravo, "Travel Report Summary," 24 November 1983, 4. L4/441/10. WHO Archives, Geneva.

74. The Brazilian National Commission on Alternative Therapy for Hansen's Disease, consisting of Drs Aguinaldo Goncalves, Cesar Bernardi, Diltor Opromolla, and Jair Ferreira.

75. "Travel Report Summary submitted by Dr S. K. Noordeen, Visit to AMRO/ PAHO, Washington and Manaus, Brazil," 11 December 1984. "Dr S. K.

Noordeen's Various Duty Travels," December 1984–October 1991. L4/441/11 J1. WHO Archives, Geneva.

76. Lopez Bravo, "Travel Report Summary," 4.

77. Noordeen, "Travel Report, 4–8 April 1988."

78. WHO, "Report of the Second Coordinating Meeting on Implementation of Multidrug Therapy in Leprosy Control Programmes," Geneva, 4–5 November 1987, 15. WHO/CDS/LEP/87.2.

79. WHO, "Report of a Consultation on Implementation of Leprosy Control Through Primary Health Care," Geneva, 16–18 June 1986. WHO/CDS/LEP/86.3.

80. "Report of a Consultation on Implementation of Leprosy Control through Primary Health Care."

81. "Report of a Consultation on Implementation of Leprosy Control through Primary Health Care," 7.

82. "Report of a Consultation on Implementation of Leprosy Control through Primary Health Care," 19.

83. "Report of a Consultation on Implementation of Leprosy Control through Primary Health Care," 12.

84. Daumerie, "Implementation of MDT," *Multidrug Therapy Against Leprosy*, 45.

85. "Report of the Second Coordinating Meeting on Implementation of Multidrug Therapy," 3.

86. "Report of the Second Coordinating Meeting on Implementation of Multidrug Therapy," 52.

87. "Report of the Second Coordinating Meeting on Implementation of Multidrug Therapy," 75.

88. Yuasa to Noordeen L4/370/7, 584, 412. WHO Archives, Geneva.

89. Daumerie, "Implementation of MDT," 45.

90. Daumerie, "Implementation of MDT."

8. ELIMINATION, THE IDEA

1. WHO, "Forty-Fourth World Health Assembly, Provisional agenda item 17.2," 5.

2. WHO, "Forty-Fourth World Health Assembly, Provisional agenda item 17.2," 4.

3. WHO, "Forty-Fourth World Health Assembly, Provisional agenda item 17.2," 8–9.

4. WHO, Executive Board, Eighty-Seventh Session, Agenda Item 5.2, "Leprosy (Draft Resolution Proposed by Professor O Ransome-Kuti," 16 January 1991, EB87/Conf. Paper No. 2; WHO, Executive Board, Eighty-Seventh Session, "Summary Records: Thirteenth Meeting," 168; WHO, "Forty-Fourth World Health Assembly, Provisional Summary of the Third Meeting," 4, A44/A/SR/3, WHO Archives, Geneva.

5. WHO, "Forty-Fourth World Health Assembly, First Report of Committee A (Draft)," (Draft) A44/49 11 May 1991, 12–13, WHO Archives, Geneva.

6. The taskforce also developed formal definitions for "eradication," "extinction", and "control". The Carter Center, Program Definitions: "International Task Force for Disease Eradication (I) 1989–1992," https://www.cartercenter.org/health/itfde/program_definition.html; 1993. Recommendations and Reports: Recommendations of the International Task Force for Disease Eradication. *Morbidity and Mortality Weekly Report*, 42 (1993): RR-16.

7. In 1997, the WHA called for the elimination of lymphatic filariasis as a public health problem, and in 1997, the WHO listed onchocerciasis and Chagas disease as candidates for elimination "as public health problems within ten years". By 1998, there were programmes for the eradication of polio and guinea worm. Walter R. Dowdle, 22. The WHA 44.9 resolution was also formulated six years before the Dahlem Workshop on the Eradication of Infectious Diseases, held in March 1997, at which the differences between control, elimination, and eradication were comprehensively delineated.

8. WHO, *Epidemiology of Leprosy in Relation to Control*, 30–1.

9. WHO, *Epidemiology of Leprosy in Relation to Control*, 33.

10. WHO, *Epidemiology of Leprosy in Relation to Control*, 35. New case detection includes cases diagnosed with onset of disease in the year in question (true incidence) and a large proportion of cases with onset in previous years (termed a backlog prevalence of undetected cases).

11. WHO, *Epidemiology of Leprosy in Relation to Control*, 36.

12. WHO, *Epidemiology of Leprosy in Relation to Control*, 39.

13. WHO, *Epidemiology of Leprosy in Relation to Control*, 40.

14. Noordeen, "The Concept of Elimination," in WHO, "Informal Consultation on the Development and Implementation of MDT," 1.

15. Author Interview; S. K. Noordeen; Geneva, 4 January 2012.

16. Author Interview; S. K. Noordeen; Oxford, 4 January 2009.

17. S. K. Noordeen, "The Concept of Elimination," 3.

18. Yo Yuasa, "Basic Paradigm Shift for Leprosy Control in the Field," Unpublished document. No page numbers.

19. Yo Yuasa, "TNF(JSIF)/SMHF's Contribution 1974–2005," 5–6.

20. Author Interview; S. K. Noordeen; Geneva, 4 January 2012.

21. Author Interview; S. K. Noordeen; Geneva, 4 January 2012, 2.

22. Sansarricq, "Lessons To Be Learned," in WHO, *Multidrug Therapy Against Leprosy: Development and Implementation*.

23. Brown et al., "The World Health Organization and the Transition from 'International' to 'Global Public Health,'" 64–5.

24. Brown et al., "The World Health Organization and the Transition from 'International' to 'Global Public Health,'" 65.

25. "Informal Consultation on the Development and Implementation of MDT," 4–5.

26. Brown, Cueto, and Fee have a great deal more to say about the role played by the latter in setting the WHO agenda, 68.

27. Brown et al., "The World Health Organization and the Transition from 'International' to 'Global Public Health,'" 68.

28. World Health Organization, Sixth Expert Committee Meeting on Leprosy, "Preliminary Review of Points for Discussion on Leprosy and Leprosy Control: Prepared by the Leprosy Unit with the collaboration of Dr H. Sansarricq, WHO Short-Term Consultant." Doc 2372F Second Draft, 17–24 November 1987. WHO Expert Committee, 1987. L4/81/6 J1. WHO Archives, Geneva.

29. *WHO Expert Committee on Leprosy: Sixth Report*, 14.

30. *WHO Expert Committee on Leprosy: Sixth Report*.

31. *WHO Expert Committee on Leprosy: Sixth Report*, 32.

32. A. Colin McDougall, Department of Dermatology, The Slade Hospital, Oxford to Dr S. K. Noordeen, Chief Medical Officer, Leprosy, Division of Communicable Diseases, 13 May 1987, 3, "WHO Expert Committee 1987," L4/81/6 J1. WHO Archives, Geneva.

33. M. O. Adeleye, the Director of Health Services, Kwara State Ministry of Health, in Nigeria, to S. K. Noordeen, Chief Medical Officer, Leprosy, Division of Communicable Diseases, 5 June 1987, 4.

34. M. O. Adeleye, the Director of Health Services, Kwara State Ministry of Health, in Nigeria, to S. K. Noordeen, Chief Medical Officer, Leprosy, Division of Communicable Diseases, 5 June 1987, 4.

35. M. O. Adeleye, the Director of Health Services, Kwara State Ministry of Health, in Nigeria, to S. K. Noordeen, Chief Medical Officer, Leprosy, Division of Communicable Diseases, 5 June 1987, 5.

36. Dr John C. Hargraves, Darwin, Northern Territory, Australia to S. K. Noordeen, Chief Medical Officer, Leprosy, Division of Communicable Diseases, 10 June 1987, in "WHO Expert Committee 1987." Ibid.

37. "WHO Expert Committee 1998," 48.

38. Professor Michel Lechat, Department d'Epidémiologie et de Médecine Préventive, Université Catholique de Louvain, to S. K. Noordeen, Chief Medical Officer, Leprosy, Division of Communicable Diseases, 3 July 1987. "WHO Expert Committee 1987." Ibid.

39. WHO, "Report of the First Meeting of the WHO Working Group on Leprosy Control, Geneva, 1–3 July 1991." WHO/CTD/LEP/91.4; WHO, "Report of the Second Meeting of the WHO Working Group on Leprosy Control, Geneva, 7–9 July 1992." WHO/CTD/LEP/92.5; WHO, "Report of the Third Meeting of the Working Group on Leprosy Control, Geneva, 14–16 July 1993." WHO/CTD/LEP/93.5; WHO, "Report of the Fourth Working Group on Leprosy Control (LWG), Hanoi, 8 July 1994." WHO/CTD/LEP/94.4; L4 522 9, J1.

40. WHO, "Report of the First Meeting," 11–12; WHO "Report of the Second Meeting," SEARO Leprosy: Group Consultation and Training Activities – General. L4 48 1. vol. 13. [HQ ref L4/522/10] and [HQ ref L4 522 9 J1]. SEARO Archives, New Delhi.

41. "Report of the Third Meeting," 3; Representatives from the following attended: ILA; ILU; ILEP; JSIF; GLRA; TLMI; AFRF; NSL; AIFO; DFB; ALM; ALES; LEPRA; and CIOMAL.

42. "Report of the Third Meeting," 7.

43. "Report of the Third Meeting," 8.

44. "Report of the Third Meeting," 9.

45. Noordeen, "Leprosy Control Through Multidrug Therapy (MDT)," 263–9.

46. Bechelli and Martínez Domínguez, "The Leprosy Problem in the World," 811–26.

47. Noordeen, et al., "Estimated Number of Leprosy Cases in the World," 7–10.

48. Noordeen, et al., "Estimated Number of Leprosy Cases in the World," 8.

49. ILEP Coordinating Bureau, "57th Meeting of the Medical Commission, Bern, 5 June 1991, Report," 4. ILEP Archives, London.

50. Fine, "Editorial: Reflections on the Elimination of Leprosy," 71–80.

51. Fine, "Editorial: Reflections on the Elimination of Leprosy," 71.

52. Diagnosis is difficult because cases are detected early, because infection with *M. leprae* is equated with clinical disease; because of misclassifications (false positives) and the impact on inaccurate results (re: vaccines) [not a reason but an effect of]; because of variations in interpretations of lesions amongst field workers; and similar disagreement over biopsies amongst histopathologists. Fine, "Editorial: Reflections on the Elimination of Leprosy," 72.

53. Fine, "Editorial: Reflections on the Elimination of Leprosy," 72.

54. Fine, "Editorial: Reflections on the Elimination of Leprosy," 73.

55. Fine, "Editorial: Reflections on the Elimination of Leprosy," 74.

56. Fine, "Editorial: Reflections on the Elimination of Leprosy," 79.

57. Fine, "Editorial: Reflections on the Elimination of Leprosy."

58. As a counter to his argument, the declining incidence in several of these countries also needs to take into account the rather draconian policies of isolation in Norway, Japan, and China, for example, as well as the rigorous rural campaign and isolation measures conducted in Portugal and possibly Venezuela. Even natural declines in leprosy can be quite complex if a truly long-term historical view is added to the epidemiological viewpoint.

59. Fine, "Editorial: Reflections on the Elimination of Leprosy," 79.

60. Fine, "Editorial: Reflections on the Elimination of Leprosy," 74.

61. Fine, "Editorial: Reflections on the Elimination of Leprosy," 79.

62. Fine, "Editorial: Reflections on the Elimination of Leprosy."

63. ILEP Coordinating Bureau, "18th General Assembly, Wurzburg, 9 June 1990, 'President's Speech Delivered by Mr Jean Loiselle at the 18th ILEP General Assembly Wurzburg, 9 June 1990,'" ILEP Archives, London.

64. ILEP Coordinating Bureau, "Cooperation Between ILEP and the WHO Leprosy Unit: Notes of a Meeting," Wurzburg, 6 June 1990. L4/372/8. WHO Archives, Geneva.

65. ILEP Coordinating Bureau, "ILEP Medical Commission: Progress Report on Activities Carried out in 1990," 1. 56MC/AGENDA/A5. ILEP Archives, London.

66. ILEP Coordinating Bureau, "ILEP Medical Commission: Tentative Programme for 1991," 1. 56MC/AGENDA/A5. ILEP Archives, London.

67. ILEP Coordinating Bureau, "ILEP Medical Commission: Tentative Programme for 1991," 1. 56MC/AGENDA/A5. ILEP Archives, London.

68. ILEP Coordinating Bureau, "Leprosy Control Expert Discipline: Expert Group on Extending the Coverage of MDT ("Filling the Gaps"): Report to the Medical Commission, 5 June 1991. 57 MC/AGENDA/A2. ILEP Archives, London.

69. ILEP Coordinating Bureau, "20th General Assembly of ILEP: Dublin, 11 July 1994: Minutes," 9. ILEP Archives.

70. ILEP Coordinating Bureau, "19th General Assembly of ILEP: Montreal, 6 June 1992: Minutes," 1 and 6. ILEP Archives, London.

71. "Dr S. K. Noordeen's Various Duty Travels," 2–5 June 1992. L4 441 11 J 2. WHO Archives, Geneva.

72. "Dr S. K. Noordeen's Various Duty Travels," 2–5 June 1992. L4 441 11 J 2. WHO Archives, Geneva.

73. "13 YEARS – Reflections by Trevor Durston," November 2006. Unpublished. TLMI Archives, London.

74. ILEP Coordinating Bureau, "21st General Assembly of ILEP: Washington, 8 June 1996: Minutes," 2. ILEP Archives, London.

75. ILEP Coordinating Bureau, "69th ILEP Medical Commission: Report, Washington, 5 June 1994"; ILEP Coordinating Bureau, "19th General Assembly of ILEP: Montreal, 6 June 1992: Minutes," 1, GA 22, Brighton, UK, 14 December 1996, 3. ILEP Archives, London.

76. ILEP Coordinating Bureau, "19th General Assembly: Speech Given by Mr André Récipon of FF: ILEP General Assembly, Montreal, 6 June 1992," 19AG/Minutes/A4. ILEP Archives, London.

77. Ecuador was the only country that had achieved elimination of leprosy through implementing MDT. The Caribbean region; Uruguay; and Rio Grande do Sul, a State of Brazil, had the potential to achieve that goal next.

78. Dr S. K. Noordeen's Various Duty Travels, 1991, 3–7 June. L4 441 11, J 1. WHO Archives, Geneva.

79. Paul Sommerfeld, "Editorial: Voluntary Donor Agencies in Anti-Leprosy Work: Present Contribution and Probable Future," *LR* 65 (1994): 1.

80. Paul Sommerfeld, "Editorial: Voluntary Donor Agencies in Anti-Leprosy Work: Present Contribution and Probable Future," *LR* 65 (1994): 3.

81. Paul Sommerfeld, "Editorial: Voluntary Donor Agencies in Anti-Leprosy Work: Present Contribution and Probable Future," *LR* 65 (1994): 5.

82. Paul Sommerfeld, "Editorial: Voluntary Donor Agencies in Anti-Leprosy Work: Present Contribution and Probable Future," *LR* 65 (1994): 7.

9. ELIMINATION, THE REALITY

1. Yo Yuasa, "TNF(JSIF)/SMHF's Contributions 1974–2005."

2. Kenzo Kiikuni, Executive Managing Director, SMHF to Hiroshi Nakajima, DG/WHO Subject: Leprosy Drug Fund, 16 August 1994. "Supply of Multidrug Therapy Drugs – Sasakawa Fund." L4 /135/2, J1. WHO Archives, Geneva.

3.   Kenzo Kiikuni, Executive Managing Director, SMHF to Hiroshi Nakajima, DG/ WHO Subject: Leprosy Drug Fund, 16 August 1994. "Supply of Multidrug Therapy Drugs – Sasakawa Fund." L4 /135/2, J1. WHO Archives, Geneva. At the same time, the Japan Shipbuilding Industries Fund continued their annual contribution of at least US$4 million to WHO.

4.   "TDRs Contribution to the Development of MDT," 19; S. K. Noordeen to the WHO Regional Directors, 26 August 1994. "Supply of Multidrug Therapy Drugs – Sasakawa Fund." L4 /135/2, J1. WHO Archives, Geneva.

5.   Dr Wim H. van Brakel, the Project Director in the International Nepal Fellowship Leprosy Control Project in the Western and Mid-Western Regions, of Pokhara, Nepal to Dr S. K. Noordeen, Chief WHO Leprosy Unit, Geneva, Switzerland, 25 October 1994. "Supply of Multidrug Therapy Drugs – Sasakawa Fund." L4 /135/2, J1. WHO Archives, Geneva.

6.   MB packs cost US$1.72 each or US$40.00 for twenty-four. PB packs cost US$0.50 each or US$3.00 for six packs. "Report of the Second Meeting of the Leprosy Elimination Advisory Group," Geneva, 14 October 1996, 6. WHO/ LEP/97.2. WHO Archives, Geneva.

7.   "Report of the Second Meeting of the Leprosy Elimination Advisory Group," Geneva, 14 October 1996, 6. WHO/LEP/97.2. WHO Archives, Geneva.

8.   "Report of the Third Meeting of the Leprosy Elimination Advisory Group," Geneva, 16–17 July 1997, WHO/LEP/97.6. WHO Archives, Geneva.

9.   The global buffer stock was 13 million blister packs, which meant 1.5 million patient years of treatment. "Report of the Second Meeting of the Leprosy Elimination Advisory Group," 5.

10. "Report of the Fourth Meeting of the Leprosy Elimination Advisory Group," Geneva, 24–25 June 1998, 11. WHO/LEP/98.3. WHO Archives, Geneva.

11. "Report of the Second Meeting of the Leprosy Elimination Advisory Group," Geneva, 14 October 1996, 2. WHO/LEP/97.2. WHO Archives, Geneva.

12. S. K. Noordeen in communication with the author, 4 January 2012; Remi Verduin, NSL Medical Consultant to S. K. Noordeen, Director Action Programme for the Elimination of Leprosy, 13 January 1997. "Leprosy General Planning." L4 370 1, J 12; S. K. Noordeen, Director Action Programme for the Elimination of Leprosy to Remi Verduin, NSL Medical Consultant, 27 January 1997. "Leprosy General Planning." L4/370/1, J 12. WHO Archives, Geneva.

13. Packard, "Malaria Dreams," 293.

14. "Draft 'Guidelines for Plan of Action for Leprosy Elimination Campaign in Priority Areas,'" (LEC) 29 August 1995. "Leprosy: General Programme Planning." L4/370/1, J8. WHO Archives, Geneva.

15. "Draft 'Guidelines for Plan of Action for Leprosy Elimination Campaign in Priority Areas,'" (LEC) 29 August 1995. "Leprosy: General Programme Planning." L4/370/1, J8. WHO Archives, Geneva.

16. Memo A/Team Coordinator LEP to Executive Director, CDS 30 March 1999. "Consultative Meeting on Leprosy Elimination Campaigns, Geneva, 14/7–15/7 1999." L4 87 48; Letter to Programme Managers re LEC in "Leprosy General Programme Planning." L4 370 1; S. K. Noordeen to Blanc RA/LEP, CHD, WPRO, re: Leprosy Elimination Campaign (LEC); World Bank, 12 Sept 1995 in "Leprosy: General Programme Planning." L4/370/1, J8; Memo LEP HQ to WPRO Blanc, October 1995. "Leprosy: General Programme Planning." L4/370/1, J9. WHO Archives, Geneva.

17. "Establishment of a Photo Library on Leprosy," January 1996. L4 158 3. WHO Archives, Geneva.

18. "Establishment of a Photo Library on Leprosy," January 1996. L4 158 3. WHO Archives, Geneva.

19. WHO, *Action Programme for the Elimination of Leprosy: Status Report 1996.*

20. WHO, "Report of the Second International Conference on the Elimination of Leprosy as a Public Health Problem"; WHO, *Global Strategy for the Elimination of Leprosy as a Public Health Problem.* The updated global strategy called particularly for increased community participation.

21. WHO, "Report of the Second Meeting of the Leprosy Elimination Advisory Group," 2–4.

22. WHO, "Report of the Second Meeting of the Leprosy Elimination Advisory Group," 8.

23. WHO, "Report of the Second Meeting of the Leprosy Elimination Advisory Group."

24. WHO, "Report of the Third Meeting of the Leprosy Elimination Advisory Group," Geneva, 16–17 July 1997. WHO/LEP/97.6.

25. ILEP Coordinating Bureau, "23rd General Assembly of ILEP: Bologna, Italy, December 13, 1997: Minutes," Item 8. ILEP Archives, London.

26. ILEP Coordinating Bureau, "23rd General Assembly of ILEP: Bologna, Italy, December 13, 1997: Minutes," Item 8. ILEP Archives, London.

27. ILEP Coordinating Bureau, "23rd General Assembly of ILEP: Bologna, Italy, December 13, 1997: Minutes," 11. ILEP Archives, London.

28. Noordeen, "The Concept of Elimination," in "WHO, Informal Consultation on the Development and Implementation of MDT," 3.

29. Geoff Warne, personal communication with author, 16 April 2021.

30. WHO, "Action Programme for the Elimination of Leprosy: Report of the Fourth Meeting of the Leprosy Elimination Advisory Group," WHO: Geneva, 1998. WHO/LEP/98.3; "Report of a Special Meeting of the Leprosy Elimination Advisory Group with Potential Partners," Geneva, 12–13 April 1999. WHO/LEP/99.1.

31. ILEP Coordinating Bureau, "24th General Assembly of ILEP: Liège, Belgium, December 12, 1998: Minutes," ILEP Archives, London.

32. Dr Melville Christian, Director, Schieffelin Leprosy Research and Training Centre, Karigiri, "Leprosy Control Based on MDT," 6, "WHO Expert Committee 1987." L4/81/6, J2. WHO Archives, Geneva.

33. Dr Melville Christian, Director, Schieffelin Leprosy Research and Training Centre, Karigiri, "Leprosy Control Based on MDT," 6, "WHO Expert Committee 1987." L4/81/6, J2. WHO Archives, Geneva, 7.

34. Dr Melville Christian, Director, Schieffelin Leprosy Research and Training Centre, Karigiri, "Leprosy Control Based on MDT," 6, "WHO Expert Committee 1987." L4/81/6, J2. WHO Archives, Geneva.

35. Dr Melville Christian, Director, Schieffelin Leprosy Research and Training Centre, Karigiri, "Leprosy Control Based on MDT," 6, "WHO Expert Committee 1987." L4/81/6, J2. WHO Archives, Geneva, 8.

10. THE GLOBAL ALLIANCE FOR THE ELIMINATION OF LEPROSY

1. Mach, "Brundtland replaces top staff at the WHO," 229.

2. Yo Yuasa, Executive and Medical Director, SMHF to David Heymann, Executive Director, CDS, 29 September 1998 in "Leprosy General Programme Planning." L4 /370/ 1, J13, WHO Archives, Geneva.

3. David Heymann to Yo Yuasa, 16 October 1998.

4. Brown et al., "The World Health Organization and the World of Global Health."

5. Director–General Gro Harlem Brundtland to Dr Daniel L. Vasella, the President of Novartis International, 15 May 1999, "Leprosy General Programme Planning," L4 /370/ 1, J13, WHO Archives, Geneva.

6. V. K. Pannikar, 12 February 1999, re: "Consultative Meeting on the Global Leprosy Situation and Status of the Elimination of Leprosy, Geneva, 29–30 March 1999"; WHO, "Report of a Special Meeting of the Leprosy Elimination Advisory Group (LEAG) with Potential Partners, Geneva, April 12 and 13, 1999," WHO/LEP/99.1, WHO Archives, Geneva.

7. Dr Yo Yuasa to Dr Ji Baohong, AFRF, 24 February 1999, arranging joint sponsorship of the Elimination meeting in Addis in 1999, "Third International Conference on Elimination of Leprosy, Addis Ababa, Ethiopia, 11/10–13/10/99," L4 87 46, WHO Archives, Geneva.

8. Dr Yo Yuasa to M. Michel Recipon, President, Association Française Raoul Follereau, 24 February 1999, "Third International Conference on Elimination of Leprosy, Addis Ababa, Ethiopia," 11/10–13/10/99, L4 87 46, WHO Archives, Geneva.

9. Memorandum from Director, CEE CDS/H, Subject: "Information Meeting on Global Alliance for the Elimination of Leprosy: Geneva, 10 September 1999," 1 September 1999, "Leprosy General Program Planning," L4 370 1, J13, WHO Archives, Geneva.

10. David Heymann to Yohei Sasakawa, 8 September 1999, "Meetings of the Leprosy Advisory Group," L4 522 11, J2, WHO Archives, Geneva.

11. "Elimination of Leprosy in Sight: Global Alliance Created to Achieve Elimination by the End of 2005," "WHO Press," Press Release WHO/70, 15 November 1999, "Third International Conference on Elimination of Leprosy, Addis Ababa, Ethiopia, 11/10–13/10/99," L4 87 46, WHO Archives, Geneva.

12. Joyce Massé to Melinda Henry, Subject: Global Alliance Press Release, 11 November 1999. Made available to the author by Dr Denis Daumerie.

13. "Notes of Informal Discussions," provided by Dr Daumerie. Six members of the first TAG meeting that met in 2–3 May 2000 were as follows: Professor Vera Andrade (Brazil), Professor M. D. Gupte (India) Chairman; Professor H. J. S. Kawuma (Uganda); Ms Santa Raye (India); Professor Oumou Younoussa Sow (Guinea); Professor W. C. S. Smith, "Notes of Informal Discussions."

14. He emphasised that a detailed situation analysis needed to be completed in order to adapt the intensified strategy to realities in the field.

15. I am indebted to Geoff Warne's explanation of this as a misunderstanding: "It seems probable that ILEP had understood that all members of the GAEL were putting all their (financial) cards on the table and this is how much they were committing to the work of leprosy – in ILEP's case, their entire budget. I think that the imbroglio about the US$19.5m was more about misunderstanding or misinterpretation than a structural issue." Geoff Warne, ILEP CEO, in personal communication to the author, 16 April 2021.

16. "Notes of Informal Discussions."

17. "Notes of Informal Discussions."

18. "Notes of Informal Discussions."

19. "First Meeting of the Global Alliance for the Elimination of Leprosy, 'The Delhi Declaration,' 30–1 January 2001." L4 372 19, WHO Archives, Geneva.

20. Étienne Declercq, Chair, ILEP Medico-Social Commission to Dr David Heymann, Executive Director, Communicable Diseases, WHO, 8 October 2001, "Global Alliance for Elimination of Leprosy," L4 372 19. WHO Archives, Geneva.

21. Étienne Declercq, Chair, ILEP Medico-Social Commission to Dr David Heymann, Executive Director, Communicable Diseases, WHO, 8 October 2001, "Global Alliance for Elimination of Leprosy," L4 372 19, WHO Archives, Geneva.

22. Dr David Heymann, Executive Director, Communicable Diseases, WHO, to Étienne Declercq, Chair, ILEP Medico-Social Commission, 18 October 2001, "Global Alliance for Elimination of Leprosy," L4 372 19. WHO Archives, Geneva.

23. It stated that "WHO is never recommending closing leprosy diagnosis and treatment activities. In fact during the second meeting TAG strongly advised on clarifying the meaning of elimination to new senior health service managers, ministers of health and administrators. Even though there is little perceived risk of resurgence, integrated disease surveillance mechanisms are expected to provide data on this critical factor." David L. Heymann, Executive Director to Dr M. D. Gupte, Director, National Institute of Epidemiology, Indian Council of Medical Research, Chennai, Subject: Global Alliance for Elimination of Leprosy, "Global Alliance for Elimination of Leprosy," 23 October 2001, L4/372/19, WHO Archives, Geneva.

24. The announcement was made at the fifty-fourth World Health Assembly on 16 May 2001, in "Special Event on Leprosy Elimination during 54th WHA";

"Global Alliance for Elimination of Leprosy," L4 372 19, WHO Archives, Geneva.

25. "WHO Leprosy Elimination Report to the Nippon Foundation 2002 and Proposal for 2003," "GAEL," L4 372 19 J2, WHO Archives, Geneva.

26. "Meeting on the Global Alliance for the Elimination of Leprosy (GAEL), WHO, Geneva, Friday, 7 December 2001." WHO Archives, Geneva.

27. Maria Neira, Director, CPE, 20 December 2001, Re: Global Alliance for the Elimination of Leprosy (GAEL). WHO Archives, Geneva.

28. Maria Neira, Director, CPE, 20 December 2001, Re: Global Alliance for the Elimination of Leprosy (GAEL). WHO Archives, Geneva.

11. A QUESTIONABLE VICTORY

1. Ji Baohong was born in Shanghai in 1936, and his participation in international health initiatives began in 1989, when he was the Medical Officer and Secretary of the THELEP Steering Committee at the WHO until 1994. After he left the WHO, he was employed as Professor of Microbiology at the Service de Bactériologie et Hygiène of the Faculté de Médecine Pitié-Salpêtrière, at the University of Paris. He was a formidable member of the ILEP Technical Commission (previously known as the Medical Commission and then the Medico-Social Commission) from 1992 to the end of 2007. He died at seventy-four years of age, from cancer, in Paris on 10 February 2010. "Obituary: Professor Ji Baohong 1936–2010," *LR* 81 (2010): 148–9.

2. Five members of the organising committee, Paul Saunderson (ALM), W. C. S. Smith (TLMI), P. Feenstra (NLR), Étienne Declercq (DF), and Ji Baohong (FRF), were nominated.

3. Baohong Ji to Paul Saunderson, W. C. S. Smith, P. Feenstra, Étienne Declercq, Yo Yuasa. 12 March 2001, Re: Operation of the Organization Committee, Damien Foundation Archives, Brussels.

4. Baohong Ji to Paul Saunderson, W. C. S. Smith, P. Feenstra, Étienne Declercq, Yo Yuasa. 12 March 2001, Re: Operation of the Organization Committee, Damien Foundation Archives, Brussels, 3.

5. Cairns Smith to Baohong Ji, Paul Saunderson, P. Feenstra, Étienne Declercq, Yo Yuasa, Re: Operation of the Organization Committee, 13 March 2001, Damien Foundation Archives, Brussels.

6. "ILA Technical Forum, Paris," 25–28 February 2002. Participants: Elizabeth Bizuneh, ALERT; Étienne Declercq; Piet Feenstra; Paul Fine; Baohong Ji; P. Krishnamurthy; Nyunt Sein Kyaw; Lou Levy; Diana Lockwood; S. K. Noordeen; Amudha Poobalan; Paul Saunderson; Cairns Smith; Wim H. van Brakel; Marcos Virmond; Yo Yuasa; invited but unable to attend: N. S. Dharmashaktu; Denis Daumerie; Howard Engers; F. M. P. Gerson; M. D. Gupte.

7. The group identified the following topics that would be reviewed by the Technical Forum and therefore were to be covered by the working document:

I.   Elimination of leprosy (Elimination and eradication; Prevalence and incidence; Case-detection rate and incidence rate; Other indicators for elimination; Backlog cases; Early detection; Leprosy Elimination Campaign (LEC); Special Action Project (SAPEL); Information, education and communication (IEC); Leprosy elimination monitoring (LEM); Evaluation; Integration of vertical program into general health services; Decentralisation; Sustainability of elimination activities; Combined program; Capacity building; and Prophylaxis)

II.   Diagnosis (Cardinal signs of leprosy; Diffuse infiltration; Sensory impairment; Nerve-trunk thickening; Skin smears; Biopsy; Sensitivity and specificity of these examinations; Serology and PCR; Lepromin test; and Classification)

III.   Treatment (Official regimens; Flexibility of drug-delivery system and its limit; Compliance of the patient and the program; Accompanied MDT (MDT-A); Defaulter; MB relapse; Rifampicin resistance; Dapsone resistance; Newer drugs and regimens; Immunotherapy)

IV.   Prevention and Management of Leprosy Reaction, Nerve Damage and Disability (Frequency and incidence; Nerve function test; Diagnosis; Management; Prednipac; Footwear; Self-care)

"Minutes of an Informal Meeting on International Leprosy Association (ILA) Technical Forum," Baohong Ji at Hotel Meridien, New Delhi, India, 31 January 2001, Damien Foundation Archives, Brussels.

8.   "Report of the International Leprosy Association Technical Forum, Paris, 25–28 February 2002," 16.

9.   "Report of the International Leprosy Association Technical Forum, Paris, 25–28 February 2002," 2.

10.   "Report of the International Leprosy Association Technical Forum, Paris, 25–28 February 2002," 37.

11.   "Report of the International Leprosy Association Technical Forum, Paris, 25–28 February 2002," 38, 39.

12.   "Evaluation of the Global Alliance for the Elimination of Leprosy: Project Description," 1 December 2002.

13.   "Evaluation of the Global Alliance for the Elimination of Leprosy: Project Description," 1 December 2002, 17, 20.

14.   Skolnik et al., "Independent Evaluation of the Global Alliance," i.

15.   Skolnik et al., "Independent Evaluation of the Global Alliance," ii.

16.   Skolnik et al., "Independent Evaluation of the Global Alliance," 11.

17.   Skolnik et al., "Independent Evaluation of the Global Alliance," 12.

18.   Skolnik et al., "Independent Evaluation of the Global Alliance," 10.

19.   Skolnik et al., "Independent Evaluation of the Global Alliance," ii.

20.   Skolnik et al., "Independent Evaluation of the Global Alliance," 11–13.

21.   Skolnik et al., "Independent Evaluation of the Global Alliance," 8, 11.

22.   Skolnik et al., "Independent Evaluation of the Global Alliance," 11–13.

23.   Skolnik et al., "Independent Evaluation of the Global Alliance," 17–18.

24. Skolnik et al., "Independent Evaluation of the Global Alliance," 17.
25. Skolnik et al., "Independent Evaluation of the Global Alliance," 8, 10.
26. C. K. Rao, WHO STC, "Report on Lessons Learnt From the Modified Leprosy Elimination Campaign in Tamil Nadu," 8. Project Number: ICP.GEE.020/97, "India PLC," l4 370 6 IND, J 10, WHO Archives, Geneva.
27. C. K. Rao, WHO STC, "Report on Lessons Learnt From the Modified Leprosy Elimination Campaign in Tamil Nadu," 8. Project Number: ICP.GEE.020/97, "India PLC," l4 370 6 IND, J 10, WHO Archives, Geneva, 3.
28. C. K. Rao, WHO STC, "Report on Lessons Learnt From the Modified Leprosy Elimination Campaign in Tamil Nadu," 8. Project Number: ICP.GEE.020/97, "India PLC," l4 370 6 IND, J 10, WHO Archives, Geneva, 6.
29. C. K. Rao, WHO STC, "Report on Lessons Learnt From the Modified Leprosy Elimination Campaign in Tamil Nadu," 8. Project Number: ICP.GEE.020/97, "India PLC," l4 370 6 IND, J 10, WHO Archives, Geneva, 2.
30. C. K. Rao, WHO STC, "Report on Lessons Learnt From the Modified Leprosy Elimination Campaign in Tamil Nadu," 8. Project Number: ICP.GEE.020/97, "India PLC," l4 370 6 IND, J 10, WHO Archives, Geneva, 6.
31. C. K. Rao, WHO STC, "Report on Lessons Learnt From the Modified Leprosy Elimination Campaign in Tamil Nadu," 8. Project Number: ICP.GEE.020/97, "India PLC," l4 370 6 IND, J 10, WHO Archives, Geneva, 7.
32. C. K. Rao, WHO STC, "Report on Lessons Learnt From the Modified Leprosy Elimination Campaign in Tamil Nadu," 8. Project Number: ICP.GEE.020/97, "India PLC," l4 370 6 IND, J 10, WHO Archives, Geneva.
33. C. K. Rao, WHO STC, "Report on Lessons Learnt From the Modified Leprosy Elimination Campaign in Tamil Nadu," 8. Project Number: ICP.GEE.020/97, "India PLC," l4 370 6 IND, J 10, WHO Archives, Geneva, 3.
34. C. K. Rao, WHO STC, "Report on Lessons Learnt From the Modified Leprosy Elimination Campaign in Tamil Nadu," 8. Project Number: ICP.GEE.020/97, "India PLC," l4 370 6 IND, J 10, WHO Archives, Geneva, 4.
35. C. K. Rao, WHO STC, "Report on Lessons Learnt From the Modified Leprosy Elimination Campaign in Tamil Nadu," 8. Project Number: ICP.GEE.020/97, "India PLC," l4 370 6 IND, J 10, WHO Archives, Geneva, 9.
36. C. K. Rao, WHO STC, "Report on Lessons Learnt From the Modified Leprosy Elimination Campaign in Tamil Nadu," 8. Project Number: ICP.GEE.020/97, "India PLC," l4 370 6 IND, J 10, WHO Archives, Geneva, 8.
37. C. K. Rao, WHO STC, "Report on Lessons Learnt From the Modified Leprosy Elimination Campaign in Tamil Nadu," 8. Project Number: ICP.GEE.020/97, "India PLC," l4 370 6 IND, J 10, WHO Archives, Geneva.
38. C. K. Rao, WHO STC, "Report on Lessons Learnt From the Modified Leprosy Elimination Campaign in Tamil Nadu," 8. Project Number: ICP.GEE.020/97, "India PLC," l4 370 6 IND, J 10, WHO Archives, Geneva, 4.
39. C. K. Rao, WHO STC, "Report on Lessons Learnt From the Modified Leprosy Elimination Campaign in Tamil Nadu," 8. Project Number: ICP.GEE.020/97, "India PLC," l4 370 6 IND, J 10, WHO Archives, Geneva.

40. C. K. Rao, WHO STC, "Report on Lessons Learnt From the Modified Leprosy Elimination Campaign in Tamil Nadu," 8. Project Number: ICP.GEE.020/97, "India PLC," l4 370 6 IND, J 10, WHO Archives, Geneva, 5.

41. C. K. Rao, WHO STC, "Report on Lessons Learnt From the Modified Leprosy Elimination Campaign in Tamil Nadu," 8. Project Number: ICP.GEE.020/97, "India PLC," l4 370 6 IND, J 10, WHO Archives, Geneva.

42. National Leprosy Eradication Programme, India: Report of the Mid-Term Appraisal of World Bank NLEP Supported Project (7–19 April 1997), 27, "India PLC," l4 370 6, IND, J 10, WHO Archives, Geneva.

43. Rao, "Report on Lessons Learnt," 12.

44. "Proposal for Establishment of LEC Cell at NLEP Headquarters," India PLC, L4 370 6 IND, J 10. WHO Archives, Geneva.

45. K. K. Thassu, Joint Director (Leprosy) Director Health Services, Bhopal and Dr A. K. Thakur, Dy. Director Leprosy, "Leprosy Elimination Campaign (LEC) in Madhya Pradesh, India," in "Programme of Leprosy Control – India," L4 370 6 IND, J 10, WHO Archives, Geneva.

46. K. K. Thassu, Joint Director (Leprosy) Director Health Services, Bhopal and Dr A. K. Thakur, Dy. Director Leprosy, "Leprosy Elimination Campaign (LEC) in Madhya Pradesh, India," in "Programme of Leprosy Control – India," L4 370 6 IND, J 10, WHO Archives, Geneva.

47. K. K. Thassu, Joint Director (Leprosy) Director Health Services, Bhopal and Dr A. K. Thakur, Dy. Director Leprosy, "Leprosy Elimination Campaign (LEC) in Madhya Pradesh, India," in "Programme of Leprosy Control – India," L4 370 6 IND, J 10, WHO Archives, Geneva.

48. "Record note for the tripartite meeting held between the representatives of the World Bank, the WHO and the Government of India to review the National Leprosy Elimination Programme of India and to discuss future strategy, Geneva, September, 1–3 1998," 3, "Programme of Leprosy Control – India," l4 370 6 IND, J 11, WHO Archives, Geneva.

49. "Note for the Record," Denis Daumerie with Dr N. S. Dharmshaktu, Deputy Director, Lep, Directorate General of Health Services, New Delhi, 14 March 2000, "Programme of Leprosy Control – India," L4 370 6IND, J12. WHO Archives, Geneva.

50. Denis Daumerie to Dharnshaktu, 7 April 2000, "Programme of Leprosy Control – India," L4 370 6IND, J12. WHO Archives, Geneva.

51. "WHO Leprosy Elimination Report to The Nippon Foundation 2002 and Proposal for 2003," 7, "GAEL," L4 372 19 J2, WHO Archives, Geneva.

52. "WHO Leprosy Elimination Report to The Nippon Foundation 2002 and Proposal for 2003," 7, "GAEL," L4 372 19 J2, WHO Archives, Geneva, 10.

53. "WHO Leprosy Elimination Report to The Nippon Foundation 2002 and Proposal for 2003," 7, "GAEL," L4 372 19 J2, WHO Archives, Geneva, 5.

54. "WHO Leprosy Elimination Report to The Nippon Foundation 2002 and Proposal for 2003," 7, "GAEL," L4 372 19 J2, WHO Archives, Geneva, 15.

55. C. K. Rao, "Report on Lessons Learnt," 10.

56. "WHO Leprosy Elimination Report to The Nippon Foundation 2002 and Proposal for 2003," 7, "GAEL," L4 372 19 J2, WHO Archives, Geneva.
57. Htoon, "Travel Report," 18 April 2000, "Programme of Leprosy Control – India," L4 370 6IND, J12. WHO Archives, Geneva.
58. Tour report from Htoon re: New Delhi, Orissa, UPm and Chhattisgarh, 15 May 2001, "Programme of Leprosy Control – India," L4 370 6IND, J12.
59. Geneva meeting GOI/WHO re: special NLEP project; meeting of partners (GOI, ILEP, SMHF/TNF/WHO) to discuss the roles of each in supporting elimination activities in India, May 2001; Maria Neira to J. V. R. Prasada Rao (MOH&FW), "New intensified NLEP Project," "Programme of Leprosy Control – India," L4 370 6IND, J12. WHO Archives, Geneva.
60. "New intensified NLEP Project," 16.
61. "New intensified NLEP Project," 18.
62. "New intensified NLEP Project," 19.
63. S. K. Noordeen to Prasada Rao, 14 August 2003, "Programme of Leprosy Control – India," L4 370 6 IND J12. WHO Archives, Geneva.
64. Travel Report Pannikar: to attend review meeting with NLEP coordinators (23 Feb.), 11 April 2005, "Programme of Leprosy Control – India," L4 370 6 IND J12. WHO Archives, Geneva.
65. Trevor Durston, "13 YEARS – Reflections by Trevor Durston," November 2006, *Leprosy Mission International* Archives, London.
66. WHO, "Report of the Global Forum on Elimination of Leprosy."
67. WHO, "Weekly Epidemiological Record," 34 (2005), 80, 289–96; 32 (2006), 81, 309–16; 25 (2007), 82, 225–32; 33 (2008), 83, 293–300; 33 (2009), 84, 333–40.
68. WHO, Leprosy https://apps.who.int/neglected_diseases/ntddata/leprosy/leprosy.html Accessed 5 August 2020.
69. WHO, "Weekly Epidemiological Record," 35 (2018) 93, 445.
70. WHO, "Weekly Epidemiological Record," 35 (2018) 93, 445.
71. WHO, "Weekly Epidemiological Record," 35 (2018) 93, 447.
72. WHO, "Weekly Epidemiological Record," 35 (2018) 93, 453.
73. WHO, "Weekly Epidemiological Record," 35 (2018) 93, 455–6.
74. https://zeroleprosy.org/ Accessed 5 August 2020.
75. Paul Saunderson, "Reflections on the 20th International Leprosy Congress held in Manila, from 10–13 September 2019," *Leprosy Review* 90 (2019), 482–6.

12. THE HUMAN RIGHTS OF LEPROSY-AFFECTED PEOPLE

1. Ghosh and Chowdhury, *Dignity Regained*, 10.
2. GRECALTES (Greater Calcutta Leprosy Treatment and Health Education Scheme) is a non-government organisation that provides health services for leprosy and TB. In operation since 1975, it pioneered urban leprosy control in Calcutta. It began as a result of a collaboration between Hermann Kober and Dr D. S. Chaudhury with financial assistance from the German Leprosy

Relief Association. https://www.chnet.com/10241/grecaltes.html Accessed 17 June 2020.

3. Ghosh and Chowdhury, *Dignity Regained,* 12.
4. Ghosh and Chowdhury, *Dignity Regained*, 16.
5. The Dr Bandorawalla Leprosy Hospital is government owned, but it is managed by Pune District Leprosy Committee. Its existence was under threat in 2001 and again in 2011. https://timesofindia.indiatimes.com/Trust-to-give-up-leprosy-home/articleshow/22352323.cms; https://www.dnaindia.com/mumbai/report-largest-govt-run-leprosy-hospital-in-dire-straits-in-pune-1594240
6. This is the premier training institution established by Robert Cochrane and Paul Brand and supported by the Leprosy Mission. Under Dr Cochrane, Christian Medical College, Vellore became a centre for research into the development of the new sulphone drugs. This is also where Dr Brand practiced reconstructive surgery. Schieffelin Leprosy Research Centre, Karigiri, Vellore (Christian Medical College and Hospital) http://leprosyhistory.org
7. Ghosh and Chowdhury, *Dignity Regained*, 20.
8. Kakar, "Medical Developments and Patient Unrest," 2.
9. Kakar, "Medical Developments and Patient Unrest," 2.
10. Kakar, "Medical Developments and Patient Unrest," 10.
11. Kakar, "Medical Developments and Patient Unrest," 14.
12. Kakar, "Medical Developments and Patient Unrest," 1.
13. Ghosh and Chowdhury, *Dignity Regained*, 37–8.
14. Ghosh and Chowdhury, *Dignity Regained*, 41.
15. Ghosh and Chowdhury, *Dignity Regained*, 43.
16. Victoria Leprosy Hospital was founded in 1911, when Dr Isabel Kerr built the first hut for people with leprosy in the mission compound, at Nizamabad. This soon attracted more patients than it could comfortably house, and in 1915 a larger and more permanent colony was established 9 miles away in Dichpalli. A report from 1961 details a daily average of 425 patients in the institution (282 men, eighty-three women, and sixty children), under the care of Medical Superintendent Dr P. S. Samuel and his staff. Dr Frank Davey worked as a Methodist Medical Missionary at Uzuakoli, Nigeria, from 1936. From 1968 to 1973, he worked as a clinical leprologist at the Dichpalli Leprosy Hospital. Today it has its own Facebook page. https://www.facebook.com/VictoriaHospitalDichpally; https://www.findhealthclinics.com/XX/Unknown/800765850021941/Victoria-Hospital-Dichpally; http://leprosyhistory.org Accessed 11 August 2020.
17. Ghosh and Chowdhury, *Dignity Regained*, 28.
18. Ghosh and Chowdhury, *Dignity Regained*, 32.
19. The affront to the human rights of leprosy-affected people is even more obvious in light of the 2006 International Convention on the Rights of Persons with Disabilities. This began with the 1975 Declaration on the Rights of Disabled Persons and the Decade of Disabled Persons from 1983–92 with its programme

of action that led to the Standard Rules on the Equalization of Opportunities for Persons with Disabilities. The 2007 declaration also includes the optional protocol permitting the treaty-monitoring body of the Committee for the Rights of Persons with Disabilities (CRPD) to receive and consider complaints. Lauren, *Human Rights*, 268.

20. Lauren, *Human Rights*, 241.
21. Lauren, *Human Rights*, 274, 249.
22. Movimento de Reintegração das Pessoas Atingidas pela Hanseníase.
23. https://www.leprosy-information.org/organization/idea-international-association-integration-dignity-and-economic-advancement Accessed 11 August 2020.
24. http://www.idealeprosydignity.org/act/act1.htm Accessed 11 August 2020.
25. http://www.idealeprosydignity.org/Mission/IDEA%20Mission%20Statement%20-%20Leprosy%20and%20Human%20Rights.html Accessed 11 August 2020.
26. http://www.idealeprosydignity.org/Exhibit/IDEA%20Quest%20for%20Dignity%20Exhibit.html Accessed 11 August 2020.
27. IDEA has branches in Angola, Brazil, China, D. R. Congo, Ethiopia, Ghana, India, Japan, Kenya, Mozambique, Nepal, Nigeria, Norway, Paraguay, Philippines, South Korea, Sudan, Taiwan, and the United States.
28. https://www.ideaadvocates.org/international-network.html Accessed 11 August 2020.
29. "Statement by Prime Minister Junichiro Koizumi Concerning the Swift and Comprehensive Solution of the Hansen's Disease Issue," 25 May 2001. http://www.kantei.go.jp/foreign/koizumispeech/2001/0525danwa_e.html Accessed 15 February 2012.
30. The Verification Committee Concerning Hansen's Disease Problem held its first meeting on 16 October 2002. The committee consisted of thirteen members: two former Hansen's disease patients, four members of the media, two lawyers, one sanatorium director, and four experienced scholars. https://www.mhlw.go.jp/english/policy/health/01/pdf/01.pdf, 7. Accessed 11 August 2020.
31. https://www.mhlw.go.jp/english/policy/health/01/pdf/01.pdf, 7.
32. https://www.mhlw.go.jp/english/policy/health/01/pdf/01.pdf, 56.
33. https://www.mhlw.go.jp/english/policy/health/01/pdf/01.pdf, 57.
34. https://www.mhlw.go.jp/english/policy/health/01/pdf/01.pdf, 58.
35. https://www.mhlw.go.jp/english/policy/health/01/pdf/01.pdf.
36. https://www.mhlw.go.jp/english/policy/health/01/pdf/01.pdf.
37. https://www.mhlw.go.jp/english/policy/health/01/pdf/01.pdf, 61.
38. https://www.mhlw.go.jp/english/policy/health/01/pdf/01.pdf, 59.
39. https://www.mhlw.go.jp/english/policy/health/01/pdf/01.pdf, 61.
40. https://www.mhlw.go.jp/english/policy/health/01/pdf/01.pdf, 64.
41. https://www.mhlw.go.jp/english/policy/health/01/pdf/01.pdf.

42. https://www.mhlw.go.jp/english/policy/health/01/pdf/01.pdf, 64–5.
43. https://www.mhlw.go.jp/english/policy/health/01/pdf/01.pdf, 66.
44. https://www.mhlw.go.jp/english/policy/health/01/pdf/01.pdf.
45. https://www.mhlw.go.jp/english/policy/health/01/pdf/01.pdf, 68.
46. Yohei Sasakawa, "Leprosy and Human Rights – My Approaches." Posted 10 December 2008. http://www.ilep.org.uk/news-events/articles/view/leprosy-and-human-rights-my-approach. This link is no longer active, but I have a hard copy in my possession.
47. Press release, "UNHCHR Acting Chair Meets With Yohei Sasakawa," 3 July 2003. http://www.nippon-foundation.or.jp/eng/leprosy/2003609/20036091.html Accessed 10 February 2009.
48. "Author interview," Yohei Sasakawa, Tokyo, 25 August 2009.
49. Dr Gopal, the President from IDEA India, spoke of his experiences as a leprosy-affected person.
50. Yohei Sasakawa, "Speech at the 55th Session of UN Human Rights Commission Sub-Commission on the Promotion and Protection of Human Rights," 3 July 2003. http://www.nippon-foundation.or.jp/eng/leprosy/2003611/200336111.html Accessed 10 February 2009.
51. Commission on Human Rights, "Prevention of Discrimination."
52. Commission on Human Rights, "Prevention of Discrimination," 5.
53. Commission on Human Rights, "Prevention of Discrimination."
54. "UN Human Rights Sub-Commission Passes Leprosy Resolution (11/08/2005)," 11 August 2005. http://www.nippon-foundation.or.jp/eng/leprosy/2005721/20057211.html Accessed 10 February 2009. This link is no longer active, but I have a hard copy in my possession.
55. He submitted a preliminary report to the Sub-Commission at its fifty-eighth session, a progress report at its fifty-ninth session and a final report at its sixtieth session. Yozo Yokota, "Report of the Sub-Commission on the Promotion and Protection of Human Rights," 17 October 2005, 48.
56. https://www.nippon-foundation.or.jp/en/what/projects/leprosy/appeal Accessed 11 August 2020.
57. In 2008, he appealed to international human rights organisations, and over the next three years to the world's religious leaders, the world's business leaders, and the world's leading universities. Next he appealed to professional organisations such as the members of the World Medical Association in 2012 and members of the International Bar Association in 2013, and so on. https://www.nippon-foundation.or.jp/en/what/projects/leprosy/appeal.
58. Submissions came from Armenia, Azerbaijan, Canada, Costa Rica, Cuba, Cyprus, Egypt, Ecuador, Estonia, Finland, France, Greece, Israel, Japan, Kazakhstan, Oman, the Philippines, Portugal, Qatar, Romania, Spain, Turkey, and the Ukraine. Human Rights Council, "Elimination of Discrimination Against Persons Affected by Leprosy and Their Family Members," February 2009.
59. "Elimination of Discrimination Against Persons Affected by Leprosy," 12.

60. Commission on Human Rights, "Prevention of Discrimination."
61. Commission on Human Rights, "Prevention of Discrimination."
62. Commission on Human Rights, "Prevention of Discrimination," 13.
63. Commission on Human Rights, "Prevention of Discrimination."
64. Commission on Human Rights, "Prevention of Discrimination."
65. Commission on Human Rights, "Prevention of Discrimination."
66. Commission on Human Rights, "Prevention of Discrimination."
67. Commission on Human Rights, "Prevention of Discrimination," 14.
68. Other non-government organisations that made submissions were Ethiopian National Association of Persons Affected by Leprosy (ENAPAL); Guangdong Handa Rehabilitation and Welfare Association; Hind Kusht Nivaran Sangh India; International Disability Alliance (IDA); Convention on the Rights of Persons With Disabilities Forum (CRPD Forum); International Federation of Anti-Leprosy Associations (ILEP); Leprosy Relief; Movement for Reintegration of People Affected by Leprosy (MORHAN); PerMaTa Organisation of People Affected by Leprosy in Indonesia; Royal Tropical Institute Netherlands; Sasakawa India Leprosy Foundation; The International Association for Integration, Dignity and Economic Advancement (IDEA); The Leprosy Mission; and The Nippon Foundation, 19. Along with other non-government organisations, ILEP also made submissions generally referring to the "legal framework offered by the Convention on the Rights of Persons with Disabilities and its Limitations" and a summary record of the newsletters of the WHO Goodwill Ambassador for the Elimination of Leprosy, and responses from individual members of ILEP to a survey. Human Rights Council, Tenth Session, Agenda Item 2, 15.
69. Relevant actors included governments, observers of the United Nations, relevant United Nations bodies, specialised agencies and programmes, non-governmental organisations, scientists and medical experts, as well as representatives of persons affected by leprosy and their family members. Human Rights Council, Fifteenth session, Agenda item 5.
70. https://www.un.org/disabilities/documents/gadocs/a_res_65_215.pdf Accessed 11 August 2020.
71. "Author interview," Yohei Sasakawa, Tokyo, 25 August 2009.
72. "Author interview."
73. Notably, ENAPAL (Ethiopian National Association of Persons Affected by Leprosy); IDEA Ghana; IDEA Kenya; IDEA Mozambique; IDEA Niger; IDEA Nigeria; TLA (Tanzania Leprosy Association); Bogra Federation, Bangladesh; DAPA (Disadvantaged People's Association) supported by The Leprosy Mission Bangladesh; HANDA Rehabilitation and Welfare Association, China; PerMaTa Indonesia; Enterprise Self-Care Group (KUK), Indonesia; MAPAL (Myanmar Association of Persons Affected by Leprosy); IDEA Nepal; CLAP (Coalition of Leprosy Advocates of the Philippines); MORHAN (Movement for the Reintegration of Persons Affected by Hansen's Disease); Felehansen, Colombia; and Sam Utthan, "Equal Development for All," Initially Bihar Kusht Kalyan Mahasangh, India.

74. The International Federation of Anti-Leprosy Associations (ILEP) and Sasakawa Memorial Health Foundation (SMHF), *Good Practices*, 16.

75. *Good Practices*, 16–17.

76. *Good Practices*, 18.

77. *Good Practices*, 17.

78. *Good Practices*, 19.

79. *Good Practices*.

80. *Good Practices*, 21.

81. *Good Practices*, 60.

82. *Good Practices*, 64.

83. *Good Practices*, 61.

84. Human Rights Council. Thirty-Eighth Session, 18 June–6 July 2018. Agenda Item 3, 16.

85. Human Rights Council Forty-Fourth Session, 15 June–3 July 2020.

CONCLUSION

1.   Packard, "Malaria Dreams," 282; Litsios, Malaria Control"; Peter J. Brown, "Malaria, Miseria"; Packard and Brown, "Rethinking Health"; Packard, *The Making of a Tropical Disease*; Birn, "The Stages of International (Global) Health."

2.   Szlezák, *Globalizing Public Policy*, 13.

3.   Packard and Brown, "Rethinking Health," 184.

4.   Packard, "Malaria Dreams," 282.

5.   From personal observation when visiting TLM India in Tamil Nadu, 2005.

6.   Birn, "The Stages of International (Global) Health," 58.

7.   Rosenberg et al., *Real Collaboration*, 22.

8.   Muraskin, *Polio Eradication and Its Discontents*.

9.   Muraskin, *Polio Eradication and Its Discontents*, 187.

10. Diana Lockwood to Salvatore Noto discussion list, "Leprosy Elimination in Brazil," 20 January 2012.

11. Cairns Smith to Salvatore Noto discussion list, "Why Brazil is doing this?" 10 December 2011.

12. Alex de Waal, "New Pathogens, Old Politics," *Boston Review*, 3 April 2020. http://bostonreview.net/science-nature/alex-de-waal-new-pathogen-old-po litics?fbclid=IwAR39lrqrfM3IG2K_82NCoGIgXAzB7zYB7HCYyzk2wmX9I poEHzdL0Rsmcbk#.XpJ9jWesN3U.facebook Accessed 11 August 2020.

13. At the time of writing, from the Johns Hopkins database, there are over 216 million infected and over 4.5 million dead. https://coronavirus.jhu.edu/map.html. Accessed 30 August 2021.

14. South Korea has managed to avoid a lockdown because of their efficient use of a tracing app, but are now facing a new wave with highly contagious variants.

15. Pankaj Mishra, "Flailing States."

16. Carrington, "Pandemics Result From Destruction of Nature."

BIBLIOGRAPHY

Archival Sources

Australia
    Queensland Institute of Medical Research, Brisbane.
        Douglas Russell Collection.
Belgium
    Damien Foundation, Brussels.
France
    Follereau Foundation, Paris.
    Follereau Foundation Archives, St Étienne, France.
Geneva, Switzerland
    WHO Archives, Geneva.
        Official Records of the World Health Organization 1948–2005.
        Communicable Diseases: Leprosy Series, L4.
    League of Nations Archives, Geneva.
        Bulletin de L'Organisation D'Hygiène, Bibliographie des Travaux Techniques de L'Organisation d'Hygiene de la Societé des Nations, 1920–1945. Vol. 11 (1945), Lèpre.
India
    South East Asia Regional Office Archives, New Delhi.
        Regional Committee SEA/RC35.
Philippines
    Western Pacific Regional Office Archives, Manila.
    Leonard Wood Memorial Archives, Cebu.
    Culion Archives, Culion Island, Palawan Group.
United Kingdom
    The International Federation of Anti-Leprosy Associations, London (now Geneva).
    The British Leprosy Relief Association, Colchester.
    The Leprosy Mission International Archives, Brentford, London.
    Wellcome Library, London.
        Stanley Browne Collection.

BIBLIOGRAPHY

Published Sources

Adams, Francis. *The Seven Books of Paulus Ægineta*, translated from the Greek with a Commentary, "Embracing a Complete View of the Knowledge Possessed by the Greeks, Romans, and Arabians on Subjects Connected with Medicine and Surgery," in three volumes. London: Sydenham Society, 1844.

Anderson, Warwick. "Leprosy and Citizenship." *Positions* 6, no. 3 (1998): 707–30.

Anderson, Warwick. *Colonial Pathologies: American Tropical Medicine, Race, and Hygiene in the Philippines*. Durham and London: Duke University Press, 2006.

Antia, N. H. "Leprosy and Primary Health Care: the Mandwa Project, India." *Leprosy Review* 53 (1982): 205–9.

Arnold, David. *Gandhi: Profiles in Power*. Essex, UK: Longman, 2001.

Askew, A. D. "The Leprosy Mission – A Crucial Dimension of Service." *Leprosy Review* 44, no. 4 (1973): 168–71.

Askew, Eddie. *Edge of Daylight: Memoirs of a Life With the Leprosy Mission*. Brentford, UK: Leprosy Mission, 2000.

Bechelli, L. M. "Advances in Leprosy Control in the Last 100 Years." *International Journal of Leprosy* 41, no. 3 (1973): 285–97.

Bechelli, L. M. and V. Martínez Domínguez. "The Leprosy Problem in the World." *Bulletin WHO* 34 (1966): 811–26.

Berthelsen, June. Ed. Anne Ross. *The Lost Years: A Story of Leprosy*. Chipping Norton, Australia: Surrey Beatty & Sons, 1996.

Bijleveld, I. "In Reality: A Medical Anthropologist's Reservations About the Viability of Leprosy Control With Primary Health Care." *LR* 53 (1982): 181–92.

Birn, Anne-Emanuelle. "The Stages of International (Global) Health: Histories of Success or Successes of History?" *Global Public Health: An International Journal for Research, Policy and Practice* 4, no. 1 (2009): 50–68.

Black, Maggie. *The Children and the Nations: The Story of UNICEF*. Sydney, Australia: UNICEF, 1986.

Black, Maggie. *Children First: The Story of UNICEF, Past and Present*. Oxford: Oxford University Press, 1996.

Brand, Jeanne L. "The United States Public Health Service and International Health 1945–1950." *Bulletin of the History of Medicine* 63, no. 4 (1989): 579–98.

Brown, Peter J. "Malaria, Miseria, and Underpopulation in Sardinia: The 'Malaria Blocks Development' Cultural Model." *Medical Anthropology: Cross-Cultural Studies in Health and Illness* 17, no. 3 (1997): 239–54.

Brown, Theodore M., Marcos Cueto, and Elizabeth Fee. "The World Health Organization and the Transition from 'International' to 'Global Public Health.'" *American Journal of Public Health* 96, no. 1 (2006): 62–72.

Browne, S. G. "Ernest Muir: Obituary." *Leprosy Review* 46, no. 1 (1975): 1–3.

Buckingham, Jane. *Leprosy in Colonial South India: Medicine and Confinement*. Basingstoke, UK: Palgrave, 2002.

Buttle, G. A. H. "Viewpoint: A Full Circle." *TIPS* (December 1980): 443.

Camus, Albert. *The Plague.* Trans. Stuart Gilbert. New York: Vintage Books, 1991.

Carrington, Damien. "Pandemics Result From Destruction of Nature Say WHO and UN." *The Guardian*, 17 June 2020. https://www.theguardian.com/world/2020/jun/17/pandemics-destruction-nature-un-who-legislation-trade-green-recovery?CMP=share_btn_fb&fbclid=IwAR1I8ky VHkRzKh1sGFsvlTU6i2QzRhGwqS4BdcE8jRv DSXKwDsrYD_g9Bxo

Cochrane, R. G. *The Epidemiology, Pathology and Diagnosis of Child Leprosy (being the Dr Elizabeth Mathai Endowment Lectures, 1942–43, Delivered at the Medical College, University of Madras).* Madras, 1943.

Cochrane, R. G. "Correspondence to the Editor: 'The Use of Diaminodiphenyl Sulfone.'" *International Journal of Leprosy* 18, no. 1 (1950): 91–8.

Cochrane, R. G. Ed. *Leprosy in Theory and Practice.* Bristol, UK: John Wright & Sons, 1959.

Cochrane, Robert. "Correspondence: To the Editor: 'First Use of DDS by Injection; Recommendations.'" *International Journal of Leprosy* 24, no. 2 (1956): 195.

Cochrane, Robert. *Leprosy in Relation to Public Health: Being a Course of Lectures Delivered at the Course of Training for Health Officers Held at the Lady Willingdon Leprosy Sanatorium, Chingleput.* Madras, India: Superintendent Government Press, 1941.

Cochrane, Robert. "Opportunity in India." *Lancet* 250 (23 August 1947): 286.

Cochrane, Robert. "The Campaign Against Leprosy." *British Medical Journal* (18 April 1931): 681.

Commission on Human Rights. "Prevention of Discrimination: Preliminary Working Paper on Discrimination Against Leprosy Victims and Their Families, Submitted by Yozo Yokota." Commission on Human Rights, Sub-Commission on the Promotion and Protection of Human Rights, Fifty-Seventh Session, Item 5 of the Provisional Agenda. E/CN.4/Sub2/2005/WP.1, 14 July 2005.

"Coordination of Medical Congresses." *IJL* 17, nos. 1&2 (1949): 130–1.

Cueto, Marcos. "The Origins of Primary Health Care and Selective Primary Health Care." *American Journal of Public Health* 94, no. 11 (2004): 1864–74.

Danielssen, D. C. and C. M. Boëck. *Traite de la Spedalskhed ou Elephantiasis de Grecs.* Bergen, Norway: D. Bayer, 1847.

Denny, Oswald E., Ralph Hopkins, and Frederick A. Johansen. "Recoveries From Leprosy: An Analysis of the Records of 65 Cases." *Public Health Reports* 45, no. 13 (1930): 667–88.

de Waal, Alex. "New Pathogens, Old Politics." *Boston Review* 3 (April 2020). http://bostonreview.net/science-nature/alex-de-waal-new-pathogen-old-politics?fbcl id=IwAR39lrqrfM3IG2K_82NCoGIgXAzB7zYB7HCYyzk2wmX9IpoEHzdL0 Rsmcbk#.XpJ9jWesN3U.facebook

Di Giacomo, Susan M. "Metaphor as Illness: Postmodern Dilemmas in the Representation of Body, Mind and Disorder." *Medical Anthropology* 14 (1992): 109–37.

BIBLIOGRAPHY

Diwan, M. B. "The Three All India Leprosy Workers Conferences." *Leprosy in India* (1951): 127–31.

Douglas, Mary. "Witchcraft and Leprosy: Two Strategies of Exclusion." *Man* 26, no. 4 (1991): 723–36.

Doull, James A. "Sulfone Therapy of Leprosy: Background, Early History and Present Status." *International Journal of Leprosy* 31, no. 2 (1963): 143–60.

Doull, James A. "World Health Organization: First Meeting of the Assembly." *International Journal of Leprosy* 16, no. 4 (1948): 468–72.

Dowdle, Walter R. "The Principles of Disease Elimination and Eradication," in "Global Disease Elimination and Eradication as Public Health Strategies: Proceedings of a Conference Held in Atlanta, Georgia, USA: 23–25 February 1998." Ed. R. A. Goodman, K. L. Foster, F. L. Trowbridge, and J. P. Figueroa. *Bulletin WHO* 76, no. 2, Supplement (1998).

Draper, Philip. "Editorial: The Mouse Footpad Model." *Leprosy Review* 77 (2006): 3–4.

Dyer, Isadore. "The Berlin Leprosy Conference." *New Orleans Medical and Surgical Journal* 50, no. 6 (1897): 357–68.

Editorial. "Constructive Programme and Leprosy." *Leprosy in India* (1946): 41–2.

"Editorial: Information and Comments on Development of International Leprosy Activities (November 1958–May 1960)." *Acta Leprologica* 1 (1960): 7–38.

"Editorials: Establishment of a Consultative Group of Leprosy Experts by the WHO." *International Journal of Leprosy* 19, no. 1 (1951): 75–8.

Edmond, Rod. *Leprosy and Empire: A Medical and Cultural History*. Cambridge, UK: Cambridge University Press, 2006.

Erikson, Erik H. "On the Nature of Psycho-Historical Evidence: In Search of Gandhi." *Daedalus* 97, no. 3 (1968): 695–730.

"Experimental Leprosy." *British Medical Journal* (20 April 1963): 1040–1.

Faget, G. H. "The Story of the National Leprosarium (U.S. Marine Hospital), Carville, Louisiana." *Public Health Report* 57, no. 18 (1942): 641–52.

Faget, G. H. "The Story of the National Leprosarium: The United States Marine Hospital, Carville, Louisiana." *Public Health Reports* 61, no. 52 (1946): 1871–83.

Faget, G. H., F. A. Johansen, and Sister Hilary Ross. "Sulfanilamide in the Treatment of Leprosy." *Public Health Reports* 57, no. 50 (1942): 1892–9.

Faget, G. H. and R. C. Pogge. "Penicillin Treatment of Leprosy: Clinical Note." *Public Health Reports* 60, no. 12 (1945): 324–5.

Faget, G. H. and R. C. Pogge. "The Therapeutic Effect of Promin in Leprosy." *Public Health Reports* 60, no. 40 (1945): 1165–71.

Faget, G. H., R. C. Pogge, F. A. Johansen. "Promizole Treatment of Leprosy." *Public Health Reports* 61, no. 26 (1946): 957–60.

Faget, G. H., R. C. Pogge, F. A. Johansen, J. F. Dinan, B. M. Prejean, and C. G. Eccles. "The Promin Treatment of Leprosy: A Progress Report." *Public Health Reports* 58, no. 48 (1943): 1729–1941. Reprinted in *International Journal of Leprosy* 34, no. 3 (1966): 298–310.

Fenner, F. "The Pathogenic Behaviour of *Mycobacterium ulcerans* and *Mycobacterium balnei* in the Mouse and Developing Chick Embryo." *American Review of Tuberculosis* 73 (1956): 650–73.

Fine, Paul E. M. "Editorial: Reflections on the Elimination of Leprosy." *International Journal of Leprosy* 60, no. 1 (1992): 71–80.

Gandhi, M. K. *An Autobiography: The Story of My Experiments With Truth.* Boston, MA: Beacon Press, 1993.

Gandhi, M. K. *Constructive Programme: Its Meaning and Place. Mani Bhavan Gandhi Sangrahalaya: Mahatma Gandhi Information Website.* http://www.gandhi-manibhavan.org/gandhiphilosophy/philosophy_consprogrammes_bookwritten.htm#LEPERS

Gibney, Frank. "Preface," in Sato Seizaburo, *Sasakawa Ryoichi: A Life.* Trans. Hara Fujiko. Norwalk, CT: EastBridge, 2006.

Ghosh, Rupak and Prof. Ujjwal K. Chowdhury, eds. *Dignity Regained.* Maharashtra, India: Icons Media Publication, 2005.

Greenwood, David. *Antimicrobial Drugs: Chronicle of a Twentieth Century Medical Triumph.* Oxford and New York: Oxford University Press, 2008.

Gussow, Zachary. *Leprosy, Racism and Public Health: Social Policy in Chronic Disease Control.* Boulder, San Francisco, and London: Westview Press, 1989.

Hansen, Gerhard Henrik Armauer and Carl Looft. *Leprosy: In Its Clinical and Pathological Aspects,* translated by Norman Walker. Bristol, UK: John Wright, 1895.

Harris, G. F. "LEPRA's Campaign to the World Wide Campaign Against Leprosy." *Leprosy Review* 44, no. 4 (1973): 165–6.

Hastings, Robert C. Ed. *Leprosy.* New York: Longman, 1985.

Hebra, Ferdinand and Moriz Kaposi. *On the Diseases of the Skin Including the Exanthemata.* Translated and edited by Waren Tay. London: The New Sydenham Society, 1875.

Human Rights Council, Tenth Session, Agenda Item 2. "Annual Report of the United Nations High Commissioner for Human Rights and Reports of the Office of the High Commissioner and the Secretary–General: Elimination of Discrimination Against Persons Affected by Leprosy and Their Family Members. Report of the Office of the United Nations High Commissioner for Human Rights." A/HRC/10/62. 23 February 2009.

Human Rights Council, Fifteenth Session, Agenda Item 5. Human Rights Bodies and Mechanisms. "Draft Set of Principles and Guidelines for the Elimination of Discrimination Against Persons Affected by Leprosy and Their Family Members, Submitted by the Human Rights Council Advisory Committee." A/HRC/15/30.

Human Rights Council. Forty-Fourth Session, 15 June–3 July 2020. Agenda Item 3, Promotion and Protection of All Human Rights, Civil, Political, Economic,

Social and Cultural Rights, Including the Right to Development. "Policy Framework for Rights-Based Action Plans: Report of the Special Rapporteur on the Elimination of Discrimination Against Persons Affected by Leprosy and Their Family Members." 27 April 2020.

Human Rights Council. Thirty-Eighth Session, 18 June–6 July 2018. Agenda Item 3. "Report of the Special Rapporteur on the Elimination of Discrimination Against Persons Affected by Leprosy and their Family Members," 25 May 2018.

IDEA Centre for the Voices of Humanity. *Freeing Ourselves of Prejudice: In Commemoration of the Second International Day of Dignity and Respect, March 11, 2000.* Seneca Falls, NY: IDEA, 2000.

"ILA Relationship With WHO." *International Journal of Leprosy* 21, no. 4 (1953): 549.

India Council of the British Empire Leprosy Relief Association. "All-India Leprosy Conference, Wardha." *Leprosy in India*, 20, no. 1 (Jan 1948): 1–45.

International Federation of Anti-Leprosy Associations (ILEP). "From Leprosaria to Vaccine Trials: 20 Years of Cooperation in the Service of Leprosy Patients: 1966–1986." London: ILEP, 1986.

International Federation of Anti-Leprosy Associations (ILEP) and Sasakawa Memorial Health Foundation (SMHF). *Good Practices in Strengthening Participation of Persons Affected by Leprosy in Leprosy Services.* Geneva/Tokyo, 2018.

"International Work in Leprosy, 1948–1959." *Chronicle* 14 (1960): 3–39.

Jacobson, R. R. and J. R. Trautman. "The Treatment of Leprosy With the Sulfones: 1. Faget's Original 22 Patients. A Thirty Year Follow-up on Sulfone Therapy for Leprosy." *International Journal of Leprosy* 39, no. 3 (1971): 726–37.

Jagadisan, T. N. "Ernest Muir: Obituary." *Leprosy Review* 46, no. 1 (1975): 3.

Jagadisan, T. N. *Fulfilment Through Leprosy.* India: Kasturba Kushta Nivaran Nilayam, 1988.

Janssens, P. G. and S. R. Pattyn. "Current Literature: Experiences With Mouse Inoculation of Leprosy Bacilli Originating From the Congo." *International Journal of Leprosy* 31 (1963): 522.

Joshua-Raghavar, A. *Leprosy in Malaysia: Past, Present and Future.* Ed. Dr K. Rajagopalan. Sungai Buluh, Selangor, West Malaysia: A Joshua-Raghavar, 1983.

Kakar, Sanjiv. "Medical Developments and Patient Unrest in the Leprosy Asylum, 1860 to 1940." *Social Scientist* 4–6, no. 24 (1996): 62–81.

Lauren, P. G. *The Evolution of International Human Rights: Visions Seen.* 3rd ed. Philadelphia, PA: University of Pennsylvania Press, 2011.

League of Nations, Health Organisation, Leprosy Commission, "Report on the Programme of Work of the Leprosy Commission" CH 887 (a) Geneva, 20 August 1930. League of Nations, Health Organisation. *Report of the Study Tour of the Secretary of the Leprosy Commission in Europe, South America and the Far East, January 1929–June 1930.* Official Number: CH 887. League of Nations, Geneva, 1930.

Lechat, Michel F. "Editorial." *Leprosy Review* 40 (1969): 191–3.

Leonard Wood Memorial (American Leprosy Foundation) Scientific Research Program. *Transactions of the Leonard Wood Memorial – Johns Hopkins University: Symposium on Research in Leprosy, Baltimore, Maryland, 8–10 May 1961*.

"Leprosy Activities of WHO, 1960–1961: Leprosy Control Activities." *International Journal of Leprosy* 29, no. 2 (1961): 231–3.

"Leprosy News and Notes: Fifth International Leprosy Congress." *International Journal of Leprosy* 16, no. 2 (1948): 187–244.

"Leprosy News and Notes: Sixth International Congress of Leprosy." *International Journal of Leprosy* 21, no. 4 (1953): 484–557.

"Leprosy Relief on Humane Understanding Lines." *Madras Information Fortnightly* 3, no. 14 (1949): 62–4.

"Leprosy at the Third World Health Assembly." *International Journal of Leprosy* 18, no. 3 (1950): 413–4.

Leung, Angela Ki Che. *Leprosy in China: a History*. New York: Columbia University Press, 2009.

Litsios, Socrates. "Malaria Control, the Cold War, and the Postwar Reorganization of International Assistance." *Medical Anthropology: Cross-Cultural Studies in Health and Illness* 17, no. 3 (1997): 255–78.

Loh Kah Seng. *Making and Unmaking the Asylum: Leprosy and Modernity in Singapore and Malaysia*. Petaling Jaya, Malaysia: SIRD, 2009.

Long, Esmond R. "Forty Years of Leprosy Research: History of the Leonard Wood Memorial (American Leprosy Foundation) 1928 to 1967." *International Journal of Leprosy* (1967): 241–2.

Lowe, John. "Treatment of Diamino-Diphenyl Sulphone by Mouth." *Lancet* (28 January 1950): 145–50.

Mach, Andrea. "Brundtland Replaces Top Staff at the WHO." *British Medical Journal* 317 (1998): 229.

Mark, Samuel. "Alexander the Great, Seafaring, and the Spread of Leprosy." *Journal of the History of Medicine and Allied Sciences* 57, no. 3 (2002): 285–311.

Martin, Betty. *Miracle at Carville*. New York: Doubleday, 1950.

McDougall, A. C. "Editorial: Leprosy and Primary Health Care." *Leprosy Review* 53, no. 3 (1982): 161–226.

McMillen, Christian W. *Discovering Tuberculosis: A Global History, 1900 to the Present*. New Haven, CT: Yale University Press, 2015.

Mishra, Pankaj. "Flailing States," *London Review of Books*, 16 July 2020. https://www.lrb.co.uk/the-paper/v42/n14/pankaj-mishra/flailing-states

Mouat, F. J. "Notes on Native Remedies. No. 1, Then Chaulmoogra." *Indian Annals of Medical Science* 1 (1854): 646–52.

Muir, Ernest. *Manual of Leprosy*. Edinburgh, UK: Livingstone, 1948.

Muraskin, William. *Polio Eradication and Its Discontents: A Historian's Journey Through an International Public Health (Un) Civil War*. New Perspectives in South Asian History. New Delhi, India: Orient BlackSwan, 2012.

Narayanaswamy, S. "Constructive Programme Towards Twenty First Century." *Mahatma Gandhi's One Spot Information Website.*
http://www.mkgandhi-sarvodaya.org/articles/constr.%20prog.htm

National Leprosy Control Program, Department of Health, Philippines. "Final Report: The Pilot Study for MDT Implementation in Ilocos Norte and Cebu: 1984–1988." Edited for International Release, January 1990.

"News and Notes." *International Journal of Leprosy* 43, no. 2 (1975): 159.

"News and Notes: CIBA Symposium on Pathogenesis, London, Convened by J. A. Doull." *International Journal of Leprosy* 31, no. 2 (1963): 248–9.

"News and Notes: Government-Aided Leprosy Research Projects." *International Journal of Leprosy* 28, no. 4 (1960): 471.

"News and Notes: The International Leprosy Association and the United Nations." *International Journal of Leprosy* 16.4 (1948): 480.

"News and Notes: Leprosy at the Second World Health Assembly." *International Journal of Leprosy* 17, no. 3 (1949): 321–6.

"News and Notes: Leprosy at the Third World Assembly." *International Journal of Leprosy* 18, no. 3 (1950): 411.

"News and Notes: Research Activities." *International Journal of Leprosy* 29, no. 2 (1961): 232–6.

"News and Notes: Second WHO Expert Committee on Leprosy." *International Journal of Leprosy* 27, no. 4 (1959): 389.

"News and Notes: Seventh International Congress of Leprology, Held in Tokyo, Japan, November 12 to 19, 1958." *International Journal of Leprosy* 26, no. 4 (1958): 360–409.

"News and Notes: Sixth International Congress of Leprosy Sponsored by the Government of Spain With the Collaboration of the International Leprosy Association." *International Journal of Leprosy* 21, no. 4 (1953): 484–557.

"News and Notes: WHO and Leprosy." *International Journal of Leprosy* 19, no. 2 (1951): 229–30.

Noordeen, S. K. "Leprosy Control Through Multidrug Therapy (MDT)." *Bulletin WHO* 69, no. 3 (1991): 263–9.

Noordeen, S. K., L. Lopez Bravo, and T. K. Sundaresan. "Estimated Number of Leprosy Cases in the World." *Bulletin WHO* 70 (1992): 7–10.

Obregón, Diana. "The State Physicians and Leprosy in Modern Colombia," in *Disease in the History of Modern Latin America: From Malaria to AIDS.* Ed. Diego Armus. Durham, NC: Duke University Press, 2003. 130–57.

"Obituary: James Angus Doull." *Leprosy Review* 34, no. 3 (1963): 115.

"Organisation of WHO and Its Budget." *International Journal of Leprosy* 18, no. 3 (1950): 418.

Packard, Randall M. "Malaria Dreams: Postwar Visions of Health and Development in the Third World." *Medical Anthropology: Cross-Cultural Studies in Health and Illness* 17, no. 3 (1997): 279–96.

Packard, Randall M. *The Making of a Tropical Disease: A Short History of Malaria.* Baltimore, MD: Johns Hopkins University Press, 2007.

Packard, Randall M. and Peter J. Brown. "Rethinking Health, Development, and Malaria: Historicizing a Cultural Model in International Health." *Medical Anthropology: Cross-Cultural Studies in Health and Illness* 17, no. 3 (1997): 181–94.

Parascandola, John. "Chaulmoogra Oil and the Treatment of Leprosy." *Pharmacy in History* 45 (2003): 47–57.

"Proceedings of a Conference on Research Problems in Leprosy: Sponsored by the Leonard Wood Memorial (American Leprosy Foundation) and the Armed Forces Institute of Pathology, Washington DC, May 11–14, 1965." *International Journal of Leprosy* 33, no. 3 (1965): 395–783.

Rees, R. J. "New Prospects for the Study of Leprosy in the Laboratory." *Leprosy Review* 41 (1970): 136–54.

Rees, Dr R. J. W. "'Recent Applications of Experimental Human Leprosy in the Mouse Foot-Pad': Seventh Scientific Session: Experimental Studies in Leprosy: Report of the Conference of the Indian Association of Leprologists." *Leprosy in India* 37, no. 3 (1965): 163–74.

Rees, R. J. W. and M. F. R. Waters, "Applicability of Experimental Murine Leprosy to the Study of Human Leprosy," in *Ciba Foundation Study Group No. 15: Pathogenesis of Leprosy (In honour of Professor V. R. Khanolkar).* Ed. G. E. Wolstenholme and Maeve O'Connor. London: J & A Churchill, 1963.

Rees, R. J. W. and R. C. Valentine, "The Appearance of Dead Leprosy Bacilli by Light Electron Microscopy." *International Journal of Leprosy* 30, no. 1 (1962): 1–9.

"Reports of Speciality Panels: Committee 5: Advances in Epidemiology." *International Journal of Leprosy* 41, no. 4 (1973): 461–2.

"Reprinted Article: Immunological Problems in Leprosy Research: 1 and 2." *Leprosy Review* 45 (1974): 244–72 and 257–72.

Robertson, Jo. "The Leprosy Asylum in India: 1886–1947." *Journal of the History of Medicine and Allied Sciences* 64, no. 4 (2009): 474–517.

Robertson, Jo. "The Leprosy-Affected Body as a Commodity: Autonomy and Compensation," in *The Body Divided: Human Beings and Human "Material" in Modern Medical History.* Ed. Sarah Ferber and Sally Wilde, 131–64. Farnham, UK: Ashgate Publishing, 2011.

Robertson, Jo and A. C. McDougall. "Leprosy Work and Research in Oxford, the United Kingdom: Four Decades in the Pursuit of New Knowledge about an Arcane Disease." *International Journal of Dermatology* 44, no. 8 (2005): 695–8.

Rogers, Sir Leonard and Ernest Muir. *Leprosy.* Bristol, UK: John Wright & Sons, 1946.

Ross, W. F. "Leprosy and Primary Health Care." *Leprosy Review* 53 (1982): 201–4.

Ryan, Terence J. and A. Colin McDougall, eds. *Essays on Leprosy.* Department of Dermatology, the Slade Hospital, 1988.

BIBLIOGRAPHY

Sasakawa Memorial Health Foundation. "The 1st Seminar on Leprosy Control Cooperation in Asia: Proceedings" (28 Nov–3 Dec 1974) Tokyo-Oiso-Okayama, Japan. Tokyo: SMHF, 1975.

Sasakawa Memorial Health Foundation. "The Second Seminar on Leprosy Control Cooperation in Asia: Proceedings," 20–22 August 1975, Tokyo, Japan. Tokyo: Sasakawa Memorial Health Foundation, 1975.

Sasakawa Memorial Health Foundation. "The First International Workshop on Training of Leprosy Workers in Asia," Bangkok and Pattaya, Thailand, 25–8 November 1976.

Sasakawa Memorial Health Foundation. "The 1st International Workshop on Chemotherapy in Asia," Manila, Philippines, 26–8 January 1977. Jointly Sponsored by Department of Health, Republic of the Philippines, and Sasakawa Memorial Health Foundation, Japan. Tokyo, Sasakawa Memorial Health Foundation, 1977.

Sasakawa, Ryoichi. *Sugamo Diary*. Trans. Ken Hijino. London: Hurst, 2010.

Scheper-Hughes, Nancy and Margaret M. Lock. "Speaking 'Truth' to Illness: Metaphors, Reification, and a Pedagogy for Patients." *Medical Anthropology Quarterly* 17, no. 5 (1986): 137–40.

Seizaburo, Sato. *Sasakawa Ryoichi: A Life*. Trans. Hara Fujiko. Norwalk, CT: EastBridge, 2006.

Shepard, Charles C. "Acid-Fast Bacilli in Nasal Excretions in Leprosy and Results of Inoculation of Mice." *American Journal of Hygiene* 71 (1960): 147–57.

Shepard, Charles C. "The Experimental Disease That Follows the Injection of Human Leprosy Bacilli Into Foot-Pads of Mice." *Journal of Experimental Medicine* 112 (1960): 445–54.

Shepard, Charles C. "Multiplication of *Mycobacterium Leprae* in the Footpad of the Mouse." *International Journal of Leprosy* 30, no. 3 (1962): 291–306.

Shepard, C. C., Gordon Ellard, Louis Levy, V. de Araujo Opromolla, Sefaan R. Pattyn, John Peters, R. J. W. Rees, and M. F. R. Waters. "Experimental Chemotherapy in Leprosy." *Bulletin WHO* 53 (1976): 425–33.

Skinsnes, Olaf K. "Leprosy in Society. I. Leprosy Has Appeared on the Face." *Leprosy Review* 35 (1964): 21–35.

Skinsnes, Olaf K. "Leprosy in Society. II. The Pattern of Concept and Reaction to Leprosy in Oriental Antiquity." *Leprosy Review* 35 (1964): 106–22.

Skinsnes, Olaf K. "Leprosy in Society. III. The Relationship of the Social to the Medical Pathology of Leprosy." *Leprosy Review* 35 (1964): 175–81.

Smith Kipp, Rita. "The Evangelical Uses of Leprosy." *Society of Science and Medicine* 39, no. 2 (1994): 165–78.

Sontag, Susan. *Illness as Metaphor and AIDS and Its Metaphors*. New York: Doubleday Anchor Books, 1988.

Stein, Stanley. *Alone No Longer*. Baton Rouge, LA: Franklin Press, the Star, 1963.

Sun Yunshan, Chen Rinong, and Zhou Youma, eds. *Dr Ma Haide (George Hatem)*. China: China Reconstructs Press, 1989.

Swenson-Wright, John. "Sasakawa Ryoichi: Unraveling an Enigma," in Sasakawa, *Sugamo Diary*.

Szlezák, Nicole A. *The Making of Global Health Governance: China and the Global Fund to Fight AIDS, Tuberculosis, and Malaria.* London: Palgrave Macmillan, 2012.

Thévenin, Étienne. *Raoul Follereau: Hier at Aujourd'hui.* Paris: Librairie Arthème Fayard, 1992.

"Third World Health Assembly." *International Journal of Leprosy* 18, no. 2 (1950): 273.

Tiedemann, R. G. *Reference Guide to Christian Missionary Societies in China From the Sixteenth to the Twentieth Century.* New York: An East Gate Book, Ricci Institute for Chinese–Western Cultural History, 2009.

Trivedi, Lisa N. "Visually Mapping the 'Nation': Swadeshi Politics in Nationalist India, 1920–1930." *Journal of Asian Studies* 62, no. 1 (2003): 11–41.

van den Wijngaert, Pierre. "Comment j'ai fondé 'Les Amis du Pere Damien.'" Amiens, France: COR, 1996.

Vaughan, Megan. *Curing Their Ills: Colonial Power and African Illness.* Stanford, CA: Stanford University Press, 1991.

Wade, H. W. "Editorial: The Trend to DDS." *International Journal of Leprosy* 19, no. 3 (1951): 344–9.

Waters. M. F. and R. J. Rees, A. C. McDougall, et al. "Ten Years of Dapsone in Lepromatous Leprosy: Clinical, Bacteriological and Histological Assessments and the Finding of Viable Leprosy Bacilli." *Leprosy Review* 45 (1974): 288–98.

Webb, James L. A. *The Long Struggle Against Malaria in Tropical Africa.* New York: Cambridge University Press, 2014.

Webb, James L. A. "Malaria Control and Eradication Projects in Tropical Africa," in *The Global Challenge of Malaria: Past Lessons and Future Prospects.* Ed. Frank M. Snowden and Richard Bucala, 35–56. Singapore: World Scientific, 2014.

"WHO and Leprosy." *International Journal of Leprosy* 20, no. 1 (1952): 115–6.

"WHO Program and Budget Estimates for 1950." *International Journal of Leprosy* 17, no. 1–2 (1949): 129–3.

"World Health Organization and Leprosy." *International Journal Leprosy* 21, no. 1 (1953): 78–81.

WHO Expert Committee on Leprosy, Technical Report Series No. 71. *WHO Expert Committee on Leprosy: First Report.* WHO, Geneva, September 1953.

WHO Expert Committee on Leprosy, Technical Report Series No. 189. *WHO Expert Committee on Leprosy: Second Report.* WHO, Geneva, 1960.

WHO Expert Committee on Leprosy, Technical Report Series No. 319. *WHO Expert Committee on Leprosy: Third Report.* WHO, Geneva, 1966.

WHO Expert Committee on Leprosy, Technical Report Series No. 459. *WHO Expert Committee on Leprosy: Fourth Report.* WHO, Geneva, 1970.

WHO Expert Committee on Leprosy, Technical Report Series 768. *WHO Expert Committee on Leprosy: Sixth Report.* WHO, Geneva, 1988.

Worboys, Michael. "The Colonial World as Mission and Mandate: Leprosy and Empire, 1900–1940." *Osiris* 15 (2000): 207–18.

Worboys, Michael. "Was There a Bacteriological Revolution in Late Nineteenth-Century Medicine?" *Studies in the History and Philosophy of Biological and Biomedical Sciences* 38, no. 1 (2007): 20–42.

World Health Organization. *Action Programme for the Elimination of Leprosy: Status Report 1996.* WHO/LEP/96.5.

World Health Organization. *Leprosy: A Survey of Recent Legislation.* Geneva: WHO, 1954. Reprint from the *International Digest of Health Legislation* 5, no. 6 (1954).

World Health Organization. *A Guide to Leprosy Control.* Geneva: WHO, 1959.

World Health Organization. *Primary Health Care: Report of the International Conference on Primary Health Care, Alma-Ata, USSR, 6–12 September 1978.* Geneva: WHO, 1978.

World Health Organization, Technical Report Series, 675. *Chemotherapy of Leprosy for Control Programmes*: Report of a WHO Study Group. Geneva: WHO, 1982.

World Health Organization. WHO Technical Report Series 716. *Epidemiology of Leprosy in Relation to Control: Report of a WHO Study Group.* Geneva: WHO, 1985.

World Health Organization. *Global Strategy for the Elimination of Leprosy as a Public Health Problem* (Updated 1996). Geneva: WHO, 1996. WHO/LEP/96.7.

World Health Organization. *Multidrug Therapy Against Leprosy: Development and Implementation Over the Past 25 Years.* Geneva: WHO, 2004. WHO/CDS/CPE/CEE/2004.46.

Yo, Yuasa. *Towards a World Without Leprosy: Thirty Years of Sasakawa Memorial Health Foundation.* Tokyo, Japan: Sasakawa Memorial Health Foundation, 2004.

Yozo, Yokota. "Report of the Sub-Commission on the Promotion and Protection of Human Rights on Its Fifty-Seventh Session, Geneva, 25 July–12 August 2005. Rapporteur: Mr. Yozo Yokota." Commission on Human Rights, Sub-Commission on the Promotion and Protection of Human Rights. E/CN.4/2006/2; E/CN.4/Sub.2/2005/44. 17 October 2005.

WHO Working Papers

Constitution of the World Health Organization. Basic Documents, 45th edition. Supplement October 2006. http://www.who.int/governance/eb/who_constitution_en.pdf

Eleventh World Health Assembly. "Committee on Programme and Budget Provisional Minutes of the Third Meeting." A11/P&B/Min/3, 2 June 1958.

Eleventh World Health Assembly. "Committee on Programme and Budget Provisional Minutes of the Third Meeting." A11/P&B/Min/4, 2 June 1958.

Eleventh World Health Assembly. "Committee on Programme and Budget Provisional Minutes of the Fourth Meeting." A11/P&B/Min/4, 2 June 1958.

Executive Board. "Proposed Programme and Budget Estimates for the Financial Year, 1 January–31 December 1950." EB 3/37, 17 February 1949, 288–9.

Executive Board. Seventh Session. "An Overall Discussion or Symposium on the Different Phases of the Leprosy Problem Throughout the World: Memorandum Submitted by the Government of the Republic of the Philippines." EB7/17, 15 December 1950.

Executive Board. Seventh Session, "Resolution on Leprosy." EB7/R/1, 23 January 1951.

Executive Board. Eighty-Seventh Session, Agenda Item 5.2. "Leprosy (Draft Resolution Proposed by Professor O Ransome-Kuti)" 16 January 1991. EB87/Conf. Paper No. 2.

Executive Board. Eighty-Seventh Session. "Summary Records: Thirteenth Meeting." Monday, 21 January 1991.

First World Assembly. Programme Committee: Preliminary Report 12.1.7, Other Activities. Off Rec WHO 10. A/Prog/66, 13 July 1948.

First World Assembly. Committee on Programme: Working Party and "Other Activities." 12.1.7. A/Prog/71, 16 July 1948.

First World Health Assembly. Committee on Programme: Twentieth Meeting, Monday, 19 July 1948, at 10 am. A/Prog/72, 17 July 1948. 12.1.7.4.4 Leprosy.

Forty-Fourth World Health Assembly. "Provisional Agenda, Item 17.2."

Forty-Fourth World Health Assembly. "Provisional Summary of the Third Meeting," 8 May 1991. A44/A/SR/3.

Official Records of the World Health Organization. "Proposed Programme and Budget Estimates for the Financial Year 1 January–31 December 1952 with the proposed programme and budget estimates for technical assistance for economic development of under-developed countries." March 1951, 546.

"Resolutions of the Executive Board." EB17.R29. 30 January 1956.

"Review of Work During 1956: Annual Report of the DG."

Second World Health Assembly. "Leprosy: Memorandum Submitted by the Delegation of the Government of India." A2/40. 1 June 1949. Supplementary Agenda Item 8.15.3.15.

Second World Health Assembly. Rome, 13 June to 2 July 1949: Decisions and Resolutions; Plenary meetings (Verbatim Records); Committees (Minutes and Reports). WHO, Geneva, December 1949. Fourth Plenary Meeting.

Tenth World Health Assembly. "Committee on Programme and Budget Provisional Minutes of the Second Meeting." A10/P&B/Min/2.

Tenth World Health Assembly. "Committee on Programme and Budget Provisional Minutes of the Third Meeting." A10/P&B/Min/3, 13 May 1957.

Tenth World Health Assembly. "Committee on Programme and Budget Provisional Minutes of the Fourth Meeting." A10/P&B/Min/4, 14 May 1957.

Tenth World Health Assembly. "Committee on Programme and Budget Provisional Minutes of the Eighth Meeting." A10/P&B/Min/8, 16 May 1957.

Thirteenth World Health Assembly. "Committee on Programme and Budget Provisional Minutes of the Seventh Meeting." A13/P&B/Min/7. 16 May 1960.

BIBLIOGRAPHY

UNICEF–WHO Joint Committee on Health Policy. "Fifth Session Provisional Summary Record of the Second Meeting." JC5/UNICEF–WHO/Min 2, 10 April 1952.

UNICEF–WHO Joint Committee on Health Policy. "Fifth Session Provisional Summary Record of the Third Meeting." JC5/UNICEF–WHO/Min 3, 11 April 1952.

UNICEF–WHO Joint Committee on Health Policy. "Leprosy: Note by the World Health Organization; Agenda Item 4.4." JC6/UNICEF–WHO/ 5, 20 April 1953.

UNICEF–WHO Joint Committee on Health Policy Sixth Session. "Provisional Summary Record of the Third Meeting." JC6/UNICEF–WHO/Min 3, 2 May 1953.

UNICEF–WHO Joint Committee on Health Policy Tenth Session. "Minutes of the Fourth Meeting." JC 10/UNICEF–WHO/Min 4, 23 September 1957.

UNICEF–WHO Joint Committee on Health Policy Eleventh Session. "Review of Leprosy Control Activities." JC 11/UNICEF–WHO/ 3, 1 September 1958.

UNICEF–WHO Joint Committee on Health Policy. Eleventh Session Geneva, 20–21 October 1958. "Review of Leprosy Control Activities." JC11/UNICEF–WHO/3 Rev. 1, 17 December 1958.

United Nations, World Health Organization, Interim Commission. *Official Records of the World Health Organization No 10: Report of the Interim Commission to the First World Health Assembly Part II Provisional Agenda Documents and Recommendations.* New York and Geneva: UN WHO, 1948.

United Nations, World Health Organization, Interim Commission. Minutes and Documents of the Fifth Session of the Interim Commission, held in Geneva from 22 January to 7 February 1948.

WHO. "Action Programme for the Elimination of Leprosy: Report of the Fourth Meeting of the Leprosy Elimination Advisory Group" (LEAG). Geneva: WHO, 1998. WHO/LEP/98.3.

WHO. "Global Medium-Term Programme Leprosy." LEP/MTP/80.1.

WHO. "Global Medium-Term Programme: Programme 13.9: Leprosy." LEP/MTP/83.1.

WHO, Regional Office for the Western Pacific, *Final Report on the First Regional Working Group on Leprosy Manila, Philippines, 7–12 December 1978.* Manila, Philippines, February 1979.

WHO. "Report of a Consultation on Implementation of Leprosy Control Through Primary Health Care," Geneva, 16–18 June 1986. WHO/CDS/LEP/86.3.

WHO. "Report of a Meeting on Action Plans for Leprosy Control," New Delhi, 23–5 August 1982; Action Plans for Leprosy Control (WHO/LEP/83.1).

WHO. "Report of the Second Coordinating Meeting on Implementation of Multidrug Therapy in Leprosy Control Programmes," Geneva, 4–5 November 1987. WHO/CDS/LEP/87.2.

WHO. "Report of the Second International Conference on the Elimination of Leprosy as a Public Health Problem." New Delhi, India, 11–13 October 1996. WHO/LEP/97.1.

WHO. "Report of a Special Meeting of the Leprosy Elimination Advisory Group (LEAG) With Potential Partners," Geneva, 12–13 April 1999. WHO/LEP/99.1.

WHO. "Report of the Third Meeting of the Leprosy Elimination Advisory Group." Geneva, 16–17 July 1997. WHO/LEP/97.6.

WHO. Special Programme for Research and Training in Tropical Diseases: TDR/THELEP/76.1–78.2.

WHO/UNDP. Meeting of Heads of Agencies in Connexion with the Special Programme for Research and Training in Tropical Diseases, "Strategy for A Special Programme for Research and Training in Tropical Diseases," 3. TDR/WP/75.4.

Unpublished Sources

Allen, Irene. *History of LEPRA.*

Cochrane, R. G. "Summary of the Activities of the Leprosy Research Unit From Its Foundation on 12th September, 1952 until May, 1964." Unpublished from Leprosy Research Unit collection, Osler McGovern Centre, Oxford.

"History of the Philippine Leprosy Mission, Inc: Compiled and Annotated by Soledad S. Griño," No page numbers.

"Informal Consultation on the Development and Implementation of MDT Over the Last 25 Years," 2001.

Levy, Louis. "Relationships Among Laboratory Research, Chemotherapy and the Control of Leprosy." March 2009.

Pandya, Shubha. "Ridding the Empire of Leprosy: Sir Leonard Rogers FRS (1868–1962) and the Oil of Chaulmoogra." Unpublished paper presented at "Health and Medicine in History: East–West Exchange: Third Conference of the Asian Society for History of Medicine," Jawaharlal Nehru University, New Delhi, 2–4 November 2006.

Sansarricq, Hubert. "My Interventions in Leprosy Work: 1972–1984." March 2009.

Skolnik, Richard, Florent Agueh, Judith Justice, and Michel Lechat. "Independent Evaluation of the Global Alliance for the Elimination of Leprosy," 13 June 2003.

Yo, Yuasa. "Basic Paradigm Shift for Leprosy Control in the Field."

Yo, Yuasa. "TNF(JSIF)/SMHF's Contributions 1974-2005: As Source Material for the 'Recent History of Leprosy Control.'"

Yo, Yuasa. "Synthesis of Promin in Japan and the Global Elimination of Hansen's Disease."

INDEX

Note: Page numbers followed by "*n*" refer to notes and refer to "*t*" tables.